AF412993

NEURAL TRANSPLANTATION IN NEURODEGENERATIVE DISEASE:

CURRENT STATUS AND NEW DIRECTIONS

Novartis Foundation Symposium 231

NEURAL TRANSPLANTATION IN NEURODEGENERATIVE DISEASE: CURRENT STATUS AND NEW DIRECTIONS

2000

JOHN WILEY & SONS, LTD

Chichester · New York · Weinheim · Brisbane · Singapore · Toronto

Copyright © Novartis Foundation 2000
Published in 2000 by John Wiley & Sons Ltd,
Baffins Lane, Chichester,
West Sussex PO19 1UD, England

National   01243 779777
International (+44) 1243 779777
e-mail (for orders and customer service enquiries): cs-books@wiley.co.uk
Visit our Home Page on http://www.wiley.co.uk
or http://www.wiley.com

Other Wiley Editorial Offices

John Wiley & Sons, Inc., 605 Third Avenue,
New York, NY 10158-0012, USA

WILEY-VCH Verlag GmbH, Pappelallee 3,
D-69469 Weinheim, Germany

Jacaranda Wiley Ltd, 33 Park Road, Milton,
Queensland 4064, Australia

John Wiley & Sons (Asia) Pte Ltd, 2 Clementi Loop #02-01,
Jin Xing Distripark, Singapore 129809

John Wiley & Sons (Canada) Ltd, 22 Worcester Road,
Rexdale, Ontario M9W 1L1, Canada

Novartis Foundation Symposium 231
ix+323 pages, 34 figures, 9 tables

Library of Congress Cataloging-in-Publication Data

Neural transplantation in neurodegenerative disease : current status and new directions /
[edited by Derek J. Chadwick, Jamie A. Goode].
p. ; cm. – (Novartis Foundation symposium ; 231)
Includes bibliographical references and index.
ISBN 0-471-49246-9 (alk. paper)
1. Nerve tissue–Transplantation–Congresses. 2. Central nervous
system–Transplantation–Congresses. 3. Nervous system–Degeneration–Congresses. I.
Chadwick, Derek. II. Goode, Jamie. III. Series.
[DNLM: 1. Neurodegenerative Diseases–surgery–Congresses. 2. Brain Tissue
Transplantation–Congresses. 3. Central Nervous System–physiology–Congresses. 4.
Nerve Tissue–transplantation–Congresses. WL 359 N4942 2000]
RD124.n488 2000
617.4′80592–dc21   00-043390

British Library Cataloguing in Publication Data

A catalogue record for this book is available from the British Library

ISBN 0 471 49246 9

Typeset in 10½ on 12½ pt Garamond by Dobbie Typesetting Limited, Tavistock, Devon.
Printed and bound in Great Britain by Biddles Ltd, Guildford and King's Lynn.
This book is printed on acid-free paper responsibly manufactured from sustainable forestry,
in which at least two trees are planted for each one used for paper production.

Contents

Participants

P. Aebischer   Division of Surgical Research and Gene Therapy Center, Lausanne University Medical School, Centre Hospitalier Universitaire Vaudois, Pavillon 4, CH-1011 Lausanne, Switzerland

L. Annett   Department of Experimental Psychology, University of Cambridge, Downing Street, Cambridge CB2 3EB, UK

R. A. Barker   Cambridge Centre for Brain Repair, Robinson Way, Cambridge CB2 2PY, UK

A. Björklund   Wallenberg Neuroscience Center, Department of Physiological Sciences, Lund University, Sölvegatan 17, S-223 62 Lund, Sweden

W. F. Blakemore   Department of Clinical Veterinary Medicine, University of Cambridge, Madingley Road, Cambridge CB3 0ES, UK

M. C. Bohn   Children's Memorial Institute for Education and Research, Department of Pediatrics, Northwestern University Medical School, 2300 Children's Plaza, Chicago, IL 60614, USA

S. B. Dunnett[1]   Centre for Brain Repair and Department of Experimental Psychology, University of Cambridge, Forvie Site, Robinson Way, Cambridge CB2 2PY, UK

B. Finsen   Department of Anatomy and Neurobiology, University of Southern Denmark–Odense University, DK-5000 Odense C, Denmark

T. B. Freeman   Department of Neurosurgery, Department of Pharmacology and Experimental Therapuetics and The Neuroscience Program, University of South Florida, 4 Columbia Drive, Suite 730, Tampa, FL 33606, USA

---

[1]Current address: Cardiff School of Biosciences, Cardiff University, Museum Avenue, PO Box 911, Cardiff CF10 3US, UK

R. Gadient   Novartis Pharma Research, CH-4002 Basel, Switzerland

F. H. Gage   The Salk Institute for Biological Studies, Laboratory of Genetics, 10010 North Torrey Pines Road, La Jolla, CA 92037, USA

J. A. Gray (*chair*)   Department of Psychology, Institute of Psychiatry, De Crespigny Park, Denmark Hill, London SE5 8AF, UK

H. Hodges   Department of Psychology, Institute of Psychiatry, De Crespigny Park, Denmark Hill, London SE5 8AF, UK

O. Isacson   Neuroregeneration Laboratory, Harvard Medical School, McLean Hospital, Belmont, MA 02178, USA

O. Lindvall   Section of Restorative Neurology, Wallenberg Neuroscience Center, University Hospital, SE-221 85 Lund, Sweden

L. Olson   Department of Neuroscience, Karolinska Institute, S-171 77 Stockholm, Sweden

V. H. Perry   CNS Inflammation Group, School of Biological Sciences, University of Southampton, Biomedical Sciences Building, Southampton SO16 7PX, UK

M. Peschanski   INSERM Unité 532, Neuroplasticité et Thérapeutique, Institut Mondor de Médecine Moléculaire, IM3, Faculté de Médecine, 8 Rue du Général Sarrail, 94010 Creteil Cedex, France

J. Price   Institute of Psychiatry, De Crespigny Park, Denmark Hill, London SE5 8AF, UK

G. Raisman   Division of Neurobiology, National Institute for Medical Research, The Ridgeway, Mill Hill, London NW7 1AA, UK

P. J. Reier   Department of Neuroscience, University of Florida Health Science Center, Brain Institute, PO Box 100244, Gainesville, FL 32610-0244, USA

A. E. Rosser   Cambridge Centre for Brain Repair, Forvie Site, Robinson Way, Cambridge CB2 2PY, UK

J. D. Sinden   ReNeuron Ltd., Europoint Centre, 5–11 Lavington Street, London SE1 0NZ, UK

A. Smith   Centre for Genome Research, University of Edinburgh, The King's Buildings, West Mains Road, Edinburgh EH9 3JQ, UK

W. Spooren   Novartis Pharma AG, CH-4002 Basel, Switzerland

E. Y. Snyder   Departments of Neurology, Paediatrics and Neurosurgery, Children's Hospital, Harvard Medical School, Boston, MA 02115, USA

Introduction

Jeffrey Gray

Department of Psychology, Institute of Psychiatry, De Crespigny Park, Denmark Hill, London SE5 8AF, UK

This is a timely moment to hold a meeting on neural transplantation. Although the field has a remarkably long history, stretching back to the 1890s, it has since then had only a slow build-up (see Table 1) to its current vigorous level of activity and increasingly high public profile.

The early important developments nearly all involved the introduction into a host brain of primary neural tissue taken directly from a fetal donor brain. This approach met a great deal of scepticism from those outside the field. Even as recently as the mid-1980s when, very much as latecomers, our group entered the field, we encountered this scepticism from both clinicians and other neuroscientists. The doubts of the laboratory scientists were the hardest to understand, since by that time there was very clear evidence that the transplantation of fetal tissue into the damaged adult brain in rats and other species was entirely capable of producing functional recovery (for reviews, see Dunnett & Björklund 1994). Although there were certainly questions as to how these observations might translate into clinical efficacy in human beings, the basic facts were clear. None the less, outside the circle of people actually conducting the research, the scepticism was great.

Interestingly, when we applied for our first research grant in this field, the hardest hurdle to overcome lay in the doubts of the electrophysiologists. There was already a great deal of anatomical and behavioural evidence for integration of transplanted tissue in the damaged brain together with recovery of function. However, there had been hardly any electrophysiological studies and, at least in the UK, physiology has traditionally been the queen of the neurosciences. The lack of electrophysiological investigation was taken by many to mean lack of evidence or, even worse, negative evidence. This lacuna in the evidential base is still with us today. When Steve Dunnett and I put together the programme for the symposium, we were unable to identify anyone who could adequately cover this topic. Indeed, one of the hopes that we have for the symposium is that it will stimulate a few intrepid electrophysiologists finally to enter the fray.

We are now, I believe, at a turning point in the field of neural transplantation. The first pilot clinical work dates back some fifteen years or so. Only now,

TABLE 1   Milestones in the development of neural transplantation

Author and year	*Experimental or clinical development*
Thompson (1890)	First attempt to graft adult neuronal tissue into the adult brain
Forssman (1898)	First publication on neurotrophic effects of adult neural tissue grafts
Del Conte (1907)	First attempt to graft non-neuronal embryonic tissue into the adult brain
Ranson (1909)	First graft of spinal ganglia into the brain
Tello (1911)	First graft of peripheral nerve into the brain
Dunn (1917)	First demonstration of survival of embryonic neurons after intracerebral grafting
Shirai (1921)	First demonstration of the brain as an immunologically privileged site for implantation of living material
Faldino (1924)	First graft of brain tissue into the anterior chamber of the eye
Le Gros Clark (1940)	First successful intraventricular graft of fetal neuronal tissue in a neonatal host brain
Woolsey et al (1944)	First unsuccessful attempt at medullary grafting in humans
Greene & Arnold (1945)	First graft of human cerebral tissue into an animal
Flerko & Szentagothai (1957)	First intraventricular graft of endocrine tissue
Halasz et al (1962)	First intracerebral graft of endocrine tissue followed by functional improvement
Olson & Malmfors (1970)	First histological characterization of grafted embryonic neuronal tissue using histofluorescence, histochemistry and autoradiography
Hoffer et al (1974)	First electrophysiological demonstration of conservation of functional specificity in neurons transplanted into the anterior chamber of the eye
Stenevi et al (1976)	First systematic study of conditions favourable to the survival and development of brain tissue grafts
Lund & Hauschka (1976)	First demonstration of the existence of synapses in a graft of brain tissue
Perlow et al (1979)	First demonstration of behavioural recovery due to a graft of dopaminergic cells in an animal model of Parkinson's disease (6-hydroxydopamine lesion of the nigrostriatal pathway)
Backlund et al (1982)	First unsuccessful attempt to graft catecholaminergic cells into the brain in two parkinsonian patients (published in 1985)
Madrazo (1986)	First successful attempt to graft catechomaniergic cells into the brain of parkinsonian patients (published in 1987)

Adapted with permission from Cassel (1998) and reprinted with permission from the Royal Society. For the references mentioned in the table, see Gray et al (1999).

however, are we seeing the first placebo-controlled, double-blind clinical trial of fetal tissue transplantation in Parkinson's disease. Unfortunately, this has not reached the point of formal publication — all we yet know is from press releases and a published abstract (Freed et al 1999). None the less, the fact that this trial is taking place indicates that clinical transplantation using primary fetal neural tissue has come of age. And it has been able to reach this point only because there are a sufficient number of patients from the previous pilot work who have shown significant recovery of function.

However, along with these demonstrations of potential clinical value, there has been a growing realization that, for a whole host of practical and ethical reasons (Gray et al 1999), there are serious limitations to how far one can roll out this approach — taking tissue from the fetal brain and putting it directly into a patient's brain — to conditions other than Parkinson's disease. In consequence, for a decade or more there have been attempts all over the world to develop alternative methods of sourcing tissue for repair of the damaged brain.

These approaches have now in their turn just reached the stage of the first pilot clinical work, as in the trial led by Layton Biosciences (see their website, at *http://www.laytonbio.com*) looking at implanted engineered cell lines in patients who have suffered a stroke. This is a condition for which there is at present effectively no other treatment. Thus we now see emerging on the horizon the clinical prospects for a transplantation therapy using engineered cells.

To back up these developments in basic science and its clinical application there is likely to be a need for a radically new industry implementing these novel technologies. Indeed, biotechnology companies are already starting to enter the field, and we may be witnessing the beginnings of something akin to a new pharmaceutical industry. Of course, it is not only in relation to neural transplantation that these developments are occurring. This is a period in which we are seeing very rapid advances in knowledge of developmental neuroscience generally, advances that are themselves fuelled by the tremendous discoveries that have been made in molecular genetics and in intra- and intercellular signalling processes. All of these developments in basic neurobiology and developmental neuroscience are beginning to feed into neural transplantation. Until recently, work in this field has been largely empirical, trying things out to see what will work. This approach is about to change.

It is in the light of this hopeful picture that I believe this to be an excellent moment to have the kind of in-depth discussion that only the Novartis Foundation properly manages. To prompt this discussion, here is a set of suggestions of topics that should be at the forefront of our minds — suggestions, however, that are in no way intended to be prescriptive or limiting.

First, we need to take stock of where we are in the work that has been done on primary fetal grafts. What have we learned from this work in relation to the basic

TABLE 2   New approaches to neural transplantation

Xenografts

Stem cells
    endogenous
    pluripotent
    neuroepithelial
    immortalized
    conditionally immortalized
    other genetic modification
    differentiated prior to implantation

Genetic modification of carrier cells to deliver:
    neurotrophic factors
    antioxidants
    anti-apoptotic factors

Encapsulated cells

science of neural plasticity? How much functional recovery can be achieved in this way? By what mechanisms? If we continue to go down that route, what are the clinical prospects, and what problems remain to be overcome for them to be realized?

Then there are the many new approaches (Table 2), most of which are represented among the group gathered here. These include the use of xenografts to overcome limitations on the supply of human tissue, an approach that has already reached the clinic. Then there is much excitement about stem cells. These raise many questions. Might there be a useful technology based upon the use of pluripotent embryonic stem cells, or should one focus upon stem cells already committed to a neuroepithelial fate? The recent discovery of endogenous cells of the latter kind in the adult mammalian brain has raised hopes that one might in some way be able to stimulate them so as to enhance spontaneous mechanisms of repair and functional recovery. If exogenous stem cells are to be used, should these be expanded and then implanted as they are, or should they first be immortalized or conditionally immortalized? Should they be injected into the host brain while still in the undifferentiated state in the hope that the damage they encounter there may itself provide signals to direct them down a differentiation pathway useful for repair? Or should such cells first be differentiated *in vitro* down a pathway that is known to be required for repair of the damage in the host brain? Might there be other genetic modifications that it would be useful to introduce into stem cells before they are used in the attempt to repair a damaged brain? What progress can be made using either stem cells or other types of cell, e.g. fibroblasts, as vehicles for the delivery to a host brain of potentially useful molecules such as neurotrophic factors, antioxidants or anti-apoptotic factors? How great will be the need for immunosuppression in relation to each of these novel approaches? Can one reduce this need by the use of encapsulated cells that allow through to the host brain only the required molecules?

This, then, is a partial list of the new approaches that will figure in our discussions and of the questions that they raise. In relation to each of them, we shall need to ask what scientific problems need to be overcome if they are to become realistic. It is perhaps a little early to ask whether they should be used alone or in combination, but it may well turn out that a combination of two approaches will be more effective than either alone. There are also a number of practical issues that will need to be resolved if any of these approaches is successfully to reach the clinic. These include the sources of required tissue, the role of immunosuppression, the regulatory requirements that will need to be met, and the critically important design of clinical trials. In the background to all such issues will lie the question whether this kind of scientific investment will ever be clinically justified given that, at least in the case of some conditions, there are alternative therapeutic approaches that do not involve transplantation at all. Safety issues will also need to be considered. Primary cell grafts might be the vehicle for infections; engineered cells might give rise to problems of viral transfer or tumorigenesis; and xenografts pose potential risks of transfer into human hosts of retroviruses that are endemic in the donor species. One must not forget, either, the potential ethical issues: e.g. the use of aborted tissue (whether for primary fetal grafts or as the initial source for the production of engineered cell lines); or the use of placebo controls in clinical trials of transplant surgery.

In closing, I shall make one last point. We have moved from the time when the danger lay in too great a scepticism to one in which it is that of raising false hopes. The media now pay great attention to this field, as do many patients who suffer from seriously debilitating conditions, as well as their carers. There are, indeed, real hopes for clinical progress; and I believe we are on the threshold of a technology that will bring relief to many people for whom life is otherwise at present rather bleak. However, the new treatments will not be developed overnight, and we must be cautious about raising hopes too soon. So let us be careful to strike the right balance between a legitimate optimism for the medium-to-long term and a necessary caution in the short term.

References

Cassel JC 1998 Greffes de cellules nerveuses dans l'hippocampe du rat: caractérisation neurochimique et comportementale des effets. Habilitation à Diriger des Recherches, Université Louis Pasteur, Strasbourg

Dunnett SB, Björklund A (eds) 1994 Functional neural transplantation. Raven Press, New York

Freed CR, Breeze RE, Greene PE et al 1999 Double-blind placebo-controlled human fetal
    dopamine cell transplants in advanced Parkinson's disease. Soc Neurosci Abstr 25:212
Gray JA, Hodges H, Sinden J 1999 Prospects for the clinical application of neural
    transplantation with the use of conditionally immortalised neuroepithelial stem cells. Phil
    Trans R Soc Lond B 354:1407–1421

Cell replacement strategies for neurodegenerative disorders

Anders Björklund

Wallenberg Neuroscience Center, Department of Physiological Sciences, Lund University, Sölvegatan 17, S-223 62 Lund, Sweden

Abstract. Cell transplantation has over the last two decades emerged as a promising approach for restoration of function in neurodegenerative diseases, in particular Parkinson's and Huntington's disease. Clinical trials have so far focused on the use of implants of embryonic mesencephalic tissue containing already fate-committed dopaminergic neuroblasts with the capacity to develop into fully mature dopamine neurons in their new location in the host brain. However, the recent demonstration that immature neural progenitor cells with multipotent properties can be isolated from both the developing and adult CNS and that these cells can be maintained and propagated in culture, has provided a new interesting tool for restorative cell replacement and gene transfer therapies. Embryonic stem cells, obtained from the early stages of embryonic development, and neural stem cells, obtained from the developing brain, may provide renewable sources of cells for therapeutic purposes, and could eventually offer a powerful alternative to primary fetal CNS tissue in clinical transplantation protocols. The purpose of this review is to discuss the prospects of the emerging progenitor cell technology for cell replacement and restorative therapies in neurodegenerative diseases, and consider some of the critical issues that must be solved in order to make progenitor cells useful in studies of brain repair.

2000 Neural transplantation in neurodegenerative disease. Wiley, Chichester (Novartis Foundation Symposium 231) p 7–20

Neural transplantation as a tool for replacement of lost neurons and reconstruction of damaged circuitry in the mammalian CNS is still in its infancy. Transplantation of neuronal tissue is a classic approach in neuroembryology, and this technique has been extensively used as an experimental tool for the study of neuroregeneration and repair in submammalian vertebrates. Pioneering work in amphibians and fish, which was carried out above all by Matthey, Stone and Sperry, was the first to demonstrate that grafted neurons have a capacity to substitute both structurally and functionally for lost axonal connections, and that afferent and efferent connections can be established with a high degree of specificity between grafted neurons and denervated targets in the host brain (see e.g. Björklund & Stenevi 1984, for review).

The first attempts to apply neural grafting in animal models of neurodegenerative disease were made in the late 1970s (Björklund & Stenevi 1979, Perlow et al 1979). Subsequent studies in rodents have shown that the ability of grafted neurons to become functionally integrated into the host brain depends not only on the developmental potential of the implanted cells, but also on the plasticity of the host environment, i.e. the capacity of the brain tissue to accept new cellular elements to become integrated into the developing or established neuronal circuitry. Both these factors are greatly dependent on the developmental stage of donor and host: the brain becomes less plastic as it matures, and neurons removed from their normal context survive and grow well after intracerebral transplantation only if they are immature, i.e. at the stage of their development when they have become terminally differentiated but before they have formed extensive axonal connections (see Dunnett & Björklund 1994, for review). In the adult brain the capacity of transplanted fetal neurons to grow, integrate and establish functional efferent and afferent connections is in many cases substantially increased when the host circuitry is damaged, suggesting that some of the plastic properties that are present during development, such as mechanisms that regulate and guide axonal growth and synaptogenesis, can be reactivated by lesions or neurodegenerative changes. These lesion-induced cellular and molecular changes, which have yet to be clarified, form the basis for the remarkable ability of the lesioned adult brain to incorporate new functional elements, and thus to a degree rebuild itself. Cell transplantation as an approach to replace lost or damaged brain cells, is thus in its most effective form a technique for reconstruction of damaged neuronal circuitry.

Neuronal replacement in Parkinson's disease

Parkinson's disease (PD) has come to serve as the primary test bed for the neural transplantation technique, for several reasons. One important reason is that PD affects primarily a circumscribed set of neurons in the brain (the mesencephalic dopamine neurons) whose main target, striatum, is anatomically well defined and relatively accessible surgically. Moreover, and most importantly, there are well-characterized animal models, both in rodents and primates, that mimic the cardinal features of the disease. Results obtained in these animal models have repeatedly proved to have good predictive value with respect to the symptomatology of the human disease.

Neuronal replacement may be most likely to work for those types of systems which have non-specific modulatory functions in the brain. The nigrostriatal dopamine neurons are good examples of this type. These neurons, which normally are located in the midbrain substantia nigra, provide a dense, diffuse innervation of one of the principal motor control centres of the forebrain, the striatum. Dopamine released from the nigrostriatal terminals acts in a tonic, level-setting manner to regulate motor behaviour. Lesions of the nigrostriatal dopamine neurons induce a profound akinetic state which is at least in part due to an increased threshold for activation of the striatal output system and initiation of movement.

Neural transplantation in PD is based on the idea that dopamine-producing cells implanted into the denervated striatum might be able to substitute for those mesencephalic dopamine neurons that have been lost as a consequence of the disease process. The grafted neurons are proposed to function either by a 'pharmacological' type of action, whereby the released dopamine is able to diffuse over sufficient distances to activate the denervated striatal receptors, and/or through functional reinnervation of the denervated target neurons by the outgrowing axons of the implanted neuroblasts, which allows released dopamine to exert its action at defined synaptic sites (see Björklund 1992, Herman & Abrous 1994, for review).

Intrastriatal transplants of fetal nigral neurons can reverse or ameliorate impairments in both drug-induced and spontaneous motor behaviours induced by damage to the nigrostriatal system. In rodent and primate models of PD, grafted nigral neurons can re-establish a functional dopamine innervation of the previously denervated striatal target neurons and restore dopaminergic neurotransmission in the area reached by the outgrowing axons. *In vivo* data show that the grafted neurons are spontaneously active and release dopamine in an impulse-dependent manner, at both synaptic and non-synaptic sites, although largely independent of any regulatory afferent inputs.

Reconstruction of basal ganglia circuitry by striatal transplants

The striatal GABAergic neurons provide an inhibitory control of two major striatal output structures, globus pallidus and pars reticulata of the substantia nigra. Loss of this striatal inhibitory output system, as occurs in animals with striatal lesions or in patients with Huntington's disease (HD), induces a hyperkinectic syndrome in combination with cognitive deficits. Since the striatal output neurons are functionally integrated in an intricately organized cortico-striato-thalamic circuitry, however, proper functioning of the striatal output neurons will depend not only on the establishment of appropriate efferent connections but also on their access to regulatory afferent inputs.

On the neurochemical level, striatal neuron transplants can restore GABA synthesis and release both within the lesioned striatum and within the adjacent, denervated globus pallidus. More importantly, however, the implanted striatal primordium develop a striatum-like structure at the site of implantation, and part of the cells develop into fully differentiated striatal projection neurons.

These cells, which are of the medium-size densely spiny type, grow to establish normal synaptic contacts with the output neurons in the globus pallidus, as well as appropriate afferent synaptic inputs from both thalamus, cortex and substantia nigra. Indeed, *in vivo* electrophysiological and microdialysis studies in rats show that the activity of the grafted striatal neurons is under the control of both cortical glutamatergic and nigral dopaminergic afferents (see Björklund et al 1994, Dunnett 1995, for review). There is thus compelling evidence that fetal striatal neurons, implanted into the lesioned striatum, can reconstruct at least some critical elements of the damaged striatal circuitry in animal models of HD.

Proof of concept in clinical trials

Since 1987 about 250 patients with advanced PD have received transplants of mesencephalic dopamine neurons, obtained from 6–9 week old cadaver embryos at several centres in Europe and America (Olanow et al 1996, Björklund & Lindvall 2000). There is now convincing data to show that embryonic human nigral neurons, taken at a stage of development when they have started to express their dopaminergic phenotype, can survive, integrate and function over a long time in the human brain (i.e. in a tissue environment with an ongoing disease process). Positron emission tomography (PET) scans have shown significant increases in [^{18}F]fluorodopa uptake (i.e. dopamine synthesis and retention) in the areas reinnervated by the grafted cells. This increase has been maintained for at least 6–10 years in several of the longest-studied patients. Consistent with the imaging data, good survival of grafted dopamine neurons and extensive reinnervation of the surrounding host striatum have been demonstrated by immunohistochemistry in two patients that have come to autopsy at 18 months after surgery (Kordower et al 1998). Long-lasting symptomatic improvement has been observed in about two-thirds of the grafted patients, and in the most successful cases it has been possible to withdraw L-dopa treatment (see Lindvall 1997).

In HD, clinical trials using transplants of striatal primordium, obtained from the ganglionic eminences from the developing forebrain from either human or porcine embryonic donors, have been initiated in four different centres. Although initial reports have described signs of improvements in parameters of motor function and cognition, it is still too early to tell if any of these changes indeed are due to the function of the transplanted cells. The best indications that embryonic striatal transplants may also work in the larger and more complex primate brain come from two recent studies in monkeys, which show that striatal transplants can induce significant recovery in both motor and cognitive function in animals with toxin-induced destruction of the striatum, i.e. in the best models of HD that we have available today (Palfi et al 1998, Kendall et al 1998).

Neuronal progenitors

A major limitation of the fetal cell transplantation procedure is the low survival rate of the grafted dopamine neurons (in the range of 5–20%) which makes it difficult to obtain sufficient cells for grafting in patients. Currently, mesencephalic fragments from at least 6–8 embryos are needed for transplantation in one PD patient. Moreover, the ethical, practical and safety issues associated with the use of tissue from aborted human fetuses are problematic, and severely restrict the possibility for applying the procedure outside highly specialized centres. The emerging possibilities of using stem cells or neuronal progenitors as a renewable source of cells provides an attractive approach to solve these problems (Gage 1998, Snyder 1998, Svendsen & Smith 1999, Lee et al 2000).

Differentiation of immature neural progenitors into fully mature neurons depends on an interaction between extrinsic signals, present in the cells' local environment, and intrinsic signals operating in a cell autonomous manner within the cells themselves. With time during development neural progenitors will gradually acquire independence from extrinsic signals and as the cells become more restricted in their developmental potential cell autonomous programs of differentiation will take over (see Edlund & Jessell 1999, for review). This is also observed in transplantation experiments: cells taken at a stage of development when they have become committed to a specific neuronal fate (which appears to be around the time of the last cell division in case of nigral dopamine neurons) will also carry on their normal development in the fully mature brain, or when transplanted to ectopic sites (such as the anterior eye chamber or the kidney capsule). Uncommitted neural progenitors are able to integrate, differentiate and develop appropriately after transplantation to the fetal brain (Brüstle et al 1995, Fishell 1995, Campbell et al 1995), but the capacity of the host brain environment to direct the development of uncommitted progenitors in a region-specific manner is gradually lost during the late fetal and early postnatal development in rodents. This indicates that critical extrinsic signals, necessary for terminal differentiation of neuronal precursors, are lost or down-regulated as the brain matures. There are two notable exceptions to this rule: the olfactory bulb and the dentate gyrus of the hippocampal formation where active neurogenesis continues throughout life (Gage 1998, McKay 1997). In both these regions there is a continuous production of new neurons (of the small, short-axoned interneuron type) from a pool of endogenous undifferentiated progenitors located in the subventricular zone, which supplies cells to the olfactory bulb, and in the subgranular zone of the dentate gyrus. Indeed, undifferentiated progenitors transplanted into either of these sites will migrate, integrate and differentiate, along with the endogenous cells (Lois & Alvarez-Buylla 1994, Gage et al 1995, Suhonen et al 1996, Flax et al 1998, Fricker et al 1999). In these two brain regions, at least, neurogenic signals of the type present during development continues to be expressed also in the adult.

Expansion of dopamine neuron precursors *in vitro*

Along the path to fully differentiated neurons the precursor cells pass a critical event, i.e. they stop dividing and cannot re-enter the cell cycle. Determination of cell fate may take place several divisions before cell cycle exit, or — as is probably the case for the mesencephalic dopamine neurons — at the time of, or shortly after, the last cell division. In the rat ventral mesencephalon dopamine neurons are generated over a 5-day period, from about embryonic day (E) 11 to about E15, and phenotypic markers (e.g. tyrosine hydroxylase, TH) are expressed at the time of, or shortly after the last cell division (see Bouvier & Mytilineou 1995). In transplants of fetal mesencephalic tissue, grafted to the adult striatum, Sinclair et al (1999) have shown that in grafts taken at E14, i.e. during active neurogenesis, virtually all surviving dopamine neurons are derived from precursors that have undergone their last cell division prior to transplantation, and hence already been committed to a dopaminergic neuronal fate. These results are consistent with the view that those extrinsic signals which are necessary for the induction of mature neuronal phenotypes from uncommitted precursors may not be present normally in mature non-neurogenic brain regions, such as the adult striatum.

Bouvier & Mytilineou (1995) and Studer et al (1998) have shown that mesencephalic dopamine neuron precursors can be expanded in a pre-differentiated state in culture provided that they are plated at a time close to their last cell division, but before they express a definitive dopaminergic phenotype (i.e. the TH enzyme). These lineage-restricted precursors do not continue to divide spontaneously in culture but can be maintained in an undifferentiated dividing state for about a week under stimulation with a growth factor, fibroblast growth factor (FGF)2. At the end of this expansion period, Studer et al (1998) estimated that the total number of cells in the FGF2-treated cultures had increased 10-fold, and upon removal of the mitogen the yield of differentiated TH-positive neurons was increased about 30-fold over the non-expanded controls. Studer and collaborators went on to show that these *in vitro* expanded precursors can survive transplantation to the dopamine-denervated striatum. However, the overall yield of surviving dopamine neurons in the grafts was very low, above all due to the excessive loss of cells in the differentiation and grafting steps of the procedure (over 95%), where the expanded cells were first removed from the culture dishes and then allowed to differentiate into dopamine neurons in free-floating aggregate cultures prior to transplantation. This cell survival problem should be possible to solve, however, by improvements in the handling of the cells in the differentiation step.

The cells expanded in the Studer et al (1998) study differentiated spontaneously to TH-positive neurons upon removal of the mitogen, which suggests that they were committed dopamine neuron precursors. Stimulation by FGF2 was able to induce cell division in this precursor cell population and delay terminal differentiation, but only for about 7–8 days (Bouvier & Mytilineou 1995). Mesencephalic progenitors can be expanded for longer periods in neurosphere cultures. The neurosphere cells express features of multipotent progenitors, and can differentiate into both neurons and glia, but they do not spontaneously differentiate into dopamine neurons when placed in monolayer cultures in the absence of the mitogen (Svendsen & Rosser 1995, Ling et al 1998). Carvey and collaborators (Ling et al 1998, Potter et al 1999) have shown that these uncommitted progenitors can be induced to differentiate into a dopaminergic neuronal fate in the presence of a combination of cytokines, mesencephalic membrane fragments and striatal culture-condition medium. About 50% of all neurons, and 20–25% of all cells, in the differentiated cultures were seen to express the TH marker. Interestingly, the cytokine effect was seen with mesencephalic but not striatal progenitors, suggesting that this combination of factors acted to induce differentiation in a lineage-restricted mesencephalic precursor cell population (Potter et al 1999). These cells expressed not only the TH enzyme but also dopa decarboxylase, the dopamine transporter and dopamine itself, suggesting that they represent a mature dopaminergic neuronal phenotype. To what extent these cells can survive and function after transplantation is not yet clear.

Engineering cells for transplantation

In vitro expanded neural progenitors may provide a highly useful source of cells for intracerebral transplantation in PD provided that we can reliably control or direct their differentiation towards a specific dopaminergic neuronal fate. Ideally, these cells should not only be dopamine-producing but they should also possess the specific features of mature nigral dopamine neurons. This implies factors that convey both region-specific and transmitter-specific identity on the developing precursors. Local extrinsic signals, such as sonic hedgehog and FGF8 (Ye et al 1998) and cell specific transcription factors, such as Nurr1 (Zetterström et al 1997), are likely to be critically involved in this process.

Wagner et al (1999) have recently reported that overexpression of Nurr1 in combination with (as yet unidentified) factors from local type 1 astrocytes is sufficient to induce a dopaminergic neuronal phenotype in undifferentiated cells from the C17-2 immortalized neural stem cell line. With the protocol used, over 80% of the induced cells expressed the TH enzyme, as well as two other phenotypic markers, ADH-2 and c-Ret, characteristic for ventral mesencephalic dopamine neurons. These results point to an important role of glia-derived factors in the process leading to the maturation of the dopaminergic neuronal phenotype. Indeed, in primary cultures the differentiation of mesencephalic precursors into dopamine neurons coincides with the appearance of astrocytes in the FGF2-treated cultures (Bouvier & Mytilineou 1995). Moreover, it has been shown that cortical astrocytes, stimulated with FGF2, secrete factors that stimulate differentiation of mesencephalic dopamine neurons (Gaul & Lübbert 1992), and that glia-conditioned media (in combination with FGF2) can induce TH expression in *in vitro* expanded neural progenitors (Daadi & Weis 1999). These data suggest that neurons and glia may cooperate in both regional specification and the induction of specific neuronal identities of developing precursors. If so, the ideal cell preparation for transplantation in the Parkinson model will consist of a mixture of committed neuronal precursors and regionally specified glial cells in a stage of development where they can help to convey regional identity to the developing neuroblasts.

References

Björklund A 1992 Dopaminergic transplants in experimental parkinsonism: cellular mechanisms of graft-induced functional recovery. Curr Opin Neurobiol 2:683–689

Björklund A, Lindvall O 2000 Cell replacement therapies for central nervous system disorders. Nat Neurosci 3:537–544

Björklund A, Stenevi U 1979 Reconstruction of the nigrostriatal pathway by intracerebral nigral transplants. Brain Res 177:555–560

Björklund A, Stenevi U 1984 Intracerebral neural implants: neuronal replacement and reconstruction of damaged circuitries. Annu Rev Neurosci 7:279–308

Björklund A, Campbell K, Sirinathsinghji DJ, Fricker RA, Dunnett SB 1994 Functional capacity of striatal transplants in the rat Huntington model. In: Dunnett SB, Björklund A (eds) Functional neural transplantation. Raven Press, New York, p 157–195

Bouvier MM, Mytilineou C 1995 Basic fibroblast growth factor increases division and delays differentiation of dopamine precursors *in vitro*. J Neurosci 15:7141–7149

Brüstle O, Maskos U, McKay RDG 1995 Host-guided migration allows targeted introduction of neurons into the embryonic brain. Neuron 15:1275–1285

Campbell K, Olsson M, Björklund A 1995 Regional incorporation and site-specific differentiation of striatal precursors transplanted to the embryonic forebrain ventricle. Neuron 15:1259–1273

Daadi MM, Weiss S 1999 Generation of tyrosine hydroxylase-producing neurons from precursors of the embryonic and adult forebrain. J Neurosci 19:4484–4497

Dunnett SB 1995 Functional repair of striatal systems by neural transplants: evidence for circuit reconstruction. Behav Brain Res 66:133–142

Dunnett SB, Björklund A (eds) 1994 Functional neural transplantation. Raven Press, New York

Edlund T, Jessell T 1999 Progression from extrinsic to intrinsic signaling in cell fate specification: a view from the nervous system. Cell 96:211–224

Fishell G 1995 Striatal precursors adopt cortical identities in response to local cues. Development 121:803–812

Flax JD, Aurora S, Yang C et al 1998 Engraftable human neural stem cells respond to developmental cues, replace neurons, and express foreign genes. Nat Biotechnol 16:1033–1039

Fricker RA, Carpenter MK, Winkler C, Greco C, Gates MA, Björklund A 1999 Site-specific migration and neuronal differentiation of human neural progenitor cells after transplantation in the adult rat brain. J Neurosci 19:5990–6005

Gage FH 1998 Cell therapy. Nature (suppl) 392:18–24

Gage FH, Coates PW, Palmer TD et al 1995 Survival and differentiation of adult neuronal progenitor cells transplanted to the adult brain. Proc Natl Acad Sci USA 92:11879–11883

Gaul G, Lübbert H 1992 Cortical astrocytes activated by basic fibroblast growth factor secrete molecules that stimulate differentiation of mesencephalic dopamine neurons. Proc R Soc Lond B Biol Sci 249:57–63

Herman JP, Abrous ND 1994 Dopaminergic neural grafts after fifteen years: results and perspectives. Prog Neurobiol 44:1–35

Kendall AL, Rayment FD, Torres EM, Baker HF, Ridley RM, Dunnett SB 1998 Functional integration of striatal allografts in a primate model of Huntington's disease. Nat Med 4:727–729

Kordower JH, Freeman TB, Chen EY et al 1998 Fetal nigral grafts survive and mediate clinical benefit in a patient with Parkinson's disease. Movement Disord 13:383–393

Lee S-H, Lumelsky N, Struder L, Auerbach JM, McKay RD 2000 Efficient generation of midbrain and hindbrain neurons from mouse embryonic stem cells. Nat Biotechnol 18:675–679

Lindvall O 1997 Neural transplantation: a hope for patients with Parkinson's disease. Neuroreport 8:iii–x

Ling ZD, Potter ED, Lipton JW, Carvey PM 1998 Differentiation of mesencephalic progenitor cells into dopaminergic neurons by cytokines. Exp Neurol 149:411–423

Lois C, Alvarez-Buylla A 1994 Long-distance neuronal migration in the adult mammalian brain. Science 264:1145–1148

McKay RDG 1997 Stem cells in the central nervous system. Science 276:66–71

Olanow CW, Kordower JH, Freeman TB 1996 Fetal nigral transplantation as a therapy for Parkinson's disease. Trends Neurosci 19:102–109

Palfi SP, Condé F, Riche D et al 1998 Fetal striatal allografts reverse cognitive deficits in a primate model of Huntington disease. Nat Med 4:963–966

Perlow MJ, Freed WJ, Hoffer B, Seiger Å, Olson L, Wyatt RJ 1979 Brain grafts reduce motor abnormalities produced by destruction of nigrostriatal dopamine system. Science 204:643–647

Potter ED, Ling ZD, Carvey PM 1999 Cytokine-induced conversion of mesencephalic-derived progenitor cells into dopamine neurons. Cell Tissue Res 296:235–246

Sinclair SR, Fawcett JW, Dunnett SB 1999 Dopamine cells in nigral grafts differentiate prior to implantation. Eur J Neurosci 11:4341–4348

Snyder EY 1998 Neural stem-like cells: developmental lessons with therapeutic potential. Neuroscientist 4:408–425

Studer L, Tabar V, McKay RDG 1998 Transplantation of expanded mesencephalic precursors leads to recovery in parkinsonian rats. Nat Neurosci 1:290–295

Suhonen JO, Petersen DA, Ray J, Gage FH 1996 Differentiation of adult hippocampus-derived progenitors into olfactory neurons *in vivo*. Nature 383:624–627

Svendsen CN, Rosser AE 1995 Neurones from stem cells? Trends Neurosci 18:465–467

Svendsen CN, Smith AG 1999 New prospects for human stem-cell therapy in the nervous system. Trends Neurosci 22:357–365

Wagner J, Åkerud P, Castro DS et al 1999 Induction of a midbrain dopaminergic phenotype in Nurr1-overexpressing neural stem cells by type 1 astrocytes. Nat Biotechnol 17:653–659

Ye W, Shimamura K, Rubinstein JLR, Hynes MA, Rosenthal A 1998 FGF and Shh signals control dopaminergic and serotonergic cell fate in the anterior neural plate. Cell 93:755–766

Zetterström RH, Solomin L, Jansson L, Hoffer BJ, Olson L, Perlmann T 1997 Dopamine neuron agenesis in Nurr1-deficient mice. Science 276:248–250

DISCUSSION

Dunnett: With the M6 antibody you have shown beautiful outgrowth from striatal grafts over long distances, even when they are implanted into the adult. We know from the retrograde tracing studies of Klas Wictorin that there is also quite long distance growth from rat-to-rat transplants, but it never comes over as rich. Is that because the marking methods are not as sensitive and can't label everything growing out of an allograft, or do you think that xenografts can grow out more extensively than allografts?

Björklund: I think it is the former. In comparing transplants of mouse or rat cells, the anterograde tracer we use, PHAL, labels a very small number of the grafted cells. PHAL is a very good tracer in that it has limited spread from the site of injection. In this way we can know for sure that the labelled cells are graft cells, but the disadvantage is that we sample a very small portion. The M6 antibody, by contrast, stains all axons in the mouse grafts.

Isacson: Is there a question about the validity of M6 as a pure neuronal fibre marker? We have data from culture that it also stains glial cells. In Brüstle et al (1995) the authors were not sure that M6 only stained glial cells, and that would give that kind of thick line of cells and fibres that make it look like a big fibre set, which I think is actually a mixture of glial cells and fibres.

Björklund: The M2 antibody is reasonably selective for glia, although it probably doesn't stain all mouse glial cells. The M6 antibody can be fairly neuron-specific under certain conditions, but in other conditions it also stains glial cells. The distinguishing feature we use is whether or not the fibres and fibre bundles are stained. We feel fairly confident that these fibres are neurites, but we cannot say for sure whether the fibres are axons or dendrites. And in those cases where we have M2 and M6 staining of adjacent sections, we can see that the glial cells can be distinguished from the fibres. It is only when outgrowing fibres and migrating glia are densely mixed where this becomes a problem.

Raisman: You showed that after embryonic transplant into an adult host, if the adult host is intact there is no outgrowth, and if there is a lesion there is outgrowth. Do you know how long that effect lasts after a lesion?

Björklund: Yes, Klas Wictorin has done an experiment where he transplanted fetal striatal neurons into a chronic striatal ibotenic acid lesion; i.e. six months after the lesion was made. These transplants were consistently smaller in size than those in acute lesions, but there was still a clear, prominent axonal projection.

Gray: When you're talking about the graft being smaller if it's six months after lesion rather than one month after lesion, are you talking about the size of the cluster, or the degree to which migration occurs?

Björklund: I'm referring to the size of the cell cluster. We think that in chronic lesions there are fewer cells inside that cluster, caused by either reduced survival or reduced cell proliferation in the original graft deposit. We know that the striatal grafts expand about eightfold in size when we implant them into a fresh lesion, whereas if the grafts are placed in an intact striatum they will stay about the same size. It appears that the lesion provides both growth space and a stimulus for cell proliferation.

Gray: Going back to Geoff Raisman's question, how long does this effect last with respect to migration after a lesion?

Björklund: In the adults, we see very little migration of cells, even in the lesioned animals.

Isacson: I have some experience relevant to the question that Geoff Raisman raised, and it also relates to Anders Björklund's paper. Anders' paper included primarily cells that have the total gestational age of 21 d, for instance from the rat donor or mouse donor. When we use a species with a total of 115 gestational days as donor, that is pig, we can get long distance growth implanting into intact striatum. The data from the slower growing donor suggest that host signals can guide most growing axons to their normal destination (Isacson et al 1995, Isacson & Deacon 1996). In contrast to rat donor tissue, there is very specific long distance growth by pig axons that also has a component of glial migration that follows white fibre bundles. These data are also relevant to what Anders Björklund discussed about whether or not the glia come first in relation to growth. We have looked at this carefully because we had a CD44 antibody against pig-specific astrocytes, and we also had a neuron-specific marker for neurofilaments in the pig. These are analogous to the M2 and M6 markers for mouse donor tissue. We find that the glial cells grow primarily in white matter in the adult rat, whereas the axons will grow in white matter and then turn to their appropriate target, but never in association with the CD44-positive porcine astrocytes. We imagined that the astrocytes would be associated with the growth into grey matter, but from our careful data analysis we never found an association, not even within the white matter tracts themselves.

Björklund: Do you see preferential pathways for cell migration in this model?

Isacson: For the axons the pathways are not predictable. The growing axons will frequently seek out their normal target through non-typical pathways. For example, when we transplanted porcine nigra to the striatum and got axonal growth into the thalamus, this was through an atypical direction and pathway for the axons. In contrast, with the glial cells it is more or less random migration. They seem to be expanding radically from the site of implantation in the adult, and then migrate into any accessible white matter tract.

Blakemore: Do you think there's something funny going on with xenografts? Could it be that the xenografts are not obeying the same rules as allografts, and the fact that human cells grow better or pig cells migrate more may simply be because you are putting them into rats? If you put the pig cells back into pigs, would they behave in the same way as when you do a rat–rat graft, for example? In other words, are the recognition molecules in a xenograft situation incorrect, so what is seen in these situations is not that they grow better, but rather that they are being allowed to perform better because they are not subjected to the same degree of inhibition?

Isacson: This is not a theoretical question and the data are relative to rodents. In the experiments the data do not indicate that the pig cells are not exposed to growth inhibition. The fetal porcine cells are transplanted to the rat brain, which is very small compared with the pig brain. The experiments demonstrate that the pig axons can grow a relatively small distance (compared with the pig brain) to reach all normal anatomical targets. This proves that targeting molecules are available in the adult host brain. If you look at the transplant literature, the early work showing specific patterned growth in the hippocampus by cholinergic axons and very specific growth in the striatum by subsets of dopaminergic cell types, fits into that same theoretical framework for explaining our data (Isacson & Deacon 1997). My feeling is that it's not aberrant axonal behaviour, but it is showing what a continuously growing axon with highly committed targeting can do in the adult brain, but the growth is not to the extent that occurs in the pig brain. I'm suggesting that if you put pig cells into a pig they will behave in the same way as allografts of rat–rat. They will grow a fairly limited distance because of the growth cone collapsing activity present in the adult (but not in neonate) brain. This would limit reconnections in larger brains.

Björklund: There could be species differences in some of these recognition molecules, also. If they are species-specific, then some of these differences in cell migration or axon growth could be explained by the inability of the grafted cells to recognize the signals from the host. The pig cells or the human cells may not recognizing the growth-inhibiting molecules in the rat brain.

Gage: One thing that needs to be done is a head-up comparison of the cell types. You are talking about preparing cells differently in comparing pig versus human, for example. These are highly propagated cells that have often seen epidermal growth factor (EGF), FGF and leukaemia inhibitory factor (LIF). Ole Isacson, what were your cells?

Isacson: Ours were primary porcine fetal cells, but human fetal primary cells behave in a similar way with respect to connectivity, i.e. recognition of appropriate synaptic contacts.

Gage: Many of those studies need to be done systematically. We need to take the same aged cells from the same brain areas, and propagate them in the same way, with the same growth factors and then graft them into the same place. As much as possible, these experiments need to be exactly in parallel, otherwise it is difficult to begin to make comparisons between species.

Isacson: The particular experiment we were referring to was very systematic and symmetrical between donor tissues used. We determined the gestational age of the lateral ganglionic eminence (striatum) in pig so that it was similar to the rat (Deacon et al 1994). The observations we have are striking: the pig axons grow further than the rat, yet growth is slow. We think it can take up to a month to reach the substantia nigra. My interpretation from the data, is not that there are missing inhibitory influences on pig or human axons, but that the intrinsic growth capacities of these neurons are important as well as the host environment.

Price: Indeed, what is obviously required is to be able to distinguish between the cell autonomous behaviour and the interaction with the environment. If we are going to try to make these comparisons, we need a set of experiments that somehow assesses the cell autonomous capacity of the cells we're dealing with.

Finsen: I have a question relating to the axonal outgrowth in the adult CNS. Do the outgrowing axons grow along axons that have degenerated as a result of the lesion, or do they find a new route to grow along?

Björklund: We don't know what trajectory they follow. By the time of grafting there are most probably no degenerating axons left. It could be that there are vacated channels which the axons grow along, but we haven't been able to show that. The alternative possibility is that the trajectory is prepared by glial cells coming from the graft. Again, there are no data to prove or disprove this.

Gray: Would you like to try to extrapolate what you're saying to comment on the likely clinical wisdom of one strategy that is currently being used that is, to differentiate cells prior to transplantation into an all-neuronal population, as in the teratocarcinoma cells being used by Layton Bioscience (*http://www.laytonbio.com*). From what you are saying, this may not be the ultimate strategy because you don't want a purely neuronal population going in.

Björklund: This is an interesting issue that needs to be clarified. It would be of great interest to be able to do an experiment where a pure neuronal population is grafted into the striatal lesion to see what that cell population can do in the absence of any transplanted glia. This would help us sort out whether the collaboration of striatal neurons with immature glia is essential for axonal outgrowth in this model. It may be that the migrating immature glia cells play a critical role and the neurons are unable to grow over longer distances in the adult host brain without them.

Raisman: Is it possible to get a transplant of pure neurons?

Peschanski: We have done this with motor neurons: we've actually selected pure neuronal populations and used them in transplants (Rostaing-Rigattieri et al 1997). We haven't looked at axon growth, but survival is quite good. There is a trophic effect from neuronal populations on the glia: microglia and astrocytes come in to the body of the graft and establish a kind of 'normal' parenchyma.

Perry: The degenerating fibre tract is an important pathway. It is worth remembering that in humans the debris may persist for up to two years.

Reier: With regard to the pure neuronal populations, Dr Jo Velardo in my laboratory has been working with Layton Bioscience on testing their NT cells for intraspinal transplantation after injury. In contrast to what has been reported with the use of those cells *in vitro* or in other regions of the nervous system, in acute and chronic lesions of the spinal cord they do not differentiate very well. This assessment is based on looking at neuronal markers including specific receptor sub-types. However, the cells will form a very nice cohesive mass of tissue in a contusion injury with a large cyst, which fills the space very much like primary fetal cell transplants, which is interesting in its own right. However, even at six months out, these cells don't look like neurons with respect to phenotypic markers and other criteria, except in regions where they start integrating with the host. When they integrate with the host they appear to start differentiating, and one can observe a qualitatively different subpopulation of cells adjacent to the host as opposed to those that are sitting in the cyst. There also is some suggestion that there is recruitment of host glia, but I can't tell you whether this is active or passive.

Freeman: Intrinsic to the whole discussion is whether a clinical outcome or behaviour in animals is related to a trophic response. There is certainly room for the possibility that non-specific effects of grafts or trophic mechanisms can play a part. Another area that has been explored poorly throughout the field is the importance of grafts preventing second-order degeneration as a way of arresting the neurodegenerative process. There are many possible mechanisms that may respond to trophic effects secondary to outgrowth from the graft or from fibre ingrowth from the host to the graft.

Gray: It is important to get these lessons from what we've done so far with direct transplantation as clear as we can, as all the new technologies begin to go forward.

References

Brüstle O, Maskos U, McKay RD 1995 Host-guided migration allows targeted introduction of neurons into the embryonic brain. Neuron 15:1275–1285

Deacon TW, Pakzaban P, Burns LH, Dinsmore J, Isacson O 1994 Cytoarchitectonic development, axon–glia relationships, and long distance axon growth of porcine striatal xenografts in rats. Exp Neurol 130:151–157

Isacson O, Deacon TW 1996 Specific axon guidance factors persist in the adult brain as demonstrated by pig neuroblasts transplanted to the rat. Neuroscience 75:827–837

Isacson O, Deacon T 1997 Neural transplantation studies reveal the brain's capacity for continuous reconstruction. Trends Neurosci 20:477–482

Isacson O, Deacon TW, Pakzaban P, Galpern WR, Dinsmore J, Burns LH 1995 Transplanted xenogeneic neural cells in neurodegenerative disease models exhibit remarkable axonal target specificity and distinct growth patterns of glial and axonal fibres. Nat Med 1:1189–1194

Rostaing-Rigattieri S, Flores-Guevara R, Peschanski M, Cadusseau J 1997 Glial and endothelial cell response to a fetal transplant of purified neurons. Neuroscience 79:723–734

Functional analysis of fronto–striatal reconstruction by striatal grafts

Stephen B. Dunnett*

Centre for Brain Repair and Department of Experimental Psychology, University of Cambridge, Forvie Site, Robinson Way, Cambridge CB2 2PY, UK

Abstract. Excitotoxic lesions of the neostriatum induce cognitive and motor deficits in experimental animals, and model both the neuropathology and symptoms of Huntington's disease. Striatal grafts implanted into the denervated striatum survive, differentiate into both striatal- and non-striatal like neurons, restore input and output connections of the damaged striatum, and alleviate both motor and cognitive impairments in experimental rats and monkeys. Several lines of evidence suggest that the functional recovery is mediated by the grafts providing a reconstruction of the cortico–striato–pallidal circuitries of the host forebrain, including functional mapping of circuitry by immediate early gene induction, push–pull perfusion, microdialysis, electrophysiology, the lack of efficacy of pharmacological treatments and the behavioural studies themselves. Detailed analysis of motor recovery in an operant lateralized choice reaction time test indicates that for optimal functional recovery the animals require specific retraining in the stimulus–response associations lost by the lesions, which may have important implications for optimizing the functional efficacy of striatal grafts both in experimental models and clinical trials.

2000 Neural transplantation in neurodegenerative disease. Wiley, Chichester (Novartis Foundation Symposium 231) p 21–52

Striatal lesions and grafts

With the introduction of the cell suspension method of neural transplantation, which allowed implantation of embryonic neurons intraparenchymally into deep brain sites, one of the first targets for investigation was the neostriatum, not only for implantation of dopamine neurons into their terminal area but also implantation of striatal neurons after local destruction of the intrinsic striatal neurons with excitotoxins (Björklund et al 1987, Dunnett 1990a, Schmidt et al 1981). These two models have been extensively investigated, not least because

*Present address: Cardiff School of Biosciences, Cardiff University, Museum Avenue, PO Box 911, Cardiff CF10 3US, UK

they appear to contrast different mechanisms of function of neural transplants of different types — the restitution of a diffuse isodendritic core innervation in the case of dopamine grafts, as opposed to the reconstruction of both afferents and efferent pathways in the case of striatal grafts (Björklund et al 1987, Dunnett & Björklund 1994). Since Anders Björklund discusses the functional reconstruction in forebrain dopamine systems in his accompanying chapter in this volume, I will here concentrate on the analysis of functional repair after transplantation of intrinsic striatal tissues.

Striatal lesions

To date, striatal repair has been studied almost exclusively in animals with excitotoxic lesions of the neostriatum, widely considered to be an animal model of the anatomical, biochemical and functional pathology of Huntington's disease (HD) (Sanberg & Coyle 1984, Sanberg et al 1994). Early studies used predominantly kainic acid (Coyle & Schwarcz 1976, McGeer & McGeer 1976), which has been replaced in recent years by ibotenic acid and then quinolinic acid as producing more reliable and consistent lesions (Beal et al 1986, Köhler & Schwarcz 1983, Schwarcz et al 1979, 1983), without the remote damage and epileptic side effects of kainate, and with a relative selectivity for the medium spiny neurons over the large aspiny cholinergic, neuropeptide Y and NADPH diaphorase interneurons (Beal et al 1986, Schwarcz & Köhler 1983). Although this selective profile of toxicity has been taken to mimic the profile of cell loss in HD (Beal et al 1986), it is easy to overemphasize the selectivity of the toxins, which is achieved only at a critical concentration and so may be true at the microscopic level within a narrow annulus at a certain distance from the infusion site, but is never (in our experience) reproduced throughout the lesion volume.

More recently, a number of novel toxins such as malonate and 3-nitroproprionic acid (3-NP) have been introduced. These disrupt mitochondrial energy production in a manner similar to the biochemical disturbance observed in the human disease (Beal et al 1993, Maragos & Silverstein 1995). However, although 3-NP has the advantage that striatal neurons are targeted even with peripheral administration, the metabolic toxins are generally found to be less reliable than the excitotoxins and consequently have not replaced the classic methods in most transplantation studies.

It is possible that the recent advent of transgenic models of HD in mice overexpressing expanded polyglutamine tracts or the full length huntingtin protein (Hodgson et al 1999, Mangiarini et al 1996, Reddy et al 1999), but as yet these have not been characterized in sufficient detail to know whether the cellular and functional pathology is suitable for transplantation analysis and repair.

Striatal transplantation

The techniques for effective striatal transplantation are now well worked out and relatively straightforward. In essence, embryonic striatal primordium is dissected from the developing embryo, prepared as a cell suspension by incubation in trypsin, washing and mechanical dissociation according to standard protocols (see Fig. 1A) (Dunnett et al 1999a, Schmidt et al 1981), then injected stereotaxically into the brains of the host animals—rats, mice or monkeys. In contrast to dopamine-rich nigral grafts, which typically require multiple injection sites to innervate the whole striatum, in the case of striatal grafts only one or two deposits are typically required, although this dimension of striatal transplantation has not been widely investigated.

Two particular dimensions of the preparation protocol appear critical for functional efficacy. First the donor tissue must be harvested at a particular stage of embryonic development—Carnegie stage 20–22 (13–15 mm crown rump length in rat embryos, reached at approximately embryonic day [E]15) appears optimal (Dunnett & Björklund 1992). Graft tissues harvested later in development typically survive less well, show poor differentiation of neurons with a striatal phenotype and have a reduced efficacy in tests of functional recovery (Fricker et al 1997a,b). Secondly, the optimal dissection of striatal primordium is still a matter of active debate. Early studies collected both medial and lateral ridges of the ganglionic eminence (MGE and LGE respectively) (Dunnett & Björklund 1992), but Pakzaban and Isacson (Pakzaban et al 1993) proposed that a higher proportion of striatal neurons to non-striatal-like tissue (i.e. a higher ratio of P zones to NP-zones, *q.v.*) is obtained if the dissection is restricted to the LGE, and this has been replicated by others (Nakao et al 1994, Watts et al 1997). However, this restricted dissection may omit other components of the developing striatum, such as interneurons (Olsson et al 1998). The functional benefits of a restricted LGE dissection are not yet confirmed and most functional studies reviewed below have been based on a whole ganglionic eminence (WGE) dissection. Note, however, that the term 'striatal grafts' is widely used—here as well as elsewhere—as a short-hand for grafts derived from the developing ganglionic eminence—LGE or WGE. These dissections comprise precursor cells as well as newly differentiated neurons that are destined to form a variety of lateral cortical and subcortical cell populations, and include non-striatal neurons intermixed with the striatal neurons of experimental interest.

Striatal grafts

The last decade has seen extensive studies on the anatomy, neurochemistry, physiology and function of striatal grafts. As noted above, the developing grafts

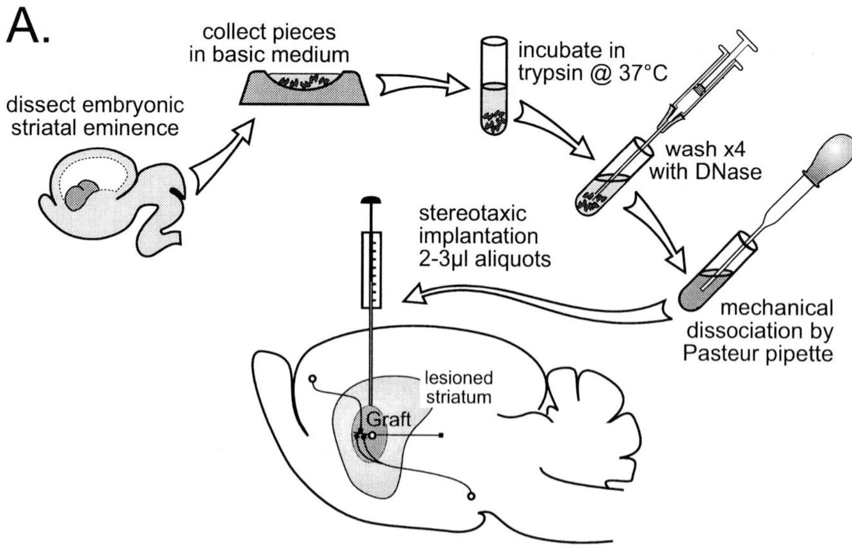

A.
dissect embryonic
striatal eminence
collect pieces
in basic medium
incubate in
trypsin @ 37°C
wash x4
with DNase
mechanical
dissociation by
Pasteur pipette
stereotaxic
implantation
2-3µl aliquots
lesioned
striatum
Graft

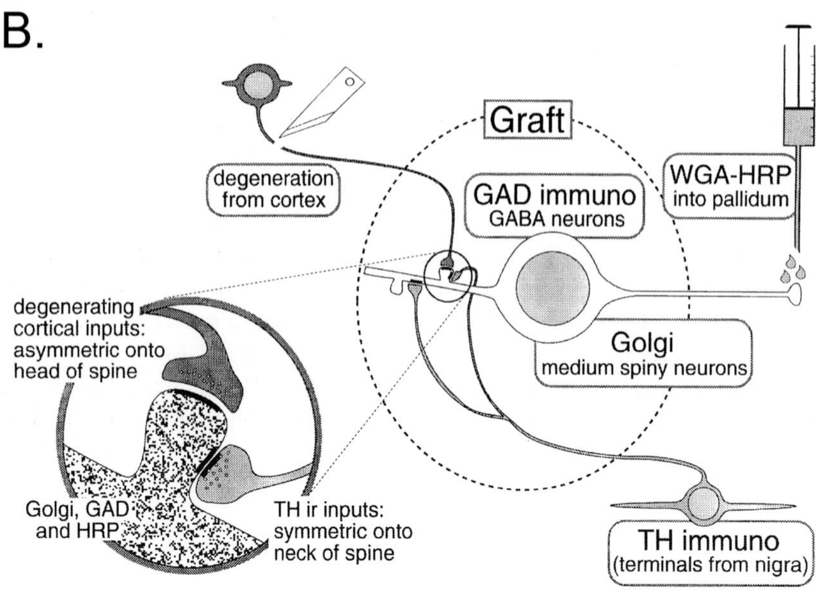

B.
degeneration
from cortex
Graft
GAD immuno
GABA neurons
WGA-HRP
into pallidum
degenerating
cortical inputs:
asymmetric onto
head of spine
Golgi
medium spiny neurons
Golgi, GAD
and HRP
TH ir inputs:
symmetric onto
neck of spine
TH immuno
(terminals from nigra)

develop a patchy pattern of staining for a variety of markers of striatal neurons, such as acetylcholinesterase, DARPP-32, Ca^{2+}-binding proteins, and opiate, dopamine or serotonin receptors (Björklund et al 1994, Graybiel et al 1989, 1990, Isacson et al 1987). These labels each co-localize in a compartment of the striatal grafts that has come to be known as the 'patches' or 'P-zones', interspersed with tissue that is negative for striatal markers but which contain neurons of non-striatal morphology in Golgi and which stains for markers of cortical, pallidal and other non-striatal areas of the forebrain derived from the ganglionic eminences (Graybiel et al 1989). Moreover, tracing of connections into and out of striatal grafts at both light and electron microscopic levels has revealed the reformation of normal striatal afferents from the neocortex, thalamus, substantia nigra and raphe nucleus, and the development of efferent projections to normal striatal targets in the globus pallidus, entopeduncular nucleus and substantia nigra (Clarke & Dunnett 1993, Wictorin et al 1988). Notably, the newly formed input and output connections with the host brain are established in particular with the GABAergic medium spiny striatal-like neurons of the P-zone compartment within the grafts (Fig. 1B). Moreover, as determined by both electrophysiological and *in vivo* neurochemical methods, these connections appear to have the capacity to transmit functional information from the host brain into the grafts and relay that information back to the host brain (Sirinathsinghji et al 1988).

Bilateral striatal lesions induce a range of functional deficits in rats and monkeys that reproduce many of the key features of HD in both the motor and cognitive realms. The different classes of functional lesion deficits will be surveyed as we consider in turn the efficacy and mechanisms of striatal transplantation repair.

FIG. 1.   (A) Schematic illustration of the protocol for striatal graft preparation, involving dissection, collection, enzymatic digestion in trypsin, washing, dissociation and stereotaxic implantation of dissociated cell suspension into the host brain (for details see Dunnett et al 1999a). (B) Schematic illustration of the tracing of neuronal connections into and out of striatal grafts, at the ultrastructural level. Cortical afferents were marked by undercutting the cortico–striatal projection and degenerating terminals identified in the grafts; dopaminergic terminals of nigral afferents were identified in the grafts by immunohistochemical labelling of tyrosine hydroxylase (TH); synapses were identified as being located on medium spiny neurons by Golgi impregnation; synapses that were GABAergic were identified by glutamic acid decarboxylase immunohistochemistry; and synapses that projected to the host globus pallidus were identified by retrograde labelling with wheat germ agglutinin-horseradish peroxidase. Examples of all double-labelled, and many triple-labelled combinations were observed (based on Clarke & Dunnett 1993).

Recovery of striatal motor functions

Rotation and activity

The most obvious symptom of striatal degeneration in humans, for example in HD, is a release of uncontrollable movements, typically chorea and other forms of dyskinesia (Harper 1996). Similarly, in animals, striatal stimulation induces 'arrest' whereas striatal lesions produce hyperactivity (Mason et al 1978, Sanberg et al 1979). Measurement of spontaneous locomotor activity thus became one of the first functional tests to be applied to animals with striatal grafts. There are now multiple replications of the observation that bilateral striatal grafts alleviate the hyperactivity seen in rats with bilateral lesions (Deckel et al 1983, Isacson et al 1984). The level of activity is dependent on the animal's motivational state; hyperactivity is more apparent both during the active nocturnal phase of the diurnal cycle and when the animals are food-deprived, and it is at these times that the grafts are most effective in restoring normal levels of spontaneous activity (Isacson et al 1986). Moreover, since the striatum is topographically organized, with ventral striatum in particular being implicated in regulation of global activation, the hyperactivity is most marked in animals in which both the lesions and the grafts are placed ventrally in the nucleus accumbens (Reading et al 1995).

A second simple measure of activation is provided by rotation. Unilateral striatal lesions induce an asymmetry of striatal outputs and a postural bias in the animals which is translated into head-to-tail turning — 'rotation' — when the animals are active. This is particularly marked when the animals are activated pharmacologically, e.g. using the dopamine stimulant amphetamine or the dopaminergic agonist apomorphine. Again, the asymmetry in rotation is alleviated by striatal grafts (Dunnett et al 1988, Norman et al 1988). Moreover, the two drugs cited have different implications for graft integration. Thus, apomorphine binds to dopamine receptors, which have been shown to be present on grafted neurons. Recovery of apomorphine-induced rotation suggests that the grafted neurons can transduce the pharmacological stimulation and so influence the striatal output targets to which they project. Conversely, amphetamine acts directly on host dopamine terminals, which innervate the grafts. Recovery of amphetamine-induced rotation therefore suggests that the grafted neurons can transduce information provided by an afferent input from the host which is then relayed back to the host. Indeed, this hypothesis has been confirmed directly by push–pull perfusion to monitor GABA release derived from grafted neurons and projecting to the host pallidum in response to pharmacological stimulation of graft afferents (Sirinathsinghji et al 1988).

Skilled paw reaching

Both nigral and striatal grafts can alleviate motor deficits in rotation induced by unilateral nigrostriatal and striatal lesions, respectively. However, there are other more complex motor deficits, in particular associated with more co-ordinated or skilled movements in tests such as paw reaching, extinction between competing stimuli or hoarding, that are not alleviated by nigral grafts. We have hypothesized that the critical feature that differentiates these latter tests is their dependence not just on the restoration of a dopaminergic activation at striatal terminals, but rather on the relay of functional information via the nigrostriatal projection, the integrity of which is not restored by nigral grafts implanted into an ectopic striatal location (Dunnett et al 1987). It is therefore noteworthy that striatal grafts can restore similar deficits in rats with striatal lesions (Dunnett et al 1988, Montoya et al 1990). Thus, for example, as shown in Fig. 2, both 6-hydroxydopmaine (6-OHDA) nigrostriatal and excitotoxic striatal lesions induce marked deficits in reaching with the contralateral paw to retrieve food pellets from the steps of a lateralized 'staircase' test. However, whereas nigral grafts have no effect on the nigrostriatal lesion deficit, the striatal grafts produce a substantial and significant recovery in the animals with intrinsic striatal lesions (Montoya et al 1990). The recovery is specific not only to the striatal lesion model but also to the matching of striatal tissues. It is noteworthy that only in this combination of lesion and graft do we see an anatomical reconstruction of the input and output connections of the striatum, supporting the initial hypothesis regarding failure in the nigral graft model.

Choice reaction time

Recently we have begun to develop a number of operant tests that allow particular features of the selection, initiation and execution of lateralized movements to be analysed. Based on a design originally introduced by Carli et al (1985), we have used two different operant apparatuses to analyse the choice reaction time to make lateralized responses to brief visual stimuli.

The first test is conducted in a Skinner box with two retractable levers, one on either side of a central food panel. The rat is required to hold its nose in the central panel while the two levers are extended into the chamber, and then after a variable delay a light flashes briefly above one of the levers. The animal is required to rapidly press the lever under the light signal in order to gain a food pellet reward. Unilateral striatal lesions impair accuracy in responding in particular on trials on the contralateral side, and even when the animals do respond correctly the speed of the response is markedly slowed (Döbrössy & Dunnett 1997). This deficit is significantly alleviated by a striatal graft (Döbrössy & Dunnett 1998). In particular, whereas some measures of accuracy and side bias were also alleviated

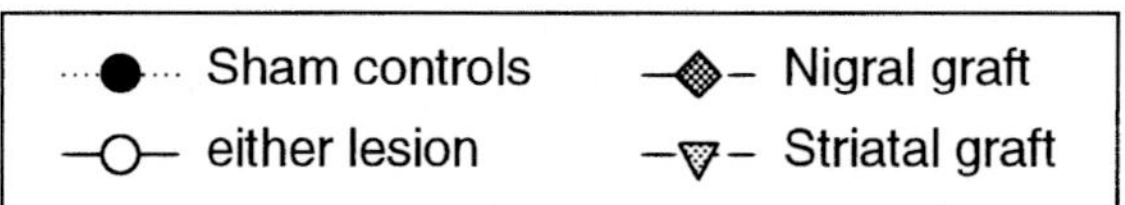

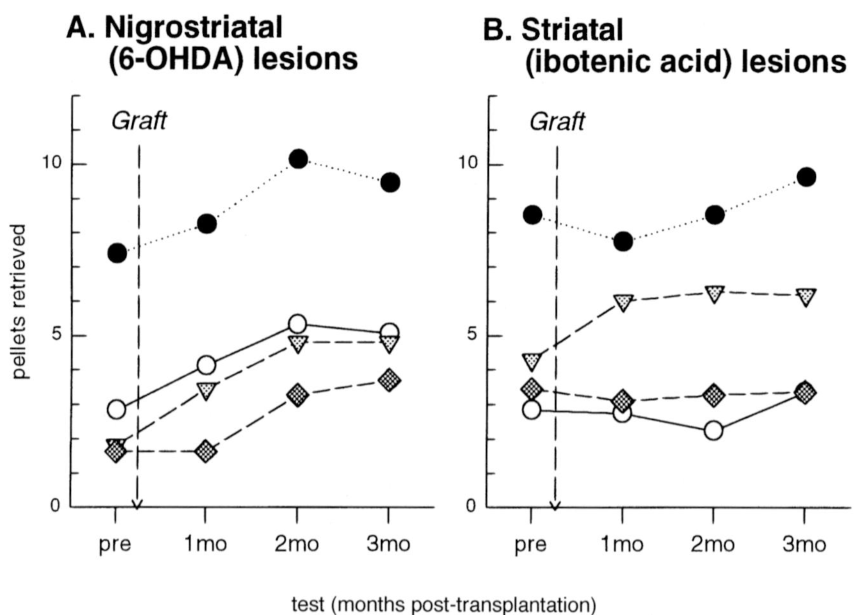

test (months post-transplantation)

FIG. 2.   Skilled paw reaching in the staircase test. (A) Four groups of rats received either control or 6-OHDA lesion of the nigrostriatal pathway. One of the lesion groups received nigral grafts (the experimental group for the nigrostriatal lesion) and a second received striatal grafts (the control graft for this lesion). (B) A further four groups received either control or ibotenic acid lesion of the striatum. One of these lesion groups also received nigral grafts (which should not affect the striatal lesion damage) and a second received striatal grafts (the experimental graft for this lesion). Both lesions produced marked deficits in skilled reaching, but only the striatal grafts provided specific recovery of the striatal lesion deficit, whereas the nigral grafts were without effect in either lesion model and the nigral lesions was not alleviated by either graft (based on Montoya et al 1990).

by control grafts of cortical tissue, the specific deficit in the speed of movement was alleviated by the striatal grafts alone.

In the second series of tests, we have used a 'nine-hole box' apparatus, in which the rat is confronted by a horizontal array of holes in each of which a light can be illuminated briefly to signal target locations, and in each of which a photocell beam can detect nose-poke responses of the rat (Robbins et al 1993). In a task similar to that originally used by Carli et al (1985), only three holes are used, the centre hole and one on each side. Rats are trained to hold their noses in the centre hole until a light flashes briefly in either the left or right hole. Rats can be trained in two conditions: in the 'Same' condition a reward is given for responding to the hole in which the light stimulus appeared, whereas in the 'Opposite' condition the rat must respond on the other side, to the hole in which the stimulus light did not appear. Not only is the opposite condition more difficult for rats to learn — and so can provide a greater challenge to tease out small differences in performance — but more critically it allows us to distinguish the nature of the rat's impairment after a unilateral lesion. Both 6-OHDA nigrostriatal lesions and excitotoxic striatal lesions produce marked deficits in the rat's ability to respond in the holes on the contralateral side of the body, whereas there is little deficit on the ipsilateral side (Brown & Robbins 1989, Carli et al 1985). This deficit has several important features, including a decline in accuracy of responses to the contralateral side, a marked bias towards the ipsilateral side, and an impairment in the speed of the response. The deficit appears to be at an output (motor) rather than an input (sensory) level, since the stimuli that give rise to deficits appear on different sides in the two conditions — contralateral to the lesion in the Same condition but ipsilateral to the lesion in the Opposite condition (Brown & Robbins 1989, Carli et al 1985). In the nine-hole box, the apparatus can distinguish between 'reaction time' (RT), the latency for the rat to withdraw its nose from the central hole, and 'movement time' (MT), the time to execute the lateralized movement and make the nose poke into the signalled hole. It is noteworthy that both nigrostriatal and striatal lesions produce a greater impairment in RT than in MT for responses on the contralateral side, even though the RT is itself a relatively non-lateralized response. This suggests that the striatal lesion deficit is one of the planning and initiation of a contralateral movement rather than in the motor execution of the movement itself.

Again, as in the Skinner box, we have seen that striatal grafts can alleviate the ipsilateral response bias (Mayer et al 1992). In a subsequent experiment, we replicated this effect over a longer period of postoperative testing and observe that a rather comparable degree of recovery is achieved whether the striatal grafts are based on the WGE or LGE dissections of the embryonic ganglionic eminence (Brasted et al 1999a). In a further experiment we then manipulated the interval between the lesion and graft surgeries. Whereas good recovery was achieved when only 10 days separated lesion and grafting, no recovery was seen when 10 weeks separated the two surgical sessions (Fig. 3) (Brasted et al 2000). Since striatal afferents gradually retract over a period of weeks following excitotoxic lesions of the striatal neurons that are their targets, this latter result provides further corroboration for the hypothesis that functional recovery is critically dependent upon the reformation of afferent connections to, as well as efferent connections from, the grafts.

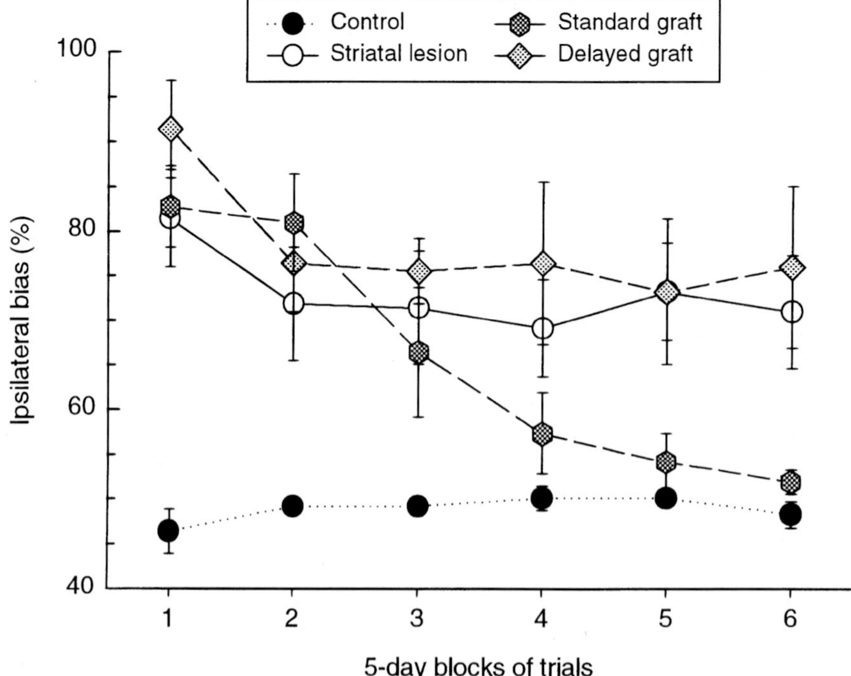

FIG. 3.   Graft derived recovery on a choice reaction time task in the nine-hole box. Unilateral lesions induced a marked ipsilateral bias in responding to stimuli on the contralateral side which is significantly alleviated by striatal grafts implanted 10 days after unilateral striatal lesion, but not when implanted 10 weeks after lesions (data from Brasted et al 2000).

Recovery of fronto–striatal cognitive functions

The neostriatum receives a rich projection from the association areas of the frontal lobe (the 'prefrontal' cortex). Associated with the highest levels of cognitive processing in the brain, damage of prefrontal cortex in rats and monkeys produces a syndrome of impairments that has been characterized as involving a disruption of 'executive' function apparent in tests of planning, spatial mapping, short-term memory and adaptation of response selection to changing stimuli and task demands. Since the classic experiments of Rosvold and Divac, it has been known that striatal lesions can reproduce deficits on the same tests (Battig et al 1960, Divac et al 1967), reflecting the involvement of the striatum in an integrated frontal–subcortical functional system. Indeed these early observations provided an important foundation for modern conceptualizations of multiple cortical–basal ganglia loops in the control of both cognition and action (Alexander et al 1986). This same association between striatum and prefrontal cortex is mirrored in the clinical realm by the observation that cognitive symptoms are as central to HD as the motor symptoms, and that the former are of the 'frontal' type (Zakzanis 1998).

T maze alternation

The first tests of cognition in rats with striatal grafts used simple maze learning tests. Bilateral striatal lesions produce a marked and lasting inability of rats to learn a delayed alternation task in a T maze, a classic test of prefrontal deficits. This deficit can be significantly alleviated by bilateral grafts of striatal tissue implanted into the lesioned striatum but not when the grafts are implanted into the pallidum (Isacson et al 1986). Thus, recovery was only seen when the grafts were placed in a location compatible with reformation of cortico–striatal connections, but not when they were placed in an ectopic location, which would have been efficient for target reinnervation (the principle which works best in the case of nigral grafts) but would be unlikely to reconstruct the full cortical–striatal–pallidal circuitry.

Operant delayed matching

A second test that has been widely used to evaluate prefrontal-like deficits in monkeys is delayed matching to sample (D'Amato 1973, Goldman-Rakic 1989). In this test, a sample object or computer-generated stimulus is shown to the monkey, and then after a variable delay interval two different objects/stimuli are shown. In the delayed matching variation, the monkey is rewarded for responding to the sample stimulus, whereas in the delayed non-matching variation, the monkey is rewarded for responding to the novel stimulus. Although it has proved difficult to train rats to perform a similar task based on visual stimuli (at least in automated test boxes), rats will learn quickly and efficiently if spatial stimuli are used. Thus, in tests of 'delayed matching and non-matching to position' (DMTP, DNMTP), one or other of the Skinner box levers is presented in the sample phase of each trial and then, after a delay, the rat makes a choice between the two levers, being given rewards according to either a matching or a non-matching rule (Dunnett 1985). The power of DMTP and DNMTP is that many trials can be presented on each day, allowing us to construct for each rat an accurate measure of response accuracy at different delay intervals, and thereby determining the rate of forgetting as the delay lengthens. Delayed matching and non-matching tests provide an efficient and selective test of short-term memory on which rats with medial frontal lesions exhibit a specific pattern of deficit, viz. accuracy is increasingly impaired at progressively longer delays (Dunnett 1990b). This delay-dependent pattern of impairment suggests a rather specific disturbance in short-term memory. However, larger lesions that extend into the anterior cingulate cortex produces a broader impairment at all delays, reflecting a more generalized deficit in the animal's ability to perform the matching rule (Dunnett 1990b). Similarly, when we looked at impairments following striatal lesions, lesions in the ventral striatum (which receives restricted prefrontal inputs) exhibited a clear delay-dependent deficit, whereas lesions in the dorsal striatum (which receives cingulate as well as frontal inputs) disrupted animals performance at all delays (Fig. 4) (Döbrössy et al 1996, Dunnett 1990b,c).

Whereas the DMTP and DNMTP tasks have proved effective for revealing the parallel between frontal and striatal involvement in short-term memory, the test has been less efficient for evaluating the influence of striatal grafts on this aspect of frontal-type cognition. In particular, in all experiments so far, the striatal deficit is minimal when the animals are trained on acquisition following a lesion (Döbrössy et al 1996), and when pre-trained the deficits that are seen after the lesion recover rapidly with further training (Döbrössy et al 1995). This pattern of spontaneous recovery makes it difficult to evaluate the effects of grafts which require a stable baseline of deficit against which specific graft-derived recovery can be evaluated. We have therefore turned to investigation of another operant task that might prove more suitable for this purpose.

Operant delayed alternation

Since delayed alternation provides perhaps the most robust classic test of prefrontal deficits and this contingency had proved effective for revealing the effects of striatal graft in open maze tests (see section 'T maze alternation', above), we have recently developed an operant version by adaptation of the DNMTP task to the delayed alternation rule (Dunnett et al 1999b). In this task, both levers are presented on every trial and the response rule is simply to press the lever on the side opposite to that pressed on the previous trial. This turns out to be more difficult for rats to learn than the DNMTP task in which the sample and choice trials are separated and discrete. By contrast, in delayed alternation, each response is both a choice based on the previous response and the sample for the next choice, and so there is more chance for interference between successive responses. As in DNMTP, a variable interval is used between each trial in our operant delayed alternation test so as to provide additional information on short-term forgetting and interference between trials.

Lesions both of the prefrontal cortex and of the medial striatum disrupt performance on the operant delayed alternation task (Dunnett et al 1999b). Moreover, the deficit is more stable and long-lasting than that seen after striatal lesions in the delayed non-matching task. Nevertheless, with extensive training, at least partial recovery is seen on this task also. We have recently undertaken a preliminary evaluation of animals with bilateral lesions and striatal grafts and seen that over a period of 10 weeks retraining, the lesioned animals remain significantly impaired. The grafted animals appeared to show a clear improvement, their performance falling between the lesion and graft groups, but the magnitude of the baseline deficit was such that the graft groups fell in-between and differed from neither the control nor lesion animals (F. Nathwani, P.J. Brasted & S.B. Dunnett, unpublished observations). This study is therefore currently being repeated, using larger lesions to increase the separation between groups and so determine the significance of these preliminary observations.

Recovery of striatal habit learning

The motor and cognitive deficits are frequently presented as qualitatively different functional realms. However, several considerations argue against such an overt distinction. Firstly, contemporary attempts to characterize the nature of frontal cognition are emphasizing the role of the prefrontal cortex in 'executive' functions, in particular in the planning, selection and initiation of appropriate motor action (Robbins 1998, Shallice & Burgess 1999). As such the prefrontal cortex may be considered as providing the very highest level of motor control. Secondly, other theoretical considerations have emphasized the role of the striatum in motor learning, in particular in the formation and maintenance of habits (Knowlton et al 1996, Mishkin et al 1984, Packard et al 1989, White 1997). 'Habits' are motor programmes (integrated sequences of co-ordinated responses) that come under stimulus control by associative stimulus–response (S-R) learning. Once well established, they are expressed automatically under the control of the appropriate stimuli, and lie outside the realm of conscious attention or intention. This aspect of learning has been attributed to the striatum, in contrast to the more purposive, episodic aspects of learning and memory attributed to the hippocampus (Mishkin et al 1984, Packard et al 1989, Packard & Teather 1997). The ability to learn new motor skills and habits is the major aspect of learning that is spared after bilateral temporal lobe lesions in patients such as HM (Milner 1966).

As we consider the operant tasks that were developed to evaluate restoration of motor functions in rats and monkeys with striatal grafts (see 'Recovery of striatal motor functions: choice reaction time', above) it is apparent that not only the tasks themselves require extensive training to provide the measures of the rats' motor capacity, but also that the motor performance itself is profoundly influenced by learning. Indeed, the 'motor' functions assessed are highly trained and rapidly executed S-R associations that define habits, and as such they fundamentally involve learned motor skills rather than simple spontaneous motor capacity *per se*. Moreover, the use of these operant tasks to analyse striatal lesion and graft function has led to novel and unexpected insights into the nature of graft

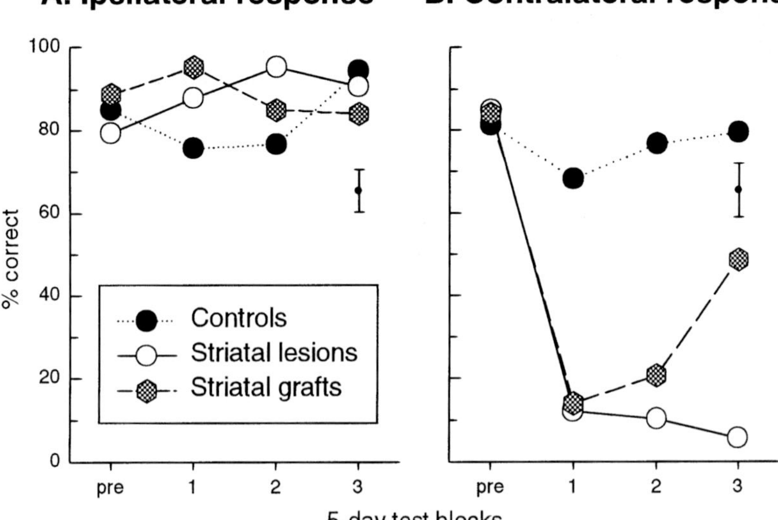

FIG. 4.   Learning to use the transplant. (A) The unilateral lesions and grafts have no effect on accuracy of performance on the ipsilateral side. (B) Striatal lesions in pre-trained rats induced a marked deficit in the accuracy of responding on the contralateral side, which did not recover with training. Rats with striatal grafts initially exhibit as big a deficit as the rats with lesions alone, but the grafted rats exhibited a significant relearning of the task contingencies over three weeks of training (data from Mayer et al 1992).

function, in particular in the phenomenon that we have labelled 'learning to use the transplant' (Brasted et al 1999b, Mayer et al 1992).

Learning to use the transplant

In the experiment by Mayer and colleagues (Mayer et al 1992) described above, striatal grafts alleviated the deficits induced by a unilateral striatal lesion in choice accuracy on the contralateral side in the opposite condition of the Carli test. However a key feature of these data was that when first tested 6 months after the lesion and graft surgery the grafted rats were as impaired as the lesion animals on the contralateral side. It was only after three weeks retraining on the task that the groups diverged: the grafted animals relearned the opposite S-R contingency, whereas the lesion animals remained profoundly impaired (Fig. 4). We reasoned that the anatomical regrowth of the grafts over six months after implantation would have reached asymptote and that it was unlikely that the 3 weeks' training provided any major change in the long-distance connections of the graft into the host circuitry. Rather, if the striatum provides a substrate for habit formation then the specific S-R contingency would have to be relearned, presumably involving some aspect of synaptic plasticity within the reconstructed integrated host and graft fronto–striatal circuits. The animals not only required the graft to replace the lost striatum, they had to learn to use the transplant by retraining in the specific habits disrupted by the lesion.

In the first study (Mayer et al 1992), retraining was terminated after 3 weeks while recovery was only partial, and the extent of the potential for relearning was not established. The two subsequent studies reported above by Brasted et al (1999b, 2000, and see Fig. 3) used the same Opposite task to replicate the effect but continued training over 6–8 weeks and established that with extensive retraining relatively complete recovery can eventually be achieved in many animals.

Lateralized two-choice discrimination

Whereas the Opposite contingency in the Carli task has been effective in demonstrating and replicating the learning to use the transplant effect, it neither establishes precisely what is relearned, nor addresses whether the relearning phenomenon is universal.

In order to cast light on the mechanism of graft function, Brasted and colleagues introduced a variation of the basic serial reaction time paradigm to assess the formation of choice S-R associations separately on the ipsilateral and contralateral sides (Brasted et al 1999b). Animals were trained to hold their nose in a central hole and then detect and respond to brief stimuli appearing laterally in near or far holes, with separate training on the ipsilateral and contralateral sides on alternate days. Unilateral striatal lesions induced marked deficits in accuracy when stimuli appeared on the contralateral side, an ipsilateral response bias to the near hole, and significant slowing of reaction and movement times for contralateral responses (Brasted et al 1997).

As in the Carli task, unilateral striatal grafts provided significant alleviation of the deficit on the contralateral side in the two choice task, and this recovery required relearning of the task (Brasted et al 1999b). However, this version of the task now allows us to probe what exactly the animal relearns, general motor activation, retraining in the general task contingencies, or relearning of the specific S-R association on the contralateral side. All animals were trained on both sides, but then after lesion and grafting half the animals were tested and retrained on the contralateral side for 30 days before retraining on the ipsilateral side, and the other half were retrained in the opposite order, ipsilateral and then contralateral (Brasted et al 1999b). As shown in Fig. 5A, the rats that were first trained on the contralateral side again replicated the learning to use the transplant effect — the control animals retained the discrimination from 4 months previously,

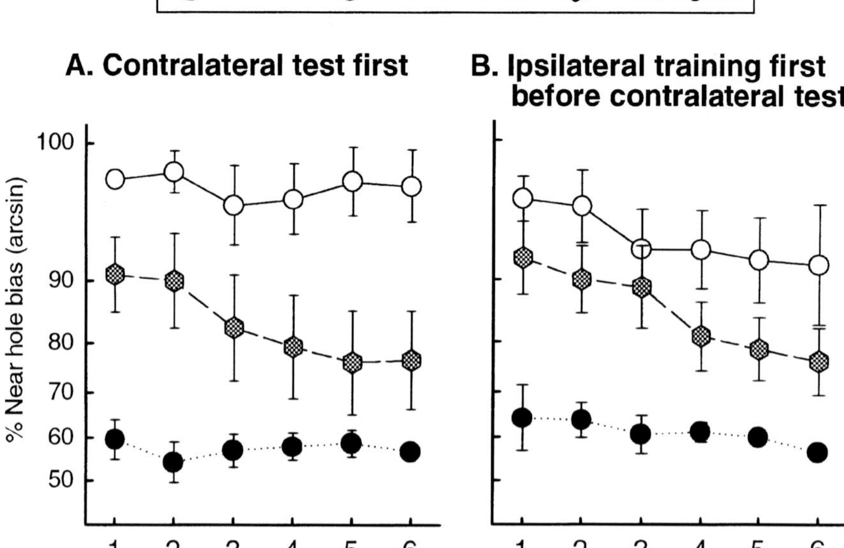

FIG. 5.   Specificity of the learning to use the transplant effect. Pre-trained rats with striatal lesions exhibit a lasting deficit in the response bias on the contralateral side, which is alleviated after relearning by rats with striatal grafts. The effect is exactly comparable whether the animals are tested first on the contralateral side (A) or whether they first receive 30 days of intensive training on the ipsilateral side (B). The absence of transfer of training between sides indicates lateralized specificity of the need for relearning to the grafted striatum (data from Brasted et al 1999b).

whereas both the lesion and graft animals exhibited profound deficits ($>90\%$ near hole bias) when first retested. Thereafter, the grafted animals showed substantial and significant relearning, whereas the lesion animals remained fully deficient. The other group of rats was retrained for 30 days on the ipsilateral side (on which both the lesion and graft rats exhibited significant but small deficits which did not change with training) before switching to the contralateral side. As shown in Fig. 5B, these latter lesion animals showed exactly the same lesion deficit and the graft animals showed exactly the same pattern of relearning on the contralateral side as the former group with no ipsilateral training (neither main effect nor any interaction with previous training were significant). Thus, the specific S-R association had to be relearned *de novo* on the lesion side — presumably within the reformed graft-host circuitry — and there was no savings whatsoever, even with extensive training of the task contingencies on the intact side.

The ambiguity on the second of the two issues raised above (the universality of relearning) relates to the question of why, if habit formation is central to striatal function, the phenomenon had not been observed in the many previous studies of striatal graft function. This could be explained by two factors, which are not mutually exclusive. First, many tests assess motor skills and habits that the animals use in the course of their normal daily lives — locomoting, exploring, picking up and manipulating food pellets, interacting with their cage partners, etc. All of these activities will therefore be retrained in the normal passage of time between surgery and retest. Second, in many other tests that are more complex, such as recovery of delayed alternation, the animals are tested under acquisition of the task contingencies, i.e. lesion, graft and control animals are trained *de novo* on the test once the grafts are already established. To reveal the learning to use the transplant effect we require specific S-R habits that are pre-trained prior to lesion and graft surgery and which involve specific associations that are not otherwise encountered in the course of the animal's daily lives. This is clearly true of the somewhat 'unnatural' opposite contingency in the Carli task, but does not apply to most other tests which are often chosen for their ecological validity but which thereby excludes their relevance in this context.

These considerations have several implications (Brasted et al 1999b, Marshall 1999). First, if the host — whether a rat or a patient — is to gain maximum benefit from a graft it is not sufficient simply to maximize graft survival and anatomical integration. We must also consider whether specific training or retraining is required to relearn previously established habits of relevance to the animal's (or patient's) contemporary environment, needs and demands. This may suggest the benefit of environmental enrichment conditions for animals throughout the recovery phase, or specific programmes of physiotherapy or occupational therapy for patients in transplantation programmes. Conversely, the fact that rats do in fact show good recovery on many tests in the absence of specific retraining suggest that although relearning may be required the grafted striatum has considerable plasticity and there are many ways this may be acquired.

Conclusions

Striatal grafts can alleviate deficits induced by striatal lesions in diverse aspects of normal striatal function, including simple motor responding, cognition on functions of the frontal type, and skilled habit formation and motor learning. Detailed analysis does not indicate a simple association between graft survival and recovery, as might be suggested by a simple pharmacological mode of action. Rather, recovery depends both on the reformation of grafts into the anatomical circuitry of the host brain and on the relearning of the specific S-R associations within an integrated graft-plus-host fronto–striatal system.

References

Alexander GE, DeLong MR, Strick PL 1986 Parallel organization of functionally segregated circuits linking basal ganglia and cortex. Annu Rev Neurosci 9:357–381

Battig K, Rosvold HE, Mishkin M 1960 Comparison of the effects of frontal and caudate lesions on delayed response and alternation in monkeys. J Comp Physiol Psychol 53:400–404

Beal MF, Kowall NW, Ellison DW, Mazurek MF, Swartz KJ, Martin JB 1986 Replication of the neurochemical characteristics of Huntington's disease by quinolinic acid. Nature 321:168–171

Beal MF, Brouillet EP, Jenkins BG et al 1993 Neurochemical and histologic characterization of striatal excitotoxic lesions produced by the mitochondrial toxin 3-nitropropionic acid. J Neurosci 13:4181–4192

Björklund A, Lindvall O, Isacson O et al 1987 Mechanisms of action of intracerebral neural implants: studies on nigral and striatal grafts to the lesioned striatum. Trends Neurosci 10:509–516

Björklund A, Campbell K, Sirinathsinghji DJS, Fricker RA, Dunnett SB 1994 Functional capacity of striatal transplants in the rat Huntington model. In: Dunnett SB, Björklund A (eds) Functional neural transplantation. Raven Press, New York, p 157–195

Brasted P, Humby T, Dunnett SB, Robbins TW 1997 Unilateral lesions of the dorsal striatum in rats disrupt responding in egocentric space. J Neurosci 17:8919–8926

Brasted PJ, Watts C, Torres EM, Robbins TW, Dunnett SB 1999a Behavioural recovery following striatal transplantation: effects of postoperative training and P-zone volume. Exp Brain Res 128:535–538

Brasted PJ, Watts C, Robbins TW, Dunnett SB 1999b Associative plasticity in striatal transplants. Proc Natl Acad Sci USA 96:10524–10529

Brasted PJ, Robbins TW, Dunnett SB 2000 Behavioral recovery following transplantation into a rat model of Huntington's disease requires both anatomical connectivity and extensive postoperative training. Behav Neurosci 114:431–436

Brown VJ, Robbins TW 1989 Elementary processes of response selection mediated by distinct regions of the striatum. J Neurosci 9:3760–3765

Carli M, Evenden JL, Robbins TW 1985 Depletion of unilateral striatal dopamine impairs initiation of contralateral actions and not sensory attention. Nature 313:679–682

Clarke DJ, Dunnett SB 1993 Synaptic relationships between cortical and dopaminergic inputs and intrinsic GABAergic systems within intrastriatal striatal grafts. J Chem Neuroanat 6:147–158

Coyle JT, Schwarcz R 1976 Lesions of striatal neurons with kainic acid provides a model for Huntington's chorea. Nature 263:244–246

D'Amato MR 1973 Delayed matching and short-term memory in monkeys. Psychol Learn Motiv 7:227–269

Deckel AW, Robinson RG, Coyle JT, Sanberg PR 1983 Reversal of long-term locomotor abnormalities in the kainic acid model of Huntington's disease by day 18 fetal striatal implants. Eur J Pharmacol 92:287–288

Divac I, Rosvold HE, Szwarcbart MK 1967 Behavioral effects of selective ablation of the caudate nucleus. J Comp Physiol Psychol 63:184–190

Döbrössy MD, Dunnett SB 1997 Unilateral striatal lesions impair response execution on a lateralised choice reaction time task. Behav Brain Res 87:159–171

Döbrössy MD, Dunnett SB 1998 Striatal grafts alleviate deficits in response execution in a lateralised reaction time task. Brain Res Bull 47:585–593

Döbrössy MD, Svendsen CN, Dunnett SB 1995 The effects of bilateral striatal lesions on the acquisition of an operant test of short-term memory. Neuroreport 6:2049–2053

Döbrössy MD, Svendsen CN, Dunnett SB 1996 Bilateral striatal lesions impair retention of an operant test of short-term memory. Brain Res Bull 41:159–165

Dunnett SB 1985 Comparative effects of cholinergic drugs and lesions of nucleus basalis or fimbria-fornix on delayed matching in rats. Psychopharmacology (Berl) 87:357–363

Dunnett SB 1990a Functional analysis of neural grafts in the neostriatum. In: Björklund A, Aguayo AJ, Ottoson D (eds) Brain repair. Macmillan, Basingstoke, p 355–373

Dunnett SB 1990b Role of prefrontal cortex and striatal output systems in short-term memory deficits associated with ageing, basal forebrain lesions, and cholinergic-rich grafts. Can J Psychol 44:210–232

Dunnett SB 1990c Is it possible to repair the damaged prefrontal cortex by neural tissue transplantation? Prog Brain Res 85:285–297

Dunnett SB, Björklund A 1992 Staging and dissection of rat embryos. In: Dunnett SB, Björklund A (eds) Neural transplantation: a practical approach. IRL Press, Oxford, p 1–19

Dunnett SB, Björklund A 1994 Mechanisms of function of neural grafts in the injured brain. In: Dunnett SB, Björklund A (eds) Functional neural transplantation. Raven Press, New York, p 531–567

Dunnett SB, Whishaw IQ, Rogers DC, Jones GH 1987 Dopamine-rich grafts ameliorate whole body motor asymmetry and sensory neglect but not independent limb use in rats with 6-hydroxydopamine lesions. Brain Res 415:63–78

Dunnett SB, Isacson O, Sirinathsinghji DJS, Clarke DJ, Björklund A 1988 Striatal grafts in rats with unilateral neostriatal lesions. III. Recovery from dopamine-dependent motor asymmetry and deficits in skilled paw reaching. Neuroscience 24:813–820

Dunnett SB, Boulton AA, Baker GB 1999a Neural transplantation methods. Humana Press, Totowa, NJ (Neuromethods 36)

Dunnett SB, Nathwani F, Brasted PJ 1999b Medial prefrontal and neostriatal lesions disrupt performance in an operant delayed alternation task in rats. Behav Brain Res 106:13–28

Fricker RA, Sirinathsinghji DJS, Torres EM, Hume S, Dunnett SB 1997a The effects of donor stage on the survival and function of embryonic striatal grafts in the adult rat brain. I. Morphological characteristics. Neuroscience 79:695–710

Fricker RA, Torres EM, Hume SP et al 1997b The effects of donor stage on the survival and function of embryonic striatal grafts. II. Correlation between positron emission tomography and reaching behaviour. Neuroscience 79:711–721

Goldman-Rakic PS 1989 Circuitry of primate prefrontal cortex and regulation of behavior by representational memory. In: Handbook of physiology: the nervous system, vol V. American Physiological Association, Baltimore, NJ, p 373–417

Graybiel AM, Liu FC, Dunnett SB 1989 Intrastriatal grafts derived from fetal striatal primordia. I. Phenotypy and modular organization. J Neurosci 9:3250–3271

Graybiel AM, Liu FC, Dunnett SB 1990 Cellular reaggregation *in vivo*: modular patterns in intrastriatal grafts derived from fetal striatal primordia. Prog Brain Res 82:401–405

Harper PS 1996. Huntington's disease. WB Saunders, London

Hodgson JG, Agopyan N, Gutekunst CA et al 1999 A YAC mouse model for Huntington's disease with full-length mutant huntingtin, cytoplasmic toxicity, and selective striatal neurodegeneration. Neuron 23:181–192

Isacson O, Brundin P, Kelly PAT, Gage FH, Björklund A 1984 Functional neuronal replacement by grafted striatal neurons in the ibotenic acid lesioned rat striatum. Nature 311:458–460

Isacson O, Dunnett SB, Björklund A 1986 Graft-induced behavioral recovery in an animal model of Huntington disease. Proc Natl Acad Sci USA 83:2728–2732

Isacson O, Dawbarn D, Brundin P, Gage FH, Emson PC, Björklund A 1987 Neural grafting in a rat model of Huntington's disease: striosomal-like organization of striatal grafts as revealed by acetylcholinesterase histochemistry, immunocytochemistry and receptor autoradiography. Neuroscience 22:481–497

Knowlton BJ, Mangels JA, Squire LR 1996 A neostriatal habit learning system in humans. Science 273:1399–1402

Köhler C, Schwarcz R 1983 Comparison of ibotenate and kainate neurotoxicity in rat brain: a histological study. Neuroscience 8:819–835

Mangiarini L, Sathasivam K, Seller M et al 1996 Exon 1 of the HD gene with an expanded CAG repeat is sufficient to cause a progressive neurological phenotype in transgenic mice. Cell 87:493–506

Maragos WF, Silverstein FS 1995 The mitochondrial inhibitor malonate enhances NMDA toxicity in the neonatal rat striatum. Brain Res Dev Brain Res 88:117–121

Marshall JF 1999 The education of a brain transplant. Proc Natl Acad Sci USA 96:9976–9978

Mason ST, Sanberg PR, Fibiger HC 1978 Kainic acid lesions of the striatum dissociate amphetamine and apomorphine stereotypy: similarities to Huntington's chorea. Science 201:352–355

Mayer E, Brown VJ, Dunnett SB, Robbins TW 1992 Striatal graft-associated recovery of a lesion-induced performance deficit in the rat requires learning to use the transplant. Eur J Neurosci 4:119–126

McGeer EG, McGeer PL 1976 Duplication of the biochemical changes of Huntington's choreas by intrastriatal injection of glutamic and kainic acids. Nature 263:517–519

Milner B 1966 Amnesia following operation on the temporal lobes. In: Whitty CWM, Zangwill OL (eds) Amnesia. Butterworths, London

Mishkin M, Malamut B, Bachevalier J 1984 Memories and habits: two neural systems. In: Lynch G, McGaugh JL, Weinberger NM (eds) Neurobiology of learning and memory. Guilford Press, New York, p 65–77

Montoya CP, Astell S, Dunnett SB 1990 Effects of nigral and striatal grafts on skilled forelimb use in the rat. Prog Brain Res 82:459–466

Nakao N, Odin P, Brundin P 1994 Selective sub-dissection of the striatal primordium for cultures affects the yield of DARPP-32-containing neurons. Neuroreport 5:1081–1084

Norman AB, Calderon SF, Giordano M, Sanberg PR 1988 Striatal tissue transplants attenuate apomorphine-induced rotational behavior in rats with unilateral kainic acid lesions. Neuropharmacology 27:333–336

Olsson M, Björklund A, Campbell K 1998 Early specification of striatal projection neurons and interneuronal subtypes in the lateral and medial ganglionic eminence. Neuroscience 84:867–876

Packard MG, Teather LA 1997 Double dissociation of hippocampal and dorsal-striatal memory systems by posttraining intracerebral injections of 2-amino-5-phosphonopentanoic acid. Behav Neurosci 111:543–551

Packard MG, Hirsh R, White NM 1989 Differential effects of fornix and caudate nucleus lesions on two radial maze tasks: evidence for multiple memory systems. J Neurosci 9:1465–1472

Pakzaban P, Deacon TW, Burns LH, Isacson O 1993 Increased proportion of acetylcholinesterase-rich zones and improved morphological integration in host striatum of fetal grafts derived from the lateral but not the medial ganglionic eminence. Exp Brain Res 97:13–22

Reading PJ, Dunnett SB 1995 Embryonic striatal grafts reverse the disinhibitory effects of ibotenic acid lesions of the ventral striatum. Exp Brain Res 105:76–86

Reddy PH, Charles V, Williams M, Miller G, Whetsell WO Jr, Tagle DA 1999 Transgenic mice expressing mutated full-length HD cDNA: a paradigm for locomotor changes and selective neuronal loss in Huntington's disease. Philos Trans R Soc Lond B Biol Sci 354:1035–1045

Robbins TW 1998 Dissociating executive functions of the prefrontal cortex. In: Roberts AC, Robbins TW, Weiskrantz L (eds) Prefrontal cortex: executive and cognitive functions. Oxford University Press, Oxford, p 117–130

Robbins TW, Muir JL, Killcross AS, Pretsell D 1993 Methods of assessing attention and stimulus control in the rat. In: Sahgal A (ed) Behavioural neuroscience, vol 1. IRL Press, Oxford, p 13–47

Sanberg PR, Coyle JT 1984 Scientific approaches to Huntington's disease. CRC Crit Rev Clin Neurobiol 1:1–44

Sanberg PR, Pisa M, Fibiger HC 1979 Avoidance, operant and locomotor behavior in rats with neostriatal injections of kainic acid. Pharmacol Biochem Behav 10:137–144

Sanberg PR, Wictorin K, Isacson O 1994 Cell transplantation for Huntington's disease. RG Landes, Austin, TX

Schmidt RH, Björklund A, Stenevi U 1981 Intracerebral grafting of dissociated CNS tissue suspensions: a new approach for neuronal transplantation to deep brain sites. Brain Res 218:347–356

Schwarcz R, Köhler C 1983 Differential vulnerability of central neurons of the rat to quinolinic acid. Neurosci Lett 38:85–90

Schwarcz R, Hökfelt T, Fuxe K, Jonsson G, Goldstein M, Terenius L 1979 Ibotenic acid-induced neuronal degeneration: a morphological and neurochemical study. Exp Brain Res 37:199–216

Schwarcz R, Whetsell WO Jr, Mangano RM 1983 Quinolinic acid: an endogenous metabolite that produces axon-sparing lesions in rat brain. Science 219:316–318

Shallice T, Burgess PW 1999 Deficits in strategy application following frontal lobe damage in man. Brain 114:727–741

Sirinathsinghji DJS, Dunnett SB, Isacson O, Clarke DJ, Kendrick K, Björklund A 1988 Striatal grafts in rats with unilateral neostriatal lesions. II. *In vivo* monitoring of GABA release in globus pallidus and substantia nigra. Neuroscience 24:803–811

Watts C, Dunnett SB, Rosser AE 1997 Effect of embryonic donor age and dissection on the DARPP-32 content of cell suspensions used for intrastriatal transplantation. Exp Neurol 148:271–280

White NM 1997 Mnemonic functions of the basal ganglia. Curr Opin Neurobiol 7:164–169

Wictorin K, Isacson O, Fischer W, Nothias F, Peschanski M, Björklund A 1988 Studies on host afferent inputs to fetal striatal transplants in the excitotoxically lesioned striatum. Prog Brain Res 78:55–60

Zakzanis KK 1998 The subcortical dementia of Huntington's disease. J Clin Exp Neuropsychol 20:565–578

DISCUSSION

Gray: Was I correct in seeing that there was a difference in the performance of the lesion-only animals, depending on whether they were using their lesioned versus non-lesioned side?

Dunnett: Yes, there's a massive difference between the deficit on the ipsilateral side and the deficit on the contralateral side. These animals are showing 95% bias in responding on the ipsilateral side, so they have a very high rate of correct detections when the stimulus is presented ipsilateral to the lesion, but a very low rate on the opposite side.

Gray: What I meant was, did the training alter the extent of the lesion-only deficit?

Dunnett: The standard multiway analysis of variance (whether using transformed or non-transformed data) showed no difference in any main effect or interaction between the top left and the bottom right-hand panel. Thus the non-specific training had no effect on the lesion-only rats, and specific training had only modest benefit in comparison to the large effect of specific training on the grafts.

Gray: These results provide a nice illustration of the way training actually affects the graft.

Gage: Is your measure a reaction time?

Dunnett: Each of these tasks has a reaction time, movement time, accuracy and bias. All I presented here is the bias, which is symmetrical to accuracy. There are parallel data on the effects on the graft having small effects on the reaction time and on movement time. Interestingly, these are apparent immediately you go back and test. There are some aspects of performance where the graft simply being in place enhances recovery on the speed of the movement, but doesn't enable them to make the specific choice discrimination.

Freeman: You pointed out how a graft into the pallidum was not effective for behavioural recovery. You have reported in primates that grafts that were closest to the pallidum provided improved behavioural responses. Do you have any further development of the role of graft proximity to the pallidum in behavioural response?

Dunnett: I don't have any further development. It is likely that where the graft is positioned influences its capacity both to project to the target and to attract host afferents. This is certainly the way our thinking is going, but we don't have hard evidence to support this hypothesis.

Hodges: If you train the animals very intensively after the lesion but before the graft, and then put the graft in and look, would you expect that prior training would actually speed up recovery with the graft, or would you expect the animals to do worse because they started to learn a different strategy?

Dunnett: That's a nice experiment I haven't thought of.

Perry: With regard to the training issue and its specificity, the experiments that Alan Cowey did many years ago on monkeys with striate cortex lesions are relevant (Cowey & Weiskrantz 1963). The animals have scotoma, and they can be left for more than a year, but they apparently have no information they can use coming from the scotoma. However, you can then train them to use information from a scotoma to detect a spot of light falling on the scotoma. In a series of experiments we trained monkeys with motor cortex lesions to use the contralateral hand to do quite sophisticated recovery tasks for a food reward (Passingham et al 1983). They never used that hand in the cage to feed.

Gray: I'm not sure I correctly understand the implication of what you're saying. In the scotoma experiments you talk about, the inference from the work on blind sight is that it is not that damaged bit of the cortex that is being retrained, but rather the rest of the visual system is taking over a function that it wouldn't normally have. This would leave open the possibility that in Steve Dunnett's experiments it is not the graft itself that is being retrained, but some other bit of that hemisphere.

Perry: It is the point that Fred Gage made: is it the whole brain, or is it that bit? The importance lies in the fact that you can train animals to use information arising from the scotoma, for the animal to get used to using an aberrant, unusual form of information. The motor experiments then tell you that even though the animal can learn to use a hand in a state-dependent fashion, in its home cage it does not use it. The interesting problem is whether in the grafted animal there is a state-dependent learning that shows that any transfer. Is there an unlearned behaviour you could assay that also shows some benefit of the training procedure? This would be interesting.

Dunnett: I think this is the first experiment in what must be a series, because it's setting up a transfer of training hypothesis. We now need to think of all the clever variants — not just to think of the alternatives, but select exactly which ones to do, because they're very time-consuming experiments. My reason for presenting the first set of data is to stimulate discussion. What is being learned, and how can you get at whether it's actually going on within the transplant circuitry, as opposed to the transplant providing enhanced plasticity in the adjacent areas?

Perry: You need to inactivate your transplant to find out.

Gray: If my interpretation of what you're saying here is correct, you would expect to see some improvement also in the lesion-only group.

Perry: It may just be a matter of time.

Dunnett: We did 30 days of 150–200 trials per day.

Perry: The experiments I mentioned were very long, and involved months and months of trials.

Raisman: If you train, for example, one hand in human, does the other hand improve when it later has to do that task? In other words, does the training transfer from one side to the other?

Dunnett: The human equivalents that I know of are the Taub experiments, which are to do with stroke. When patients neglect and do not use one hand, extensive forced training will eventually lead to improvement, but it takes a lot of forced training to get there.

Raisman: What about in a non-lesioned situation? If you train up a hand for one skill, will the untrained hand have profited?

Peschanski: It is actually very selective. Mike Merzenich can teach monkeys to differentiate two very close vibrations on a small part of one finger. If he tries on the next finger, it doesn't work.

Steve Dunnett, how would you adapt your findings to the way that clinical trials should be carried out in patients? You say that learning is necessary to get the graft to work. I really wonder how you can adapt this type of thing. If you don't you may miss the benefit of the graft.

Dunnett: I think that's absolutely right. This relates to the point that was made earlier, which is that this sort of phenomenon is apparent when you're probing the animal on something it doesn't normally do. If you are testing the animals on simpler motor responses, then the grafted rats show recovery without explicit retraining because they're doing that sort of thing in their day-to-day life. The message to the neurologists and other members of the clinical team is that they should look at the range of skills that a patient is missing out on, that they used to be able to do, and encourage the patients to practise these tasks.

Gray: That would have to be standardized across any control group.

Dunnett: There is a difference between what's going on in an experimental context and what constitutes practical clinical rehabilitation. One can in principal design experiments to test whether this sort of phenomenon is relevant: half the patients could learn a motor skill *de novo*, to be compared with others that have been given extensive practice. A more fundamental question concerns what impact this has for present and forthcoming clinical trials. It says to the clinical teams that there are data coming through from the labs indicating that they should at least consider whether the post-operative care with which the patients are being provided is optimal.

Peschanski: Perhaps we should introduce to the clinical trials a completely different task that is repeated over a week of sessions just to see whether there is some learning effect within that week. Whether or not they are grafted, the patient will try to practice other tasks at home.

Dunnett: The hypothesis is that if you had a series of comparable motor tasks as available within a test battery, then at monthly intervals the patient can be trained intensively on a new one over, say, a period of a week. Then, with a dysfunctional striatum, we predict that the patient is not going to be able to learn that skill to a high level in the course of a week, whereas once the graft is well established he or she should show a much greater capacity to learn it. So I think rather than looking at the same test and comparing learning in different patients, if you could have a series of separate motor tasks which could be trained before, immediately after and some time after transplantation, it may reveal the hypothesized loss and recovery of a capacity for motor skill learning.

Isacson: I'm interested in the question that you started your presentation with, namely fetal graft connectivity and other functional recovery. There are some data we haven't talked about here. You did a delayed grafting, and you referred to some earlier work we did, where the dopaminergic afferents die back after striatal lesions (Isacson et al 1985). But what do you think is happening there? In this model of HD they have had the lesion for a while, then you transplant — how do you think that informs us about a potential clinical scenario? Further, does the experiment give specific evidence about connectivity, or could it be that the trophic projection by the fetal striatal grafts is more active in the first week after lesion when there is more retrograde axon degeneration?

Dunnett: In the third experiment, which I didn't have time to explain in detail, we were trying to get at the issue of whether connections are important. We know that cortico–striatal systems are involved in alternation learning. What we are looking at the moment is whether a bilateral striatal lesion and a bilateral cortical lesion would impair automation learning. If we have a bilateral striatal lesion and implant a graft on one side, and if delayed alternation recovers, I predict that a lesion of the contralateral cortex will have no effect, but a lesion of ipsilateral cortex will disrupt recovery. The idea behind such a 'cross-over' experiment is that we need an intact cortex on the same side as the graft, whereas if the cortex projecting to a graft is lesioned and the intact contralateral cortex projects to a striatal lesion, then the required cortico–striatal circuit is disrupted bilaterally and the animal will remain unable to learn or perform the alternation rule. This would then provide direct evidence that the graft is functionally integrated into a circuit.

Gray: Is that an experiment that is planned?

Dunnett: It's in progress, and I've got some preliminary data.

Sinden: Steve, in your experiments examining learning to use the transplants, did you have a control tissue graft, using a cell type from the brain that would never integrate in the striatum?

Dunnett: We have other experiments that had a cortical graft, but these weren't the ones I presented.

Sinden: The reason I asked is because clinically, after a unilateral lesion there is a period in which rehabilitation will work, and then there is a period when it has no further effect. Presumably, these changes reflect some reorganization in the undamaged brain, such as in the opposite side of the brain.

Dunnett: In terms of control tissues, there are two experiments, one that is published and one that is in press. These are based on the lateralized discrimination task (go left, go right), where cortical tissue does not provide the same pattern of recovery as is provided by striatal grafts.

Sinden: So it is not just the preserved new graft, allowing the tissue to again reorganize itself, introducing a period where plasticity is possible.

Björklund: Talking about transfer experiments, Peter Coffey has done some interesting experiments with retinal transplants placed over the tectum. Could you comment on what these experiments tell us?

Dunnett: Peter Coffey had two experimental set-ups. One was an arena, half of which was covered over. Normal rats avoid light and prefer to sit in the dark area. An animal with a retinal transplant that reinnervated the tectum showed no indication of whether they were in the light or dark area. He then took the animals into a conditioned avoidance paradigm, where a flash of light was followed by foot-shock. He trained the animals to associate light with a shock and then put them back into the arena and found that they now avoided the light. This experiment indicates that you have to train the animal to use or recognize information coming in from the graft. What this particular experiment does not resolve is whether what the animal is learning is to see or whether it is learning that some sensation is associated with foot-shock and therefore is to be avoided. This can be addressed by training the animals also to recognize light but with a positive reinforcement. Then, if they were learning that light was good, they would spend all their time in the light side in the arena, whereas if they were learning through the training to actually recognize the input as a visual stimulus, they would still go to the dark side. He didn't report that second situation that would tease out the nature of exactly what was being learned. This experiment is addressing some very similar questions in what superficially seems to be a very different system.

Björklund: This experiment appears to demonstrate transfer in the sense that once the animal has learned to use the transplant in a particular situation it can use it in a quite different one.

Perry: They have never taught them to do a visual discrimination.

Björklund: Yes, but it is not clear that the rats perceive the information coming from the retinal transplant as light.

Perry: As far as the rats are concerned it is 'information' that will give rise to a foot-shock, and when it arrives they know it is time to get out of the way.

Björklund: If you remove the transplant, it would be expected that the rats are no longer able to see, thus demonstrating that the information is coming from the grafted retina.

Dunnett: You shouldn't have to remove the transplant; you can just put a window over it.

Lindvall: I would like to discuss some clinical implications of this work. What we're talking about is functional integration of the graft in a more broad sense, which means that the patient's brain can make use of the graft. Do you foresee a difference between different types of graft? You used striatal grafts, but if you use nigral transplants instead, would there also be an element of training or learning to use the graft in an optimal way? In my paper tomorrow I will present data indicating that there is a time lag between when dopamine is first secreted from the intrastriatal nigral transplants, and when we observe optimal functional recovery. This may be due to several different mechanisms, including the functional integration of the graft. I wonder whether one could envisage a situation in which the patient's brain needs to re-learn things, irrespective of whether it's a nigral transplant with tonic dopamine release or a striatal graft.

Dunnett: I suspect there's some of each. In many contexts when the situation changes an organism adapts to cope with that change. When you change it back again presumably the animal will have to adapt back again, but there's also a specific sense in which these data are clearly fitting within an experimental framework that sees the striatum as not just involved in simple motor control, but also habit formation, habit learning and setting up the motor routines. These functions are specific to the striatum. The equivalent in the nigral graft would be to ask: what is the nigral system doing in the normal animal and to what extent is that restored by putting in a nigral graft? In our standard nigral context we are dealing with ectopic grafts where you get recovery on those things that can be restored by providing a dopaminergic reactivation of the striatum. There remain aspects that, in animals and patients alike, are not as well recovered as the simple motor activation-type deficits. This presumably relates to the fact that the nigrostriatal pathway is not being restored. I suppose I think that the equivalent question if you're interested in nigral grafts is to what extent just putting back a terminal innervation restores what is lost by the disrupted circuitry, and to what extent are we going to have to move towards circuit reconstruction. Once you have got to that point and you can actually put cells in the nigra to reconstruct the nigrostriatal projection, then you're going to have to address the questions as to what is the patterned information that this system is providing in the normal brain. Is a grafted cell able to feed that information into a plastic striatum?

Lindvall: Take a patient, for example, who has had severe motor problems for several years and who has lost the capacity to select and plan different motor functions. Then you transplant dopamine neurons in an ectopic site (striatum). Is there an element that the patient has to relearn to have maximum symptomatic relief?

Björklund: Guido Nikkhah has performed an experiment involving paw reaching in rats that is relevant here. Multiple nigral transplants, in unilateral 6-OHDA lesioned rats, induced a partial recovery of skilled paw use in the paw reaching test. They continued to train these animals for four or five months, but did not observe any further training effect over and beyond that seen in the initial sessions of the test.

Freeman: The lesioned rat model for HD is quite a profound lesion, whereas in reality, particularly for early HD, a partial lesion model would be more relevant. Can partial-lesioned animals be retrained?

And to take Mark Peschanski's question further, from the clinical trial point of view, wouldn't we actually be confounding our trial results if we retrained our patients after a transplant?

Dunnett: We don't have any data on retraining partial lesioned animals. You are raising a more general point, and this applies equally to nigrostriatal lesioned rats. To what extent can we go from very simple model systems designed for experimental purity? We make relatively complete unilateral nigrostriatal lesions in rats so there is no prospect for spontaneous recovery. This is a powerful model to see what a dopamine cell do in a totally dopamine-deficient brain, but we cannot pretend that it closely mimics or is directly relevant to Parkinson's disease (PD) in humans. Similarly the excitotoxic lesions have different time-courses to human HD. It is a model system for teasing out basic principles of the relationship between graft survival, growth and functional effects. It is very seductive to try to draw implications for patients and of course that is a constant pressure. But at the same time as trying to understand the basic principles we need to develop better models.

Freeman: Just a caveat: in the reports by Madrazo and colleagues there were many criticisms of their trials. One of them was that these patients came from poorly medically managed communities into a medical centre where they not only received adrenal transplants but three months of post-operative care, including readjustment of medications and physical therapy. Teasing out the information in that model became, of course, impossible. For clinical trials, it is very important to separate out the science from the clinical aspects of getting clean data that's interpretable.

Björklund: The relationship between the magnitude of the lesion and extent of spontaneous recovery has been addressed following lesions of the nigrostriatal system in rats. Interestingly, deficits in initiation of movement in the stepping task are stable over time, provided that the size of the lesion exceeds a critical threshold. These partially lesioned animals are only partially impaired in the test, but they nevertheless show no spontaneous recovery. In the paw reaching test, by contrast, there is a clear training-dependent recovery in animals with partial lesions. Training may help to promote functional recovery, up to a point, although the rats will remain impaired in the test.

Gage: The question that seems important here concerns whether or not the graft itself is contributing to the recovery, and to what extent, versus the function of the host cells. We sometimes set these up as a dichotomy: but isn't it fundamentally an interaction of the two? There will probably not be a functional integration of the graft into the host unless the host is reorganizing simultaneously with the graft. To try to tease these things out and parcel them out exclusively into attributes of the graft and the host may not be possible. When we look at a control graft, such as a cortical graft into this lesioned area, there may be re-organizational events that are occurring in the host, but they're a different sort of re-organizational event responding to this intrusion into its environment which are completely different than a striatal graft.

Price: That's a very important point, and there are some developmental studies that might be relevant. There is evidence that if you graft in a piece of tissue that is very closely related to a piece a tissue that you have otherwise removed or lesioned, you can actually make things worse. There are studies involving different areas of cortex in development, and if for example you transplant a piece of occipital cortex into a motor field, you can actually make things worse, presumably because what's actually happened is that this piece of cortex has been recognized as cortex and has wired up, but something about its intrinsic organization isn't correct (Barth & Stanfield 1994). It is not a question of 'there's the host and there's the graft': one is going to become integrally involved in the other.

Reier: The issue of grafting into a setting of intrinsic plasticity is an important consideration from a couple of perspectives. In our study of transplants in patients with progressive post-traumatic syringomyelia, we've seen a couple of people who are very similar to some others that have been described in the literature, but here I'll just describe one. This is a gentleman who sustained a T_{12} spinal injury 30 years ago. He has an unusual paralysis in that he mostly exhibits lower extremity paralysis and is thus ambulatory with bracing and use of a cane. Despite this he's been ranching several hundred acres for the last 30 years. He came to our neurosurgeon, Dr Richard Fessler, complaining about a progressive upper extremity weakness which usually signifies that something in terms of chronic tissue damage may be ascending. In this case, we would usually suspect that the cyst, which was originally at T_{12}, may be enlarging. We initially thought that there was perhaps a little ascending cavitation. Upon looking at his magnetic resonance imaging (MRI) scan, however, we found a huge cyst that extended from T_{12} continuously to C_2. The lesion is asymmetric, off to one side, which some feel is a pathological configuration that some feel may predispose a person to chronic post injury pain, but not in this case. The point of mentioning this is that we are really working with a black box when we talk about how we are going to bring a graft in under various pathological conditions, because we don't know the background of plasticity, which may set the threshold in terms of behavioural outcomes. Here's an individual who, in principle, should not be breathing, but who does fine and has the strongest grip I've ever seen: he should have virtually minimal cervical innovation of his upper extremity. I suspect he is using every last bit of circuitry that he has against a dynamic background of intrinsic repair. I think this example illustrates a need to be aware both from a safety and therapeutic efficacy perspective that we need eventually to have some clue how to interface whatever we do, whether it is grafting, gene therapy or a combination, with this background in order not to compromise inherent repair while at the same time taking more advantage of these mechanisms to optimize therapeutic benefit.

Gray: There's another case like that. Jonathan Cole (1991) has published a book about one particular patient who had lost all proprioceptive feedback from below the neck to indicate any movement that had been made. Without any help from anybody, this patient has been able after many years to recover a great deal of ability to move including walking and driving a car.

Perry: This business of slowly evolving lesions is an entirely different business from the acute lesions. There is a whole literature about what happens if you make partial or serial lesions. Slowly evolving degenerative diseases evoke a completely different response from the brain when compared with acute lesions.

Isacson: From a pre-clinical point of view, the basic experiments we did in the 1980s were not very predictive for the kind of recovery that eventually would occur in patients. For example, the patients are on L-dopa and our rats are not on L-dopa; the patients had dyskinesias, our rats didn't have dyskinesias, and the patients that we've seen recover have recovered on tasks that we did not simulate in the rats. Even beyond that, each patient is different, whereas in rats, with inbreeding and appropriate lesions we can more or less create a cohort of identical group neuropathology. It really requires an analysis beyond that to see what type of patient recovers with what type of transplant, and even for PD that to me looks very complex — each PD patient is going to be slightly different in his or her response to implanted cells.

Gray: But there's a whole bunch of entangled difficulties in doing what you suggest, even though it clearly would be desirable. You could only approach that kind of question with an enormously large sample so that you can at least begin to look for similarities between subsets of patients. To gather a large sample, if we use properly controlled trials of the kind Tom Freeman has been talking about, raises substantial problems with an untried therapy.

Barker: In PD, in some ways we almost have to go back to the original disease to try to define exactly what we mean by 'PD' in terms of the heterogeneity of the disorder. It's quite clear there are many different subtypes of PD, and simply transplanting into patients with PD might not actually be the most useful way forward. I think we have to try to classify a subtype of patient that we actually wish to transplant. Then we have to ask specific questions about what is it within that patient that we think will actually recover, given the sort of clinical responses that we've seen with transplants.

Gray: Is heterogeneity also a problem in HD?

Rosser: There is certainly a degree of heterogeneity in HD, but not to the extent seen in PD.

Gray: And of course when you move on to stroke, which is coming into focus as a target for therapy, the heterogeneity is greater still.

Gage: The number of CAG repeats is dramatically different between HD patients, and the onset is different in terms of age.

Rosser: There is heterogeneity that can be attributed to CAG repeat number, but it is also clear that there is heterogeneity outside the number of CAG repeats.

Peschanski: The heterogeneity of HD might even be worse than in PD. The people we want to transplant who have PD are at a certain stage of evolution of the disease. You don't take people who are still in the steep curve of the evolution of the disease. With HD we want to graft people who are entering the disease. We are opposing the process after just one or two years of evolution, and we don't know where on the curve we are, which might be steep or shallow. In the patients we have grafted there were four who were at the starting place, stage one, with problems but not yet stage two. We were not expecting to have major atrophy of the striatum. Then, one had no posterior putamen on the left side and another one had no caudate nucleus on the right side. A third one had half the caudate nucleus on both sides. It was completely heterogeneous (Bachoud-Lévi et al 2000).

Freeman: From the clinical perspective, I agree that HD is more heterogeneous. In addition to Marc Peschanski's point, as the disease progresses there's much more gliosis, which may provide a worse host milieu for transplant survival. There is also more atrophy which from a surgical perspective leads to targeting difficulties and post-operative subdural haematoma risks.

In addition to the six mechanisms that Steve Dunnett outlined in his talk, we now see a seventh mechanism from the Gainesville group: there may be mechanical mechanisms, and just plugging up a hole may be all that is required of the transplant. Our surgical treatment of syringomyelia is to put a tube in to drain the syrinx: the patients get better as you just remove the mass effect of the syrinx on the remaining spinal cord. In a similar fashion, it may be that the graft is performing nothing more than a mechanical function. The conclusion is that these mechanistic discussions have to be disease-specific.

Spooren: With regard to the issue about the rewiring, in PD one usually transplants a defined patient group: as a rule they are relatively young and no longer responding to L-dopa. I would be interested to see the effect of transplantation in relatively unaffected patients and then to see the progression of the disease. In these cases would you then see a complete reorganization, retraction of striatal input, or a slower or faster rate of disease progression?

Gray: This is to some extent a chicken and egg problem: until one can demonstrate sufficient clinical benefit from the transplantation approach, one isn't going to want to operate on patients at a still-early stage of disease, but in principle if it's working we should presumably in the end want to tackle patients at an early stage rather than later.

References

Bachoud-Lévi A-C, Bourdet C, Brugières P et al 2000 Safety and tolerability assessment of intrastriatal neural allografts in five patients with Huntington's disease. Exp Neurol 161:194–202

Barth TM, Stanfield BB 1994 Homotypic, but not heterotypic, fetal cortical transplants can result in functional sparing following neonatal damage to the frontal cortex in rats. Cerebral Cortex 4:271–278

Cole J 1991 Pride and a daily marathon. Duckworth, London

Cowey A, Weiskrantz L 1963 A perimetric study of visual field defects in monkeys. Q J Exp Psych 15:91–115

Isacson O, Brundin P, Gage FH, Björklund A 1985 Neural grafting in a rat model of Huntington's disease: progressive neurochemical changes after neostriatal ibotenate lesions and striatal tissue grafting. Neuroscience 16:799–817

Passingham RE, Perry VH, Wilkinson F 1983 The long-term effects of removal of sensorimotor cortex in infant and adult rhesus monkeys. Brain 106:675–705

Functional reconstruction of the hippocampus: fetal versus conditionally immortal neuroepithelial stem cell grafts

H. Hodges*†, P. Sowinski*†, D. Virley*, A. Nelson*, T.R. Kershaw†, W. P. Watson†, T. Veizovic†, S. Patel†, A. Mora†, T. Rashid†, S. J. French†, A. Chadwick†, J. A. Gray*† and J. D. Sinden†

*Department of Psychology, Institute of Psychiatry, De Crespigny Park, Denmark Hill, London SE5 8AF and †ReNeuron Ltd., Europoint Centre, 5–11 Lavington Street, London SE1 0NZ, UK

Abstract. Late fetal CA1 hippocampal grafts and stem cell grafts from the conditionally immortal MHP36 clonal line derived from the H-2K^b-tsA58 transgenic mouse neuroepithelium both improved spatial deficits in rats with ischaemic CA1 damage induced by four-vessel occlusion (4VO). However, the distribution of fetal and MHP36 grafts differed. Fetal cells lodged in clumps around the implant sites and along the corpus callosum, whilst MHP36 grafts infiltrated the area of CA1 ischaemic damage, achieving apparent architectural reconstruction of the hippocampus. The migration of MHP36 cells is damage-dependent. Few cells were found in intact brain; after 15 min of 4VO cells repopulated only the discrete area of CA1 cell loss, whereas with more extensive damage after 30 min occlusion cells migrated to all hippocampal fields and to cortex. A higher proportion of grafted MHP36 cells differentiated into neurons in the host CA1 field than grafts of striatal or cortical expanded cell populations. Cortical population grafts were as effective as MHP36 grafts in improving water maze learning, whereas striatal or ventral mesencephalic cells were ineffective, indicating a degree of stem cell specificity. The efficacy of MHP36 cells extends to primates. In marmosets with profound impairments in conditional discrimination tasks after lesions of the CA1 field, MHP36 cells improved performance as effectively as fetal grafts and migrated evenly through the CA1 field, in contrast to clustered fetal cells. These findings suggest that MHP36 stem cell grafts are as effective as fetal grafts in functional repair of hippocampal damage, and that their preference for areas of cell loss and adoption of appropriate morphologies is consistent with a point-to-point repair mechanism.

2000 Neural transplantation in neurodegenerative disease. Wiley, Chichester (Novartis Foundation Symposium 231) p 53–69

Introduction: clinical amnesia

Clinical amnesia has been associated with a variety of conditions including traumatic brain injury, encephalitis, chronic alcohol consumption, neuro-degenerative diseases, temporal lobe epilepsy and surgery for epilepsy, and ageing. Damage to the hippocampus and/or its inputs has been implicated in all these conditions but they may have little else in common (Rose & Symonds 1960, Scoville & Milner 1957, Arendt et al 1983). The most selective damage to the hippocampus associated with marked memory deficits occurs after interruption of cerebral blood flow (global ischaemia) during cardiac arrest, coronary artery occlusion or heart bypass surgery, since this region, particularly the CA1 field, is highly sensitive to effects of reduced oxygen (Schmidt-Kastner & Freund 1991). Patient RB (Zola-Morgan et al 1986), for example, was unable to recall day-to-day events, and to learn any kind of new information following massive loss of 5000 ml of blood during heart bypass surgery, though language, skills and information acquired prior to surgery were preserved. Up to 40% of patients recovering from out-of-hospital heart attack have been shown to have moderate to severe memory deficits (Grubb et al 1996), suggesting that amnesia is a relatively common though largely unrecognized consequence of improvements in the treatment of cardiac arrest (Roine et al 1992). Neuroimaging studies have revealed relatively discrete hippocampal lesions in patients showing memory loss after ischaemic episodes (Kartsounis et al 1995, Rempel-Clower et al 1996).

The four-vessel occlusion model of global ischaemia

Global ischaemia induced by four-vessel occlusion (4VO) in rats provides a well-validated model for the pathophysiological and cognitive consequences of global ischaemia. The extent of damage is related to the duration of the occlusion: with 15 min of 4VO cell loss is largely limited to the CA1 and hilar hippocampal fields, but after longer durations it extends to the CA3 field and also to cortex and striatum (Pulsinelli et al 1982). Memory deficits following 4VO have been most clearly demonstrated in tasks involving spatial learning and spatial working memory (Nunn & Hodges 1994, Nelson et al 1997a,b). Although extrahippocampal damage is likely to contribute to cognitive deficits induced by global ischaemia (Nunn & Hodges 1994), positive correlations between the extent of spatial impairments and of hippocampal cell loss suggest that damage to the hippocampus, particularly the CA1 field, is associated with these deficits (Olsen et al 1994, Nelson et al 1997a, Block & Schwarz 1998). The 4VO model provides a clinically relevant, reproducible and widely used method for looking at both histological and functional outcomes of neuroprotective drug or graft strategies designed to rescue or to repair hippocampal damage. However, graft strategies have attracted increasing attention, since it has become clear that the time window for cerebroprotective drug action is quite narrow, that drugs cannot diminish damage that has already occurred, and that histological evidence for cell survival in treated rats killed shortly (e.g. 3–7 days) after ischaemia rarely predicts clinical efficacy in patients (Hunter et al 1995).

Fetal grafts for hippocampal repair

With its well-defined circuits and prominent role in memory processes, the hippocampus is a structure of choice for the study of graft-induced functional reconstruction. Initial experiments using mixed fetal cells from all hippocampal regions demonstrated a degree of electrophysiological connectivity and functional recovery in rats (Mudrick et al 1989, Mudrick & Baimbridge 1991, Sprick 1991). However, Field et al (1991) using a fine microdissection technique to separate fields in the late embryonic (embryonic day [E]18–19) hippocampus, demonstrated that homotypic replacement of damaged cells is required for re-establishing normal laminar connections. CA3, but not CA1 cells implanted in the lesioned CA3 field attracted host mossy fibres to form appropriate juxtacellular synapses. Dawe et al (1993) confirmed that long-term potentiation could be elicited only from CA3, but not CA1 cells in rats with CA3 lesions, following tetanic stimulation of the host perforant path. Cognitive consequences of appropriate fetal cell replacement were then demonstrated by Netto et al (1993) and Hodges et al (1996) in rats with spatial learning deficits and CA1 cell loss induced by global ischaemia. Only grafts of CA1 cells, but not structurally and pharmacologically similar CA3 cells, improved spatial learning and working memory in water maze and three-door runway tasks. In the extent of thigmotaxis, CA3 grafts made the performance of ischaemic rats worse than that of ischaemic controls. These findings have suggested that conditions for functional repair of damage within the hippocampus are strictly defined and are consistent with a point-to-point mechanism, in contrast to the ameliorative effects of a variety of cell types that reduce deficits arising from damage to hippocampal cholinergic inputs (Sinden et al 1995).

Conditionally immortal neuroepithelial stem cell grafts for hippocampal repair

Despite their functional efficacy, late fetal grafts would not be practically or ethically feasible for repair of the human hippocampus. We have therefore developed alternative neuroepithelial stem cell lines for grafting, with four key advantages: (1) they are conditionally immortalized by a temperature-sensitive oncogene (*tsA 58*) so that they can be grown indefinitely in culture at 33 °C, but on implantation into a higher brain temperature (37–38 °C) cease dividing and differentiate into mature cells; (2) they are multipotential, able to differentiate into neurons, glia or oligodendrocytes according to signals from the host brain *in vivo*, or trophic agents *in vitro*; (3) they are highly migratory and head specifically towards regions of brain damage; (4) they are multifunctional, able to promote recovery from several different types of brain damage. These properties were initially demonstrated using grafts of a clonal cell line, MHP36, derived from the H-2k^b-tsA58 transgenic mouse neuroepithelium (Jat et al 1991), which were found to be just as effective as fetal CA1 grafts in improving spatial learning in rats with ischaemic CA1 cell loss after 15 min of 4VO (Sinden et al 1997).

Gross histological comparisons of fetal and stem cell grafts

Examination of the distribution of fetal and MHP36 grafts after injection into the alveus above the region of ischaemic cell loss in rats suggest that their patterns of connectivity may differ in detail, though both appear to restore sufficient hippocampal activity to sustain functional recovery. Fetal grafts remain in clumps close to the sites of injection and are found most frequently in the corpus callosum, whereas MHP36 cells, labelled by β-galactosidase (βgal) align compactly in the region of CA1 cell loss and also migrate along white matter tracts (see Plate 1). In morphology, grafted fetal CA1 cells are similar to normal host pyramidal cells, MHP36 cells adopt a variety of phenotypes, notably glial and neuronal. These findings suggest that MHP36 cells meet the specificity for functional repair suggested by effects of fetal grafts, and they also appear to be much more integrated into the host hippocampus; indeed the architecture of the damaged CA1 field is to a greater or lesser extent reconstructed. Limited electrophysiological evidence to date (G. Dawe, E. Sametsky, J. D. Stephenson, unpublished data) suggests that grafted MHP36 pyramidal-like cells fire relatively normally after depolarization, indicating the capacity for structural repair. Of the

---

PLATE 1.   Photomicrographs of the CA1 region of ischaemic rat hippocampus following transplantation of MHP36 cell line grafts (A, B) and fetal (E18–19: C, D) rat tissue from the CA1 field. (A) β-Galactosidase immunohistochemistry with haematoxylin counterstaining of nuclei shows positive transplanted MHP36 cells in the ischaemic CA1 field under the site of injection. (B) At higher magnification MHP36 cells (brown) are seen as large bipolar and multipolar cells against the background of haematoxylin-stained host cells (blue). (C) Cresyl fast violet stained section of fetal CA1 transplanted cells (arrows) above the area of ischaemic CA1 cell loss (arrowheads), showing that fetal grafts do not migrate into the denervated host CA1 layer, but form a mass above it, chiefly in the corpus callosum. (D) Glial fibrillary acid protein immunohistochemistry counterstained with haematoxylin of a serial section to C, shows a strong astrocytic reaction to the ischaemic damage in the CA1 field (arrowheads), but only a few astocytes at the margins of the fetal transplant especially near the injection site (arrows). Scale bar = 400 μm for A, C and D; 100 μm for B.

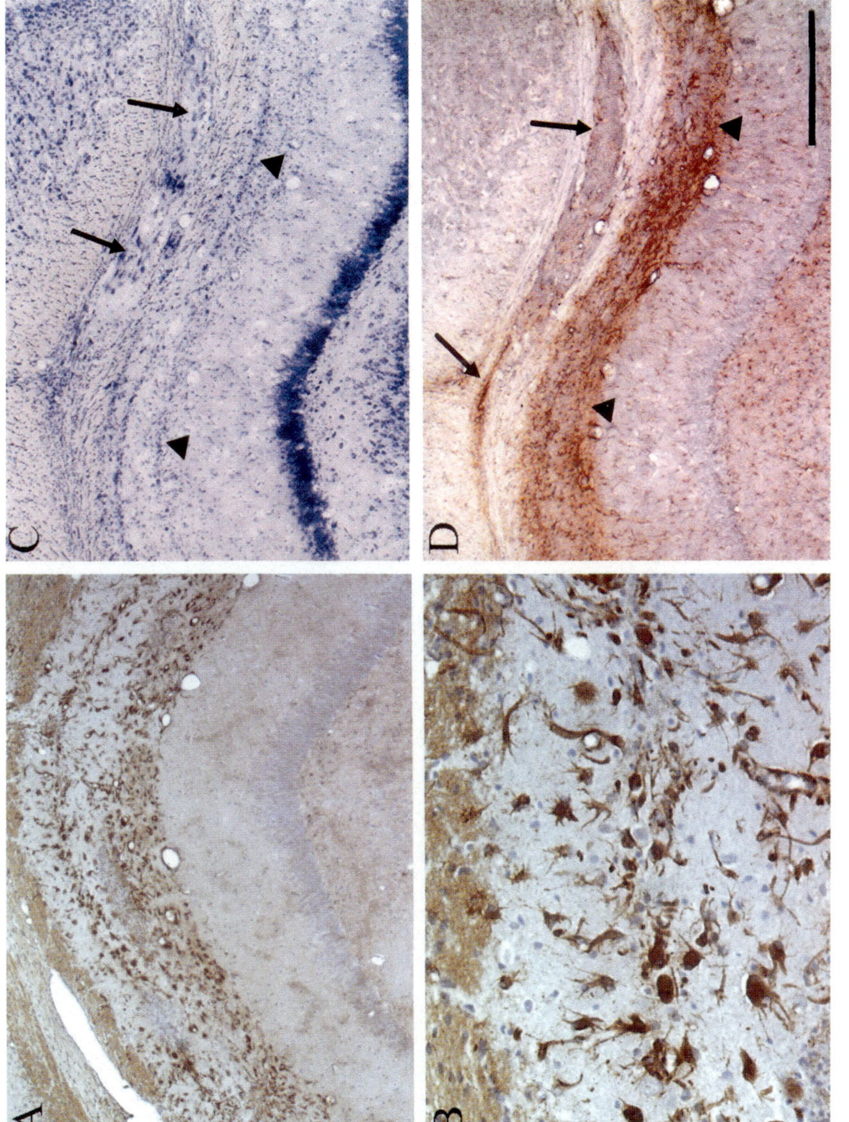

Plate 1

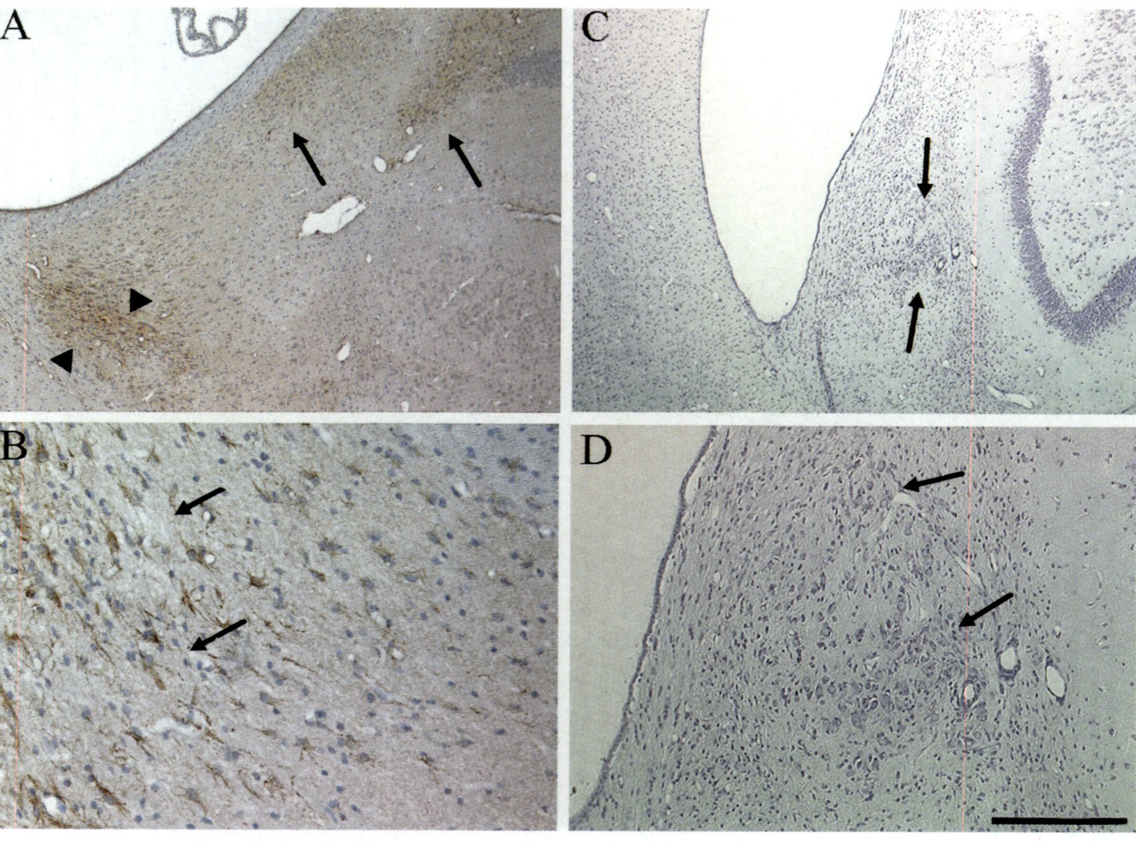

Plate 2

many questions about the mechanisms and extent of functional repair of the hippocampus, particularly by conditionally immortalized neuroepithelial stem cells, we have examined three issues: (1) Is stem cell migration within the hippocampus injury-dependent? (2) Are stem cells from any immortomouse brain region equally effective for hippocampal repair? (3) Does the efficacy of mouse-derived stem cell grafts extend to primates? These questions will be examined in turn.

Stem cell migration within the 4VO model

To establish whether MHP36 cells do in fact migrate, rather than being passively pushed through hippocampal cleavage planes by the pressure of the injection, we compared the extent of migration of MHP36 cells and cell-sized beads implanted unilaterally at two sites in the alveus above the denervated CA1 field of rats subjected to 15 min of 4VO two weeks earlier, and in intact sham-operated controls. Cell/bead density was 25 000 cells/μl, and all grafts were labelled with PKH26 for fluorescence microscopy. By two weeks after grafting, MHP36 cells were seen aligned in the host CA1 field, were numerous in the corpus callosum, and some had already crossed the midline, heading towards the contralateral CA1. In contrast, fluorescent beads remained clumped in the alveus, having moved at most a distance of 1.0 mm from the injection site and thus resembled clustered fetal grafts. We are currently looking in more detail at the time-course of contralateral migration of cells in rats with unilateral lesions of the CA1 field and grafts on the other side. In controls, the appearance and distribution of bead grafts were similar to those seen in ischaemic rats, but very few MHP36 cells were visible. These results indicate that MHP36 grafts showed true migration towards the sites of injury, and confirmed our previous observations that MHP36 cells do not survive well in intact brain (Sinden et al 1997).

To examine the influence of the extent of injury on MHP36 cell migration we subjected rats to 15 and 30 min of 4VO, and grafted 1.0 μl of cells (25 000 cells/μl) at the standard two alvear sites, bilaterally. Grafts were identified by βgal immunoreactivity and ischaemic cell loss by Nissl staining, at 1, 4 and 8 weeks

---

PLATE 2. Photomicrographs of β-galactosidase-positive MHP36 grafts (A, B) and fetal (E94–96) CA1 grafts stained with Cresyl fast violet (C, D) in the NMDA-lesioned CA1 field of marmosets. (A) MHP36 cells (brown) transplanted at the subicular end of the CA1 region (arrowheads) appear to migrate in two broad bands throughout the CA1 region (arrows). (B) A higher-power image of MHP36 cells near the injection site (arrows) shows good integration into the surrounding host tissue. (C) Fetal CA1 cells (arrows) remain in clumps near the injection site in the lesioned CA1 field. (D) A higher power image shows that clusters of grafted pyramidal cells (arrows) appear healthy but less well integrated than MHP36 cells. Scale bar = 400 μm for A and C; 100 μm for B and D.

after implantation. 4VO for 15 min resulted in cell loss largely confined to the CA1 field, but with some variable damage in the striatum and frontal cortex. After 30 min of 4VO cell loss in the hippocampus was more extensive, included the CA3 field, and was much more evident in striatum and cortex than with 15 min occlusion. In rats with 15 min occlusion MHP36 cells were seen in the CA1 field as early as one week after grafting, and with no further increase after 4 and 8 weeks. Few cells were visible elsewhere. In rats with 30 min occlusion, MHP36 cells also densely engrafted the CA3 field, and to a lesser extent infiltrated the cortex and striatum, in line with the greater neuronal loss in these regions (see Fig. 1). These results clearly indicated that the extent of migration of MHP36 cells depends on the degree of cell loss in the 4VO model.

Functional effects of stem cell populations in the 4VO model

Our experience with fetal grafts suggested that functional recovery is specific to cell type — only CA1, but not CA3 grafts improved water maze learning in rats showing CA1 cell loss and deficits after 4VO (Hodges et al 1996; see above). The efficacy of MHP36 cells derived from the neuroepithelial region destined to form the hippocampus suggested that they differentiated into cells that sufficiently met the strict requirements for functional repair. However, stem cells are multipotential, and it is possible that progenitors from any brain region could be induced to develop into cell types appropriate to the region in which they were grafted. In other words, stem cells from the developing ventral mesencephalon, striatum or cortex might be just as effective in repairing 4VO damage as those from the neuroepithelium. Since we did not have clonal lines from these immortomouse brain regions, we expanded nestin-positive populations of cells dissected from these regions at E14 through a minimum of five passages, labelled them with the fluorescent marker PKH26 and implanted them at our standard sites and concentrations in rats subjected to 15 min of 4VO. PKH26-labelled MHP36 grafts were used as a positive control.

An initial histological study compared the number of cells co-labelled with PKH26 and reactivity to the neuronal nuclear marker NeuN in 4VO rats with striatal, cortical or MHP36 grafts. Populations derived from the striatum migrated chiefly to the striatum, but were also plentiful in the denervated CA1 field. Cortical populations migrated widely to many anatomical regions, but preferentially moved towards the frontal cortex. MHP36 cells showed their usual preference for the CA1 field. The proportion of cells that differentiated into neurons in the CA1 field was calculated as the percentage of NeuN to total PKH-labelled cells within equivalent selected sections across graft groups. With MHP36 grafts on average $38 \pm 4.0\%$ were neuronal (i.e. PKH and NeuN positive), whereas significantly smaller proportions, $18 \pm 4.4\%$ of striatal and $23 \pm 3.9\%$ of cortical

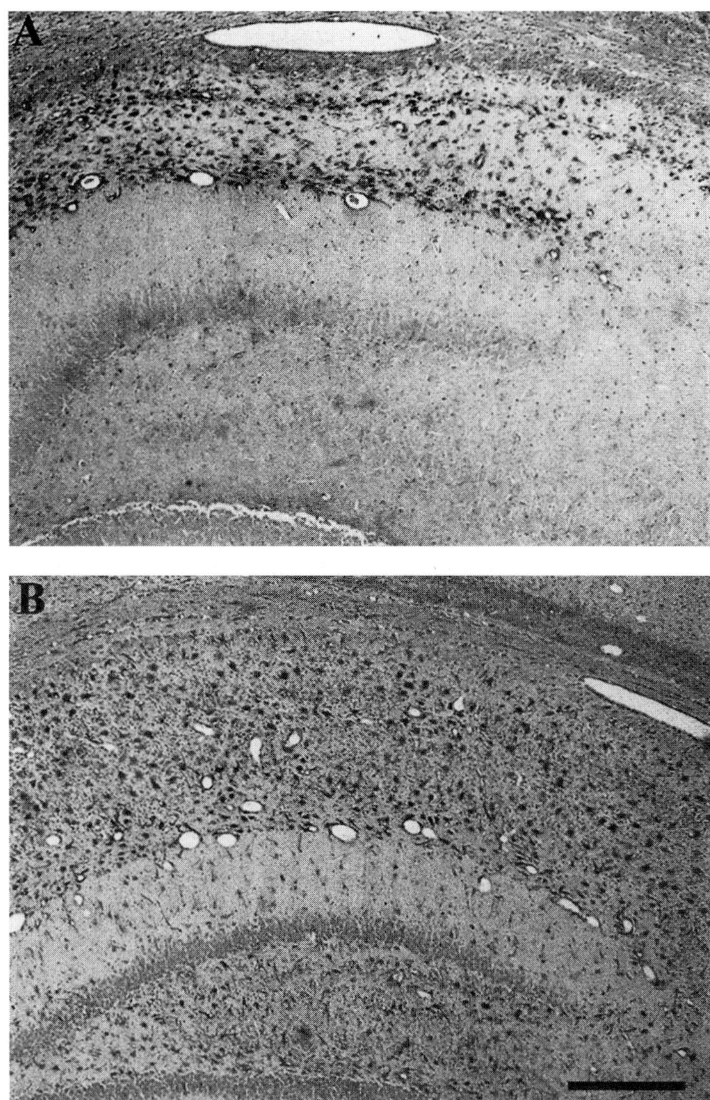

FIG. 1. Photomicrographs showing duration-related migration of MHP36 cells in the ischaemic rat hippocampus. (A) After 15 min of 4VO β-galactosidase-positive cells are seen chiefly in the CA1 field and the hippocampal fissure beneath. Few cells are seen in the hilus. (B) After 30 min of 4VO cells are distributed more diffusely through the dorsal hippocampus, and extensively colonize the hilus. Staining as in Plate 1. Scale bar = 400 μm.

cell populations, were neuronal. These findings suggested that hippocampal neuroepithelial clonal cells had a more selective preference for the CA1 field, and differentiated more readily into neurons within this field than populations from the immortomouse cortex and striatum.

Would these differences affect the capacity for functional repair? To answer this question we compared 4VO (15 min) rats with cortical, striatal or ventral mesencephalic population grafts or MHP36 grafts with sham grafted ischaemic and intact controls (n per group=9–10) on learning to find a submerged platform in the water maze (two trials a day for 12 days followed by a probe trial with the platform removed: see Hodges et al 1996 for details of our standard acquisition task). Groups differed significantly in latency to find the platform (F[5,110]=5.63, $P<0.01$: see Fig. 2). Ischaemic controls were impaired relative to intact controls, as were ischaemic groups with striatal and ventral mesencephalic grafts, which did not differ. However, groups with MHP36 grafts and those with cortical population grafts both showed comparable improvement and performed significantly better than ischaemic controls, at the level of intact controls. Thus there was a dissociation between the efficacy of stem cell grafts derived from the mid- and hindbrain as opposed to the forebrain. Positive effects of cortical cells were somewhat surprising in view of their reduced ability to differentiate into neurons, in comparison with MHP36 grafts, so that it may be that we supply cells in excess of requirement for repair. These findings suggest that there is some specificity of stem cells in functional repair: cells from any region cannot be used to repair damage in any other. This is in agreement with our failure (S. B. Dunnett, unpublished results) to reduce amphetamine and apomorphine-induced asymmetric rotation in rats with unilateral nigrostriatal lesions using MHP36 grafts implanted in striatum, substantia nigra or both regions. However, even stem cells from the immortomouse ventral mesencephalon have not proved efficacious in this rodent Parkinson's disease model (G. A. Grigoryan, unpublished results).

Fetal versus stem cell efficacy in primates following CA1 hippocampal lesions

Demonstration of neuroepithelial stem cell efficacy in a primate model of selective hippocampal damage would provide an important further proof of principle relevant to their therapeutic application to amnesia. Since there is no reliable primate model of global ischaemia, Ridley et al (1995) have developed a selective N-methyl-D-aspartate (NMDA) lesion of the CA1 field in marmosets as a model for the effects of global ischaemia, and shown that late (E94–96) fetal grafts of CA1 cells ameliorate the deficits in recall and learning of conditional visuo-spatial discriminations induced by this lesion (Ridley et al 1997). We (Virley et al 1999)

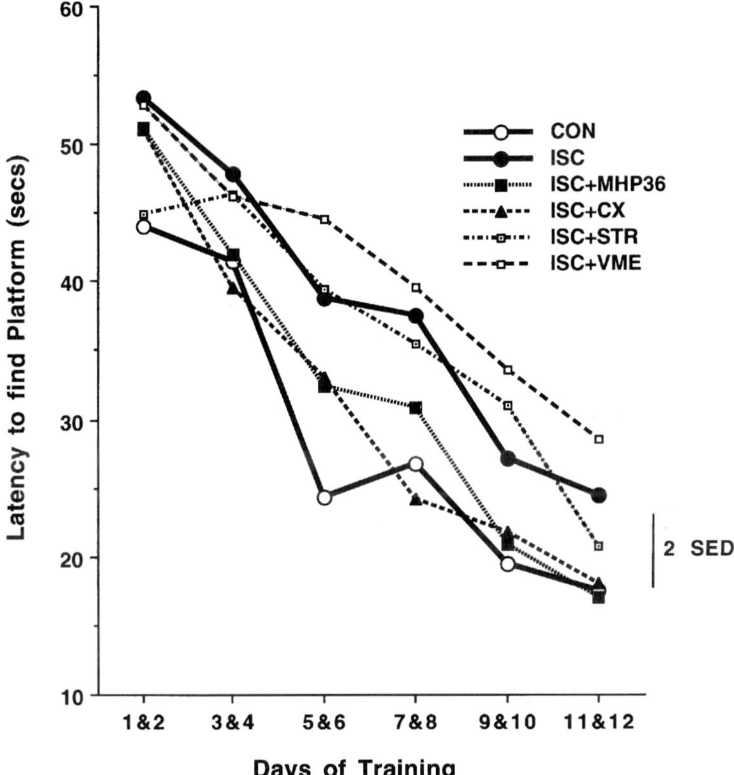

FIG. 2. Latency to find the submerged platform in the water maze in non-ischaemic and ischaemic controls (CON, ISC), and ischaemic rats grafted with and MHP36 (ISC+MHP36) cell line grafts and with immortomouse cortical (ISC+CX), striatal (ISC+STR) and ventral mesencephalic (ISC+VME) expanded cell population grafts. Non-ischaemic control rats found the platform significantly more rapidly over days of training than ischaemic controls. Rats with MHP36 and cortical grafts were as efficient as non-ischaemic controls and significantly superior to rats with striatal and ventral mesencephalic grafts that were as impaired as ischaemic controls. Bar shows twice the standard error for the difference in means for the Groups × Days interaction.

therefore compared fetal and MHP36 grafts in lesioned marmosets that showed comparable severe deficits in the recall of conditional discriminations in which the reward was always on the right with one pair of identical objects in the Wisconsin General Test Apparatus (WGTA) and on the left with a second pair. The monkeys were not impaired in simple discriminations between rewarded and non-rewarded objects, indicating that sensory, motor or motivational response was not affected by the lesion. Both fetal and MHP36 grafts improved recall of conditional discriminations learned prior to lesioning. Grafted marmosets were

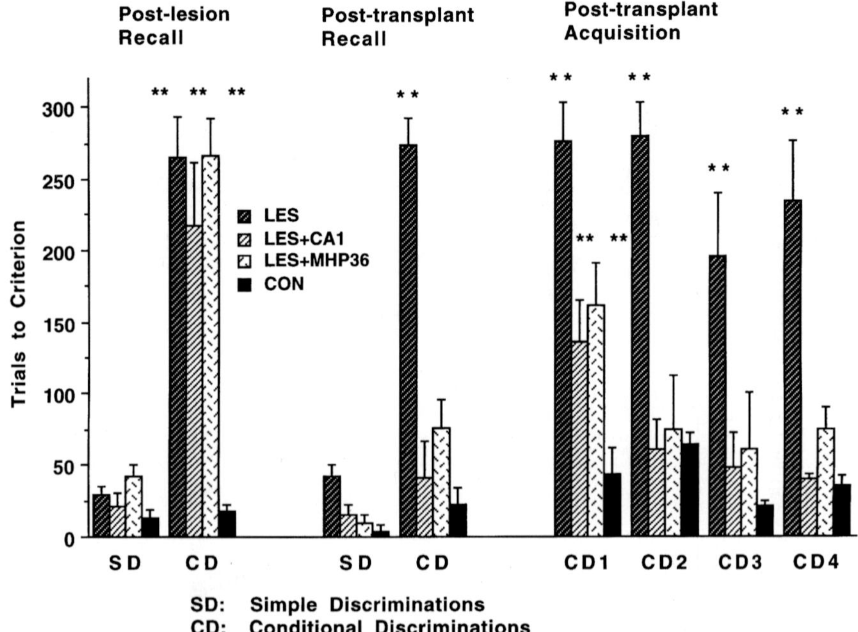

FIG. 3.   Recall of simple and conditional discriminations after CA1 lesions and after transplantation, and learning of new conditional discriminations in control (CON) and lesioned (LES) marmosets, and lesioned marmosets with fetal CA1 (LES+CA1) or MHP36 cell line (LES+MHP36) grafts. Lesioned marmosets did not differ from controls in recall of simple discriminations, but were substantially impaired in remembering conditional discriminations. Marmosets assigned to lesion-only or to graft groups did not differ in the extent of impairment after lesioning. However, when tested after transplantation, grafted groups recalled conditional discriminations as readily as control animals, while the lesion-only marmosets remained impaired. Lesioned marmosets found it difficult to learn new conditional discriminations throughout testing, whereas grafted monkeys, though impaired on the first new task, learned the remaining conditional discriminations in as few trials as controls. There were no significant differences between monkeys that received fetal and MHP36 cell line grafts.

initially impaired in learning new conditional discriminations, but improved to control level over a series of tasks, suggesting that time or training was required for full functional integration of both fetal and MHP36 grafts (Fig. 3). Lesioned marmosets with sham grafts were substantially impaired throughout testing. Histological examination showed that fetal grafts formed dense irregular masses either within the CA1 field, or clinging to its margins. MHP36 cells migrated evenly through the CA1 field, showing pyramidal and astrocytic morphology (Plate 2). The nuclei of mouse-derived pyramidal-like grafted MHP36 cells were only about half the size of normal marmoset pyramidal cells, whereas granular-type

MHP36 cells, in the host dentate granule layer in monkeys with additional dentate damage, were similar in size to normal marmoset granule cells. Interestingly, the sparse and even distribution of MHP36 cells through the broad CA1 field in marmosets was like the normal primate hippocampus, and differed from the compact alignment of these cells in rat hippocampus. Thus mouse-derived CA1 cells are functionally effective in both rats and primates with hippocampal damage, and appear to reconstitute the damaged CA1 fields in a species-appropriate manner.

Conclusions

Graft-induced functional recovery in animals with hippocampal damage offers a promising opportunity to investigate point-to-point repair mechanisms, given the integrated and laminar nature of the circuitry involved. However, much remains to be done before this connectivity can be fully demonstrated. In particular graft–host connections need to be studied by electrophysiological methods, by tract tracing, and by visualization of synapses at the electron miscroscope level. The damage-related and species-specific reconstruction of the hippocampal CA1 field by conditionally immortal stem cell lines exemplified by MHP36 grafts provides a powerful tool for mapping functional reconstruction of the hippocampus, with potential clinical relevance.

Acknowledgements

We wish to thank the Wellcome Trust and the British Heart Foundation for supporting our work on global ischaemia and fetal grafts and ReNeuron Ltd. for support of work on MHP36 grafts.

References

Arendt T, Bigl V, Arendt A, Tennestedt A 1983 Loss of neurons in the nucleus basalis of Meynert in Alzheimer's disease, paralysis agitans and Korsakoff's disease. Acta Neuropathol (Berl) 61:101–108

Block F, Schwarz M 1998 Global ischaemic neuronal damage relates to behavioural deficits: a pharmacological approach. Neuroscience 82:791–803

Dawe GS, Gray JA, Sinden JD, Stephenson JD, Segal M 1993 Extracellular recordings in the colchicine-lesioned rat dentate gyrus following transplants of foetal dentate gyrus and CA1 hippocampal subfield tissue. Brain Res 625:63–74

Field PM, Seeley PJ, Frotscher M, Raisman G 1991 Selective innervation of embryonic hippocampal transplants by adult host dentate granule cell axons. Neuroscience 41:713–727

Grubb NR, O'Carroll R, Cobbe SM, Sirel J, Fox KAA 1996 Chronic memory impairment after cardiac arrest outside hospital. BMJ 313:143–146

Hodges H, Sowinski P, Fleming P et al 1996 Contrasting effects of fetal CA1 and CA3 hippocampal grafts on deficits in spatial learning and working memory induced by global cerebral ischaemia in rats. Neuroscience 72:959–988

Hunter AJ, Green AR, Cross AJ 1995 Animal models of acute ischaemic stroke: can they predict clinically successful neuroprotective drugs? Trends Pharmacol Sci 16:123–128

Jat PS, Noble MD, Ataliotis P et al 1991 Direct derivation of conditionally immortal cell lines from an H-2K^b-tsA58 transgenic mouse. Proc Natl Acad Sci USA 88:5096–5100

Kartsounis LD, Rudge P, Stevens JM 1995 Bilateral lesions of the CA1 and CA2 fields of the hippocampus are sufficient to cause a severe amnesic syndrome in humans J Neurol Neurosurg Psychiatry 59:95–98

Mudrick LA, Baimbridge KG 1991 Hippocampal neurons transplanted into ischemically lesioned hippocampus: anatomical assessment of survival, maturation and integration. Exp Brain Res 86:233–247

Mudrick LA, Baimbridge KG, Peet MJ 1989 Hippocampal neurons transplanted into ischemically lesioned hippocampus: electroresponsiveness and re-establishment of circuitries. Exp Brain Res 76:333–342

Nelson AJ, Lebessi A, Sowinski P, Hodges H 1997a Comparison of effects of global ischaemia on spatial learning in the standard and radial water maze: relationship of hippocampal damage to performance. Behav Brain Res 85:93–115

Nelson A, Sowinski P, Hodges H 1997b Differential effects of global ischaemia on delayed matching- and non-matching-to-position in the water maze and Skinner box. Neurobiol Learn Mem 67:228–247

Netto CA, Hodges H, Sinden JD et al 1993 Effects of fetal hippocampal grafts on ischemic-induced deficits in spatial navigation in the water maze. Neuroscience 54:69–92

Nunn J, Hodges H 1994 Cognitive deficits induced by global cerebral ischaemia: relationship to brain damage and reversal by transplants. Behav Brain Res 65:1–31

Olsen GM, Scheel-Krüger J, Møller A, Jensen LH 1994 Relation of spatial learning of rats in the Morris water maze task to the number of viable CA1 neurons following four vessel occlusion. Behav Neurosci 108:681–690

Pulsinelli WA, Brierley MD, Plum F 1982 Temporal profile of neuronal damage in a model of transient global ischemia. Ann Neurol 11:491–498

Rempel-Clower NL, Zola SM, Squire LR, Amaral DG 1996 Three cases of enduring memory impairment after bilateral damage limited to the hippocampal formation. J Neurosci 16:5233–5255

Ridley RM, Timothy CJ, Maclean CJ, Baker HF 1995 Conditional learning and memory impairments following neurotoxic lesion of the CA1 field of the hippocampus. Neuroscience 67:263–275

Ridley RM, Pearson C, Kershaw TR et al 1997 Learning impairment induced by lesion of the CA1 field of the primate hippocampus: attempts to ameliorate the impairment by transplantation of foetal CA1 tissue. Exp Brain Res 115:83–94

Roine RO, Kajaste S, Kaste M 1992 Neuropsychological sequelae of cardiac arrest. Am J Med Assoc 269:237–242

Rose FC, Symonds CP 1960 Persistent memory defect following encephalitis. Brain 83:195–212

Schimdt-Kastner R, Freund TF 1991 Selective vulnerability of the hippocampus in brain ischaemia. Neuroscience 40:599–636

Scoville WB, Milner B 1957 Loss of recent memory after bilateral hippocampal lesions. J Neurosurg Psychiat 20:11–21

Sinden JD, Hodges H, Gray JA 1995 Neural transplantation and recovery of cognitive function. Behav Brain Sci 18:10–35

Sinden JD, Rashid-Doubell F, Kershaw TR et al 1997 Recovery of spatial learning by grafts of a conditionally immortalized hippocampal neuroepithelial cell line into the ischaemia-lesioned hippocampus. Neuroscience 81:599–608

Sprick U 1991 Transient and long-lasting beneficial behavioral effects of grafts in the damaged hippocampus of the rat. Behav Brain Res 42:187–199

Virley D, Ridley RM, Sinden JD et al 1999 Primary CA1 and conditionally immortal MHP36 cell
    grafts restore conditional discrimination learning and recall in marmosets after excitoxic
    lesions of the hippocampal CA1 field. Brain 122:2321–2335
Zola-Morgan S, Squire LR, Amaral DG 1986 Human amnesia and the medial temporal region:
    enduring memory impairment following a bilateral lesion to field CA1 of the hippocampus. J
    Neurosci 6:2950–2967

DISCUSSION

Björklund: Could you elaborate on what kinds of cells are formed? In your
pictures from the βgal-stained sections, the cells seemed to be spreading over the
entire width of the CA1, and their morphologies seemed to be variable. Do they
form a mixture of different types of cells?

Hodges: They are variable. Our problem is that although we have done βgal and
glial fibrillary acid protein (GFAP) staining, we've got very little double labelling
and we've not got any cell-specific labelling. Consequently, we don't know if they
are glutamatergic or GABAergic or whatever from the *in vivo* data. But we do see
cells that look like pyramidal cells; cells that look just like glia. The proportions are
about 40% neurons and 40% glia, and we do see some oligodendrocytes but
relatively fewer. These have also been picked out in cultures by specific stains, in
similar proportions.

Björklund: If you grow these cells in culture are they multipotent? Can they form
both glia and neurons?

Hodges: Yes, there has been relatively more work done with cultures. We know
that some cells are GABAergic, for example.

Gage: Were these cells taken from an E18 mouse?

Hodges: No, the MHP36 cells were taken at about E14, so they are stem cells; they
are undifferentiated.

Gage: Where were they taken from?

Hodges: The neuroepithelial lining in the hippocampus.

Gage: What happens if you put them into the hippocampus near the granule cell
layer?

Hodges: We've only seen them when they have penetrated there when there's
been a needle-tip injured site. They do align very precisely in the injury. In old
rats without a specific lesion, a lot of them went to the granule cell layer and they
looked like granule cells. In the CA1 layer they were smaller than normal CA1 cells.

Gage: I was looking at the injury you had in which where there more βgal-
positive cells in the hilar region. It didn't look like there were any cells that had
taken on granule cell morphology.

Hodges: There weren't that many in that particular example, but the clearest
examples we have seen of them going into the granule cell layer was by accidental

injury and in the very old rats, and in rats with a cholinergic lesion. In these examples MHP36 cells looked granule-like in the granule cell layer.

Gray: Fred Gage, I imagine that behind your question is the evidence that you have concerning fresh neurogenesis in the adult rat in the granule cell layer of the dentate gyrus. What is striking is that when the lesion is, as Helen Hodges' slide showed, confined to CA1, then none of the MHP36 βgal-labelled cells end up in the granule cell layer — they end up in the CA1 layer. It is only when the lesion gets bigger as after 30 min 4VO that you get labelled cells in the granule cell layer.

Gage: Can these cells respond to normal neurogenic cues and turn into granule cells like most progenitor cells can?

Hodges: Some of them look as though they can, but we haven't done detailed enough histology to answer that.

Peschanski: I'm a little surprised by the small proportion of neurons that you got out of the fetal neuron transplants from striatum and cortex. Do you think there could be a problem with the PKH, because it's a membrane marker and you may have just lost or diluted it over time in these grafts? Perhaps with the neurogenesis taking place in these fetal transplants you may have specifically lost this type of cell.

Hodges: The experiment we did to look at the proportions of cell types, in which we did double labelling with NeuN and PKH, was actually a histological experiment. The grafts had been in place for just a couple of weeks. I agree that PKH can cause problems in behavioural experiments, where cells remain in place for a very long time.

Peschanski: Two weeks would be sufficient for dilution.

Hodges: We have to assume that dilution is constant across different cell types.

Peschanski: My point is that you can't assume this. If you decide that a membrane molecule will dilute exactly the same way for different populations of cells, you will end up with a wrong estimate. It is something you have to check. You have to use another marker in addition to PKH.

Hodges: We use βgal, and we usually use this alongside PKH. We thought that PKH would provide us with a fairly quick way of visualizing our cells.

Gray: Marc Peschanski, are you saying that the dilution might vary both as a function of different cell lines, and as a function of whether those cells then differentiate *in vivo* into neurons or glia? It is only in that way that you will get a change in the proportions.

Peschanski: It is a parameter you cannot check: you cannot control for PKH. βgal is different because it is looking at the expression of a gene.

Price: I think the important take-home message, which follows from what Helen Hodges has said, is that you can only say anything about the positive cells. You can't say anything about negative cells. What has been done in Helen's experiments is a fairly careful co-expression study with βgal and PKH, and we know to a large extent the same cells stain with both.

Freeman: Was there any temporal relationship between these findings and the time of the transplant after the lesion?

Hodges: We always try to keep the transplants to within 2–3 weeks of the ischaemia. In the only case of a 4VO experiment where we left the animals six months before grafting them, we didn't see any behavioural recovery at all.

Bohn: When you injected the MPH36 cells, you showed nicely on two dimensions the formation of a layer of cells: what are the three-dimensional aspects? Does that layer extend through the whole damaged area? I find it remarkable that you had such a good behavioural recovery in the task if the repopulation was limited in three dimensions.

Hodges: Wherever you take the slices from, you can see the cells lining up. I would say that it was a three dimensional repopulation of the whole of the layer. In some of the early experiments in rats with ischaemic CA1 damage there seemed to be patches, and also quite a lot of MHP36 cells actually went into the subiculum as well as the CA1 layer.

Dunnett: Picking up on the question about being able unequivocally to track and identify the cells, do you know if the MHP cell line is male or female, because the Y chromosome probe is one of the few relatively unequivocal markers for grafted cells that does not wash out, get down-regulated, or diluted with cell division?

Hodges: We think it is male.

Gage: An issue that is often raised is nomenclature of cell types. It would be worthwhile defining what we mean by the term 'stem cell', if we are going to be using this term during this meeting. Are you grafting stem cells or a committed population of progenitors, and to what extent even *in vitro* can we identify which of the cells is an authentic stem cell?

Price: The classical definition is that a stem cell is a cell that is multipotential and has the capacity for self regeneration. I think that should be immediately amended to the 'extended capacity' for self regeneration, i.e. the idea that a cell could potentially maintain that capacity right through the lifetime of an organ. Fred Gage is attempting to do classic adoptive transfer experiment to prove stem cell properties — namely to show that a single cell can carry over those properties, with the capacity to re-populate an entire system from one animal into another. We don't have that data for any neural stem cell, although the haematopoietic people do have these kind of data. There's a tendency at present among the neurobiological field to consider any cell that's multipotential, and has even limited capacity for self regeneration, as a stem cell. My feeling is that we should resist that temptation: if we talk about any and every embryological multipotential precursor as a stem cell, the confusion will become even more considerable. My feeling is that in the absence of the absolute acid test — *in vivo* transfer — then the best definition would be that a stem cell is a multipotential precursor cell that has an extended capacity for self regeneration.

Gray: Are you happy with that, Fred?

Gage: Not really. I suppose it is somewhat a semantic issue.

Gray: No, I don't think it's semantic; it's tremendously important to get this as clear as possible.

Gage: There is also a distinction between cells which are immortalized (carrying oncogenes) and those that aren't. But if we put that aside and lump all the cells together for a moment, within a population of plated cells there will be individuals that can self-renew and propagate an entire population. It is another thing to say that every cell in that population can do the exact same thing. If you can prove by single-cell plating that every one of those cells in your dish can self-renew and give rise to all the same type of cells, then I think you're at a point where you can say that you have a homogenous population of cells with the same properties, and therefore you have a stem cell population.

Gray: Can I clarify one point: when you talk about a stem cell population are you by implication contradicting the fact that this stem cell population is a clonal line you've made?

Gage: A cell line can be clonal — i.e. derived from single cell — but in a dish, some of those cells derived from the same cell have differentiated slightly, so at any given time you have a mixed population of cells in a dish, or you have the implication that every cell is homogeneously at a fixed stem cell state. If you don't know the difference between the two of those, then when you graft cells you don't know whether or not you've grafted even one of those stem cells, or whether or not every cell that you grafted is at some later stage of differentiation. If it's a mixed population you don't know if a stem cell has differentiated into the cell of interest, or a more committed cell has differentiated into that cell. You may have a stem cell in culture, and from that population of cells, which could be clonally derived, you may or may not have a stem cell in the population you graft. Even if you do, it may or may not be that stem cell which is giving rise to the cell of interest.

Gray: Presumably you can make some progress along that line of argument on statistical grounds. One could make statements of the kind, 'We've checked out this population of cells 500 times and 60% have turned out to be stem cells, and therefore if we graft 1000 of them, 60% of that thousand are going to be stem cells'. However, I suppose you still wouldn't know, when you look afterwards at post-mortem tissue, that any particular cell you now observe is from the 60% of the stem cells rather than the other 40%, and whether or not it might have already been a committed precursor of some kind.

Gage: The answer will likely come from marking studies, which will allow us to identify precisely the nature of the cells at various stages.

Price: I agree with that, but the problem is that in practice we don't have such a marker. These are all functional definitions: there's no point in setting up an operational definition you can't then fulfil. I would have loved to been able to say that a neural stem cell is a cell that by definition carries markers A, B, C and D. However, I can't do that, so we have to set up an operational definition we can all fulfil. You are right that there is no such thing as a population of homogeneous cells, so we have to live with heterogeneity. The virtue of the definition I offered was that we can operate with it.

Peschanski: How practical would it be to define precisely stem cells from multipotent precursors or neural systems. The practicality in the bone marrow is that people are fighting to get totipotent cells because they want to have something that they can transfuse and have all the lines expressing the same thing at the same time. Is it the same type of practicality that we are looking at in the CNS, or would it make any difference to know or not to know whether our cells are second generation multipotent cells?

Smith: Theoretically, we don't know which is the best cell to transfer. It could be a bad thing to transplant stem cells because they have proliferative potential. It might be better to transplant committed precursors. Conversely, it might be better to transplant a pure population of stem cells, because they may have more plasticity and thus respond better to the environment. As I understand it, we don't know at this point. We are transplanting heterogeneous mixtures of cells and I think one ought to be clear about that and not be claiming that we are transplanting stem cells.

Gene transfer for neuroprotection in animal models of Parkinson's disease and amyotrophic lateral sclerosis

Martha C. Bohn, Bronwen Connor, Dorothy A. Kozlowski and M. Hasan Mohajeri*

*Children's Memorial Institute for Education and Research, Department of Pediatrics, Northwestern University Medical School, 2300 Children's Plaza, Chicago, IL 60614, USA, and *Department of Psychiatric Research, University of Zurich, Zurich, Switzerland*

Abstract. Glial cell line-derived neurotrophic factor (GDNF) is a potent survival factor for motoneurons (MN) and dopaminergic (DA) neurons, neurons which selectively die in amyotrophic lateral sclerosis (ALS) and Parkinson's disease (PD). GDNF gene delivery has been studied in rodent models of ALS and PD. In a mouse model of ALS, implantation of myoblasts retrovirally transduced with GDNF into hindlimb muscles at 6 weeks of age, i.e. prior to the onset of disease symptoms, increased the number of large MNs that maintained projections to treated muscles at 18 weeks of age. GDNF-treated mice also performed better on tests of motor function and had a delayed onset of disease. In a progressive degeneration rat model of PD, effects of *in vivo* GDNF gene therapy using an adenoviral vector (AdGDNF) were studied in young and aged rats. AdGDNF protected DA neurons against the neurotoxin, 6-hydroxydopamine (6-OHDA), and was effective whether injected either before or after 6-OHDA damage had commenced. However, if AdGDNF was injected prior to 6-OHDA, it was most effective in protecting against DA-dependent changes in the brain when injected near the terminals of the DA neurons. In contrast, if 6-OHDA damage had already commenced, AdGDNF was most effective if injected near the DA soma. These studies suggest that GDNF gene delivery into specific sites in the CNS or into muscle where MNs have access to secreted GDNF may slow the progression of PD and ALS, respectively. Neurotrophic factor gene therapy offers novel interventions not only for PD and ALS, but also other neurodegenerative diseases and injuries to the nervous system.

2000 Neural transplantation in neurodegenerative disease. Wiley, Chichester (Novartis Foundation Symposium 231) p 70–93

Many diseases, as well as injuries, of the CNS are characterized by the death of neurons. However, there are presently no therapies that slow or inhibit neuronal cell death in humans with neurodegenerative conditions. Exciting developments in this field, so far tested only in laboratory animals, suggest that unique gene and cell therapies for neurodegenerative diseases lie on the horizon. Studies of molecules that are crucial to the development of neurons have provided candidate genes that might be used therapeutically to stimulate survival and repair of injured and diseased neurons. Knowledge of how to transfer such genes into the brain is also increasing at a rapid pace. An increased understanding of pathways involved in apoptosis or programmed cell death have also provided therapeutic targets for intervention. During development of the nervous system where neurons are produced in overabundance and then pruned back through the process of apoptosis, neurotrophic factors play an important role in determining the number of neurons that survive. Many studies have also shown that neurotrophic factors are involved in plasticity in the mature nervous system, suggesting a role for these factors in the damaged and diseased nervous system. Assuming that chronic increased levels of neurotrophic factors will be required for effective treatment of long-term neurodegenerative diseases, our recent studies have focused on ways to provide neurotrophic factors chronically to damaged neurons. Specifically we have studied the effects of glial cell line-derived neurotrophic factor (GDNF) gene transfer in rodent models of amyotrophic lateral sclerosis (ALS) and Parkinson's disease (PD). The neurotrophic factor, GDNF, is a potent survival factor for both motoneurons (MNs) and dopaminergic (DA) neurons (Henderson et al 1994, Lin et al 1993), those neurons that selectively die in ALS and PD, respectively. Following the discovery of GDNF and its potent survival activity on DA neurons in culture, numerous studies have shown that injection of GDNF protein into the nigrostriatal system ameliorates behavioural and pathological consequences of lesioning DA neurons in rodent and primate models of PD (for review see, Bohn & Choi-Lundberg 1998). Our initial gene therapy study showed that chronically increased biosynthesis of GDNF at nanogram levels effectively slows the death of DA neurons in a rat model of PD (Choi-Lundberg et al 1997). Moreover, recent studies show that DA neurons can be rescued by GDNF gene transfer even after damage has commenced. In a mouse model of ALS, long-term transgene expression of GDNF in muscle through *ex vivo* gene delivery slows the degeneration of spinal motoneurons. The pace of research in this area has progressed rapidly due in part to the excellent laboratory animal models of these diseases. However, the application of gene therapy to protect neurons from cell death or to rescue neurons that have already suffered cell damage is generally relevant to a wide array of neurodegenerative conditions including Huntington's disease, Alzheimer's disease, retinal degeneration, spinal cord injury and stroke (Table 1).

GDNF gene transfer into the striatum or substantia nigra in an aged rat model of PD

PD is a slow, progressive neurodegenerative disease that usually commences late in life. Therefore, our laboratory has studied the effects of chronically increased levels

TABLE 1   Neuroprotective factor gene therapy in neurodegenerative disorders and cerebral injury

---

Parkinson's disease (dopaminergic neurons)

In vivo

Ad, GDNF	Choi-Lundberg et al 1997
Ad, GDNF	Bilang-Bleuel et al 1997
Ad, GDNF	Lapchak et al 1997
Ad, GDNF	Kojima et al 1997
Ad, GDNF	Choi-Lundberg et al 1998
AAV, GDNF	Mandel et al 1997
Ad, TGFβ1	Sanchez-Capelo et al 1999
HSV, Bcl-2	Yamada et al 1999

Ex vivo

Chromaffin/NGF astrocyte cografts	Cunningham et al 1991
Chromaffin/NGF astrocyte cografts	Cunningham et al 1994
Chromaffin/NGF fibroblast cografts	Niijima et al 1995
Chromaffin/NGF fibroblast cografts	Date et al 1996
Rat I, BDNF	Frim et al 1994
BHK, GDNF	Lindner et al 1995
Astrocytes, BDNF	Yoshimoto et al 1995
Fibroblasts, BDNF	Levivier et al 1995
Fibroblasts, BDNF	Lucidi-Phillipi et al 1995
Fibroblasts, BDNF	Galpern et al 1996
Fibroblasts, GDNF	Trupp et al 1996
BHK, GDNF	Tseng et al 1997
BHK, NTN	Tseng et al 1998
BHK, GDNF/NTN	Akerud et al 1999

ALS (Motoneurons)

In vivo

Ad, BDNF/GDNF	Giménez y Ribotta et al 1997
Ad, CNTF/BDNF	Gravel et al 1997
Ad, NT-3	Haase et al 1997
Ad, NT-3	Haase et al 1998
Ad, CNTF	Haase et al 1999
Ad, GDNF/BDNF NGF/CNTF	Baumgartner & Shine 1997
Ad, GDNF	Baumgartner & Shine 1998a,b

Ex vivo

BHK, CNTF	Sagot et al 1995
BHK, CNTF	Aebischer et al 1996a,b
BHK, CNTF	Tan et al 1996
BHK, GDNF	Sagot et al 1996
Myoblasts, GDNF	Mohajeri et al 1999

(Continued)

TABLE 1 (*Continued*)

Huntington's disease (striatal neurons)	
Ex vivo	
Rat I, NGF	Schumacher et al 1991
Rat I, NGF	Frim et al 1993a,b
BHK, NGF	Emerich et al 1994a
BHK, CNTF	Emerich et al 1997a
BHK, CNTF	Emerich et al 1997b
BHK, CNTF/NT-4/5	Emerich et al 1998
Alzheimer's disease (basal forebrain cholinergic neurons)	
In vivo	
Ad, NGF	Castel-Barthe et al 1996
AAV, NGF/BDNF	Klein et al 1999
Ex vivo	
208F, NGF	Rosenberg et al 1988
208F, NGF	Hoffman et al 1993
BHK, NGF	Emerich et al 1994b
BHK, NGF	Winn et al 1994
BHK, NGF	Winn et al 1996
Fibroblasts, NGF	Kawaja et al 1992
Fibroblast, NGF	Dekker et al 1994
Fibroblasts, BDNF	Lucidi-Phillipi et al 1995
Fibroblast, NGF	Lucidi-Phillipi et al 1995
Fibroblasts, NGF	Chen & Gage 1995
Fibroblasts, NGF	Tuszynski et al 1996a
Progenitor, NGF	Martínez-Serrano et al 1995a,b
Progenitor, NGF	Martínez-Serrano et al 1996
Spinal cord injury (spinal cord axons)	
In vivo	
Ad, NT-3	Zhang et al 1998
Ad, NGF	Boulis et al 1999
DNA plasmid, Bcl-2	Takahashi et al 1999
Ex vivo	
Fibroblasts, NGF	Tuszynski et al 1994
Fibroblasts, NGF	Tuszynski et al 1996b
Fibroblasts, NGF	Tuszynski et al 1997
Fibroblasts, NGF	Blesch & Tuszynski 1997
Fibroblasts, NGF / BDNF NT-3 / FGF-2	Nakahara et al 1996
Fibroblasts, PDGF	Iijichi et al 1996
Myoblasts, CNTF	Déglon et al 1996
Rat I, NGF/BDNF	Kim et al 1996

(*Continued*)

TABLE 1   *(Continued)*

Sympathetic neurons
In vivo

   HSV, NGF   Federoff et al 1992

Focal ischaemia
In vivo

   HSV, Bcl-2   Linnik et al 1995
   HSV, Bcl-2   Lawrence et al 1997
   HSV, HSP72   Yenari et al 1998
   Ad, IL-1ra   Betz et al 1995
   Ad, IL-1ra   Yang et al 1997
   Ad, IL-1ra   Yang et al 1998

Auditory system (Spiral ganglion neurons)
In vivo

   HSV, BDNF   Geschwind et al 1996
   HSV, BDNF   Staecker et al 1998

Visual system (retinal ganglion cells/photoreceptors)
In vivo

   Ad, BDNF   Isenmann et al 1998
   Ad, CNTF   Cayouette & Gravel 1997
   Ad, Bcl-2   Bennett et al 1998

Abbreviations: AAV, adeno-associated virus; Ad, adenovirus; BDNF, brain-derived neurotrophic factor; BHK, baby hamster kidney; CNTF, ciliary neurotrophic factor; FGF, fibroblast growth factor; HSV, herpes simplex virus; IL-1ra, interleukin 1 receptor antagonist; NGF, nerve growth factor; NTN, neurturin; PDGF, platelet-derived growth factor; TGFβ1, transforming growth factor β1.

of GDNF through gene transfer in a progressive degeneration rat model of PD. In this model, rats are injected with 6-hydroxydopamine (6-OHDA) into the striatum, the site of DA terminals. This results in a slow degeneration of DA neurons (Sauer & Oertel 1994). In young rats with this lesion, we had observed that injection of an adenovirus harbouring a GDNF gene (AdGDNF) into the substantia nigra near the DA soma one week prior to the 6-OHDA lesion profoundly protected DA neurons (Choi-Lundberg et al 1997). In addition, AdGDNF was also effective in protecting DA neurons if injected near the terminals of DA neurons (Choi-Lundberg et al 1998). Similar effects of GDNF gene delivery have been confirmed by other groups using either adenoviral or adeno-associated viral vectors (Table 1). Since PD is a disease of ageing, these initial studies were extended to an aged rat model of PD in which the cellular and behavioural effects of injecting AdGDNF near the DA terminals (striatum) or the DA soma (substantia nigra) were directly compared. Twenty-month-old Fischer

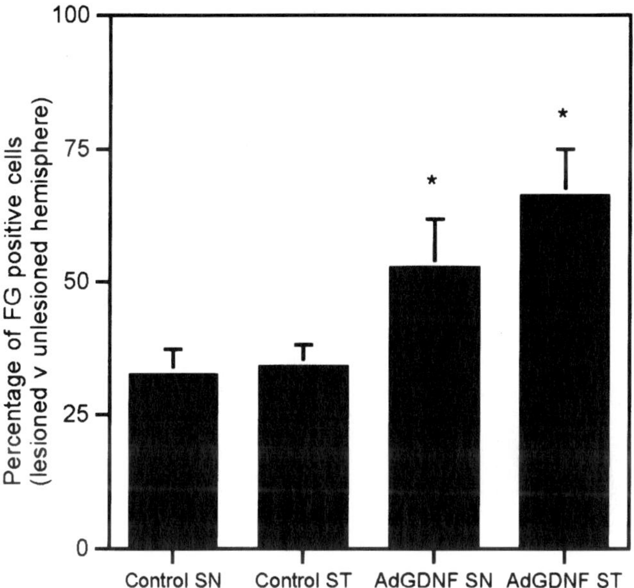

FIG. 1.   AdGDNF significantly prevents the degeneration of FG-positive DA neurons in the lesioned substantia nigra (SN) of aged rat 35 days after 6-OHDA lesioning. A significant increase in the percentage of FG-positive neurons was observed in the lesioned SN in rats injected with AdGDNF in either the striatum (ST) or the SN compared with control groups (*$P \leqslant 0.01$). There was no significant difference in the percentage of FG-positive neurons between rats injected with AdGDNF in the ST versus the SN ($P > 0.05$; reproduced with permission from Connor et al 1999).

344 rats were injected with AdGDNF or control vector into the striatum or substantia nigra 1 week prior to 6-OHDA lesioning. In addition, DA neurons that projected to the lesioned site were prelabelled with the fluorescent retrograde tracer, fluorogold (FG) as described previously (Choi-Lundberg et al 1997, Sauer & Oertel 1994). This allowed the fate of those DA neurons that projected specifically to the lesion site to be assessed without having to rely on DA phenotypic markers. As observed in the young rat, AdGDNF protected DA neurons against 6-OHDA whether the vector was placed near the cell bodies or near their terminals (Fig. 1; Connor et al 1999).

However, differential effects of the vector placed into these two sites were evident when DA-dependent behaviours and cellular changes in DA target neurons were assessed. Following a unilateral lesion of the nigrostriatal pathway, rats normally develop a preference for using their ipsilateral forelimb. While control rats and rats injected with AdGDNF in the substantia nigra showed an increased preference for ipsilateral forelimb use, rats injected with AdGDNF in

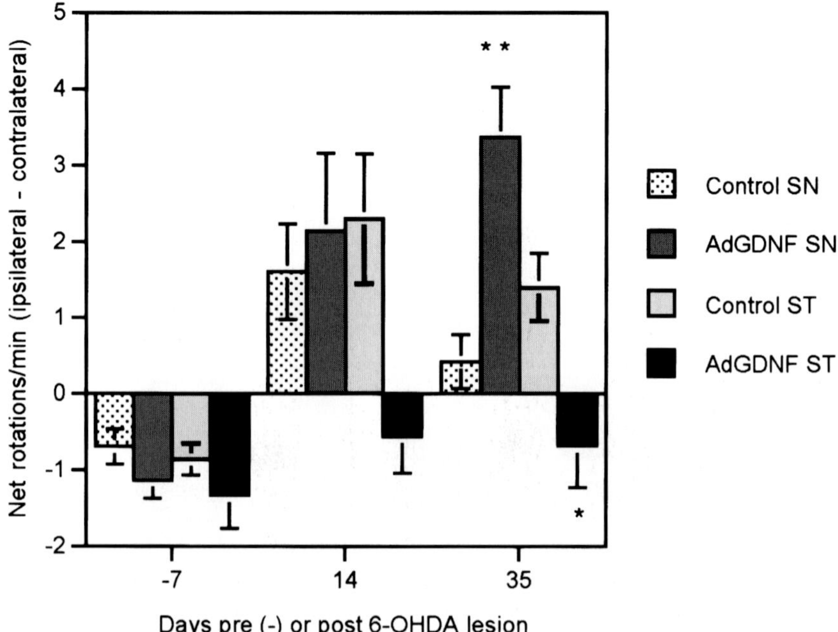

FIG. 2.　AdGDNF injected into the aged rat striatum (ST) significantly protects against the development of amphetamine-induced ipsilateral rotational behaviour observed in control rats after 6-OHDA lesioning. Rats were injected with dl-amphetamine (5 mg/kg, i.p.) and their behaviour recorded for 60 minutes. Baseline amphetamine rotation tests were performed 7 days before lesioning (-7) and the results used to assign the side of the 6-OHDA lesioning. Thirty-five days after lesioning, rats injected with AdGDNF into the striatum exhibited a significant reduction in ipsilateral rotational behaviour compared with control groups and rats injected with AdGDNF into the substantia nigra (SN) (*$P \leqslant 0.05$). In contrast, rats injected with AdGDNF into the substantia nigra exhibited a significant increase in ipsilateral rotational behaviour 35 days after lesion compared with control groups. (Reproduced with permission from Connor et al 1999.)

the striatum did not develop this deficit and at 3–4 weeks after lesioning actually showed a strong preference for using the contralateral paw (Connor et al 1999). This suggests that AdGDNF protected DA terminals and may have increased striatal DA levels above control levels in the injured nigrostriatal system. Similar findings were observed for amphetamine-induced rotation. Rats injected with control vector or AdGDNF in the substantia nigra displayed increased amphetamine-induced rotation toward the lesioned side. In contrast, rats injected with AdGDNF in the striatum did not display this behaviour (Fig. 2; Connor et al 1999).

These observations suggest that when GDNF biosynthesis is increased near the DA terminals prior to the lesion, the terminals are protected against degeneration

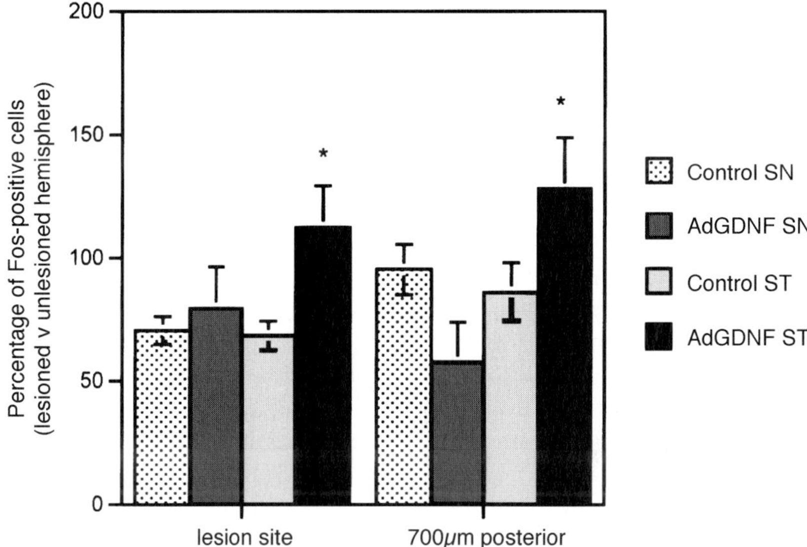

FIG. 3. The level of amphetamine-induced Fos immunoreactivity in the lesioned striatum (ST) of aged rat. Rats injected with AdGDNF in the striatum exhibit a significant increase in the percentage of Fos-IR nuclei at both the lesion site and 700 μm posterior to the lesion site compared with rats injected with AdGDNF in the substantia nigra (SN) and control groups (*$P \leqslant 0.050$). In contrast, a reduction in Fos-IR was observed both in rats injected with AdGDNF in the substantia nigra and in control rats. (Reproduced with permission from Connor et al 1999.)

and DA levels persist. On the other hand, when GDNF biosynthesis is increased near the cell bodies in the aged rat brain, levels are sufficient to inhibit cell death, but insufficient to increase DA levels at the terminals or to stimulate terminal sprouting so that behaviours indicative of a deficiency in dopamine still develop. These behavioural observations are further supported by morphological data on striatal target neurons and DA fibre density. Amphetamine-induced expression of the proto-oncogene, c-*fos*, in DA target neurons in the striatum, has been used as a measure of intact nigrostriatal input (Morgan & Curran 1991, Labandeira-Garcia et al 1996). Five weeks after 6-OHDA, the number of striatal neurons that displayed nuclear induction of immunoreactivity to Fos dropped to approximately 50%. Striatal, but not nigral, injection of AdGDNF prevented this decrease (Fig. 3; Connor et al 1999), suggesting that increased levels of GDNF near the terminals of the DA neurons increased DA levels available to target neurons. This increase could result from either an increase in DA release per terminal or an increase in the number of DA terminals. The latter possibility is supported by an assessment of the density of DA terminals in the lesion site. This assessment showed a significant increase in terminal density only in aged rats injected with AdGDNF in the striatum (Connor et al 1999). A similar protection of fibres in young adult rats 4 weeks after striatal injection of AdGDNF has been reported (Bilang-Bleuel et al 1997), but not observed at 6 weeks in another study (Choi-Lundberg et al 1998). The effects of GDNF gene delivery on metabolism of dopamine have not yet been studied, however. Taken together, our studies and those of other investigators suggest that increased levels of GDNF biosynthesis near either the DA neurons or their terminals are effective in protecting healthy DA neurons against 6-OHDA neurotoxicity in both the young and aged rat brain. Furthermore, increasing GDNF biosynthesis near the terminals but not the cell bodies of these neurons protects DA terminals from 6-OHDA-induced damage and maintains nigrostriatal function in the aged rat. A similar comparison of injecting AdGDNF into either the substantia nigra or striatum of the young rat has not been done. However, studies have been done in which GDNF protein was injected into either of these sites. In a study by Winkler and colleagues (Winkler et al 1996), long-term intranigral injections of GDNF protein protected DA neurons in the substantia nigra, but did not result in functional recovery of the forelimb akinesia test or restoration of striatal DA innervation. In contrast, several studies have observed that intrastriatal injection of GDNF or AdGDNF maintains or induces reinnervation of the denervated striatum and prevents behavioural impairment (Rosenblad et al 1998, Shults et al 1996, Bilang-Bleuel et al 1997, Choi-Lundberg et al 1998).

GDNF gene transfer rescues DA neurons
after damage has commenced

PD in humans does not result in clinical symptoms until 80% or more of the DA neurons have degenerated. In the absence of clinical symptoms or a means of early disease detection, the goal of preventing the consequences of neurodegeneration in this disease is difficult. It is interesting, however, that patients do not display behaviours indicative of a DA deficiency until such a large loss of neurons has occurred. Most likely this is due to the high capacity of DA neurons to up-regulate the synthesis of DA (Zigmond et al 1993), thus compensating during the subclinical stage for the fall out of neurons, at least until a threshold level is reached where the capacity for compensation becomes insufficient. This also implies, however, that if a therapy could slow the death of the remaining 20% of the DA neurons, up-regulate DA synthesis in remaining terminals or stimulate sprouting of DA terminals, PD patients might benefit considerably and remain without clinical symptoms for a prolonged period. It is not known how many of the remaining DA neurons are in a healthy state when symptoms occur. It is likely that a continuum of neuronal viability exists in which some neurons are healthy while others are in a compromised state. Thus, both protective and rescue-directed therapies may be valuable for PD.

To study the ability of GDNF gene transfer to rescue DA neurons, we injected 6-OHDA into the rat striatum and 1 week later injected AdGDNF into either the substantia nigra or the striatum. One month later, the retrograde tracer, FG was injected into the striatum at the lesion site to label those DA neurons that survived and maintained projections to the lesion site. AdGDNF injection into the substantia nigra significantly increased survival of such DA neurons, whereas DA neuronal survival following AdGDNF injection into the striatum was not statistically significant although it was somewhat increased (Kozlowski et al 2000). The efficacy of increased GDNF biosynthesis in the substantia nigra, but not in the striatum, also extended to DA-dependent behaviours and neurochemical changes. Both the development of ipsilateral paw preference and amphetamine-induced rotation were prevented by AdGDNF injection in the substantia nigra. Amphetamine-induction of Fos in DA target neurons in the lesioned striatum of rats injected with AdGDNF in the substantia nigra was increased above that in the unlesioned contralateral striatum, whereas striatal AdGDNF was without effect. These observations suggest that AdGDNF injected into the substantia nigra, but not into the striatum, stimulated sprouting of DA terminals after the degeneration of DA terminals had commenced.

As discussed above, in the aged rat, vector injection into the striatum prior to a 6-OHDA lesion was more effective than injection into the substantia nigra. In the young adult rat, GDNF vector or protein injection into the striatum prior to a lesion also protected neurons and ameliorated the development of DA-dependent behaviours. In contrast, when vector was injected 1 week after a 6-OHDA lesion in the young rat, only injection into the substantia nigra was effective. While these results are seemingly at odds, there are several possible explanations. In the rescue study, vector was injected 1 week after 6-OHDA during which considerable damage to terminals occurred. Therefore, there may not have been enough terminals remaining to take up sufficient GDNF for the striatal vector injections to have any significant effect. On the other hand, the effect of intranigral injection of the vector may have inhibited further degeneration of DA terminals and even stimulated sprouting. The effect of intranigral GDNF on sprouting of DA terminals might require intervention during a specific window of opportunity, or the capacity for GDNF-stimulated sprouting in the aged rat may be reduced. It is not known whether the effects observed with GDNF gene delivery on DA neurons damaged by the neurotoxin, 6-OHDA, are applicable to the disease state in humans with PD. Nevertheless, since the goal in these patients is to protect healthy DA neurons from dying, as well as to rescue compromised DA neurons, the best strategy might be to inject a GDNF vector into both the basal ganglia and the substantia nigra.

Ex vivo GDNF gene delivery in a mouse model of ALS

ALS, commonly known as Lou Gehrig's disease, is a degenerative disease of MNs characterized pathologically by an abnormal accumulation of neurofilaments (NFs) in MN perikarya and proximal axons. Patients with ALS develop severe, progressive muscular weakness and other symptoms related to the death and loss of function of both upper and lower MNs (Mulder et al 1986, Siddique et al 1989, Wong et al 1995). Most cases of ALS are sporadic, but about 10% of cases are familial (FALS). Of these, about 20% are linked to autosomal dominant mis-sense mutations in copper/zinc superoxide dismutase (SOD-1) (Deng et al 1993, Rosen et al 1993, Siddique et al 1991). Since none of these mutations is localized to the active site of SOD-1, the underlying cause of the selective MN death remains elusive. However, the elucidation of these mutations has spawned new avenues for research utilizing transgenic mouse and *in vitro* models of FALS. The Gly93Ala was the first human SOD-1 mutation to be expressed in transgenic mice (Gurney et al 1994). Mice of the G1H transgenic line expressing the mutated human SOD-1 express about five times the level of SOD-1 in wild-type mice. Spinal MNs in the G1H mouse begin to show pathological changes beginning about the fourth week of life (Mourelatos et al 1996). Early pathological signs of degeneration include fragmented Golgi, neurofilamentous inclusions and vacuoles, believed to originate from degenerating rough endoplasmic reticulum (Dal Canto & Gurney 1994, Mourelatos et al 1996). There is a subsequent loss of large spinal MNs which reaches about 50% by 18 weeks of age, as well as a severe loss of myelinated axons in ventral roots (Gurney et al 1994, Chiu et al 1995, Mohajeri et al 1999). Mice begin to exhibit tremor of the hindlimbs and become debilitated around 100 days of age (Gurney et al 1994, Mohajeri et al 1998) and die from respiratory failure by five months of age. We have used the retrograde tracer FG to follow the time-course of degeneration of MNs projecting specifically to the medial gastrocnemius (MG) muscle in the G1H mouse. This study showed that at 18 weeks of age following injection of FG into the MG one week prior to sacrifice, there were only 36% large, FG-labelled alpha MNs compared to the number of these neurons in wild-type mice (Mohajeri et al 1998). In contrast, little effect on the number of small FG-labelled MNs was observed.

The FG retrograde labelling method described was also used to determine whether GDNF gene delivery to muscles of G1H mice would slow degeneration of MNs projecting to those muscles. Myoblasts retrovirally transduced with β-galactosidase (βgal) or GDNF were injected bilaterally into the MG and lateral gastocnemius (LG) muscles at 6 weeks of age, i.e. prior to onset of neurodegeneration. At 17 weeks of age, the treated muscles were injected with FG to label viable MNs that still maintained projections to these muscles. The mice were sacrificed one week later and the total number of fluorescent MNs in the spinal cord counted. In addition, the diameter of each MN was measured to obtain a morphometric size distribution of MNs projecting to the MG and LG muscles. These analyses confirmed the marked degeneration of large MNs in untreated G1H mice, as well as in G1H mice injected with βgal-expressing myoblasts (Mohajeri et al 1999). In G1H mice that were injected with GDNF-expressing myoblasts, however, there were significantly more large MNs, although this number remained lower than that in littermate wild-type mice (Fig. 4; Mohajeri et al 1999). Interestingly, the size distribution in all experimental groups of G1H mice was shifted toward smaller MNs suggesting that many MNs shrink prior to degenerating and that increased GDNF expression at the terminals of MNs slows this shrinkage.

GDNF gene delivery to muscle also ameliorated the degeneration in motor behaviour. Around 12 weeks of age, G1H mice begin to show physical signs of MN degeneration including tremor of the hindlimbs, muscle wasting, dragging of the hindlimbs and deficits in performance on behavioural tests of motor function (Gurney et al 1994, Mohajeri et al 1998). To determine whether mice treated with GDNF-transduced myoblasts would slow the progression of these deficits, we tested mice for performance on a balance rod and an inverted screen. In the case of the balance rod test, GDNF-treated G1H mice performed as well as littermate wild-type mice through the 17th week of age, but then became debilitated (Fig. 5; Mohajeri et al 1999). Behaviour on the inverted screen test was also improved by GDNF treatment. Moreover, the atrophy of the LG and MG muscles that occurred in G1H mice was also retarded in mice injected with GDNF-transduced myoblasts. This supports the cell count data further suggesting that GDNF maintained increased innervation to these muscles. GDNF-treated mice also had a significantly delayed onset of disease symptoms compared with control G1H mice (Mohajeri et al 1999). The decline in performance at older ages in the GDNF-treated mice suggests either that GDNF is unable to protect completely against neuronal cell death that occurs as a result of the overexpression of a mutant SOD-1 gene, or that therapeutically efficacious levels of GDNF decline with time. In support of the latter possibility are data showing that the levels of mRNA and DNA of both βgal and GDNF transgenes declined to about 5% of the original levels after 12 weeks of treatment (Mohajeri et al 1999).

Summary

Studies are reviewed showing that GDNF gene transfer in rodent models of ALS and PD slows the degenerative process resulting in increased neuronal survival and function. In a mouse model of ALS, increased levels of GDNF in muscle prolongs the survival and function of spinal MNs. In a rat model of PD, increased levels of

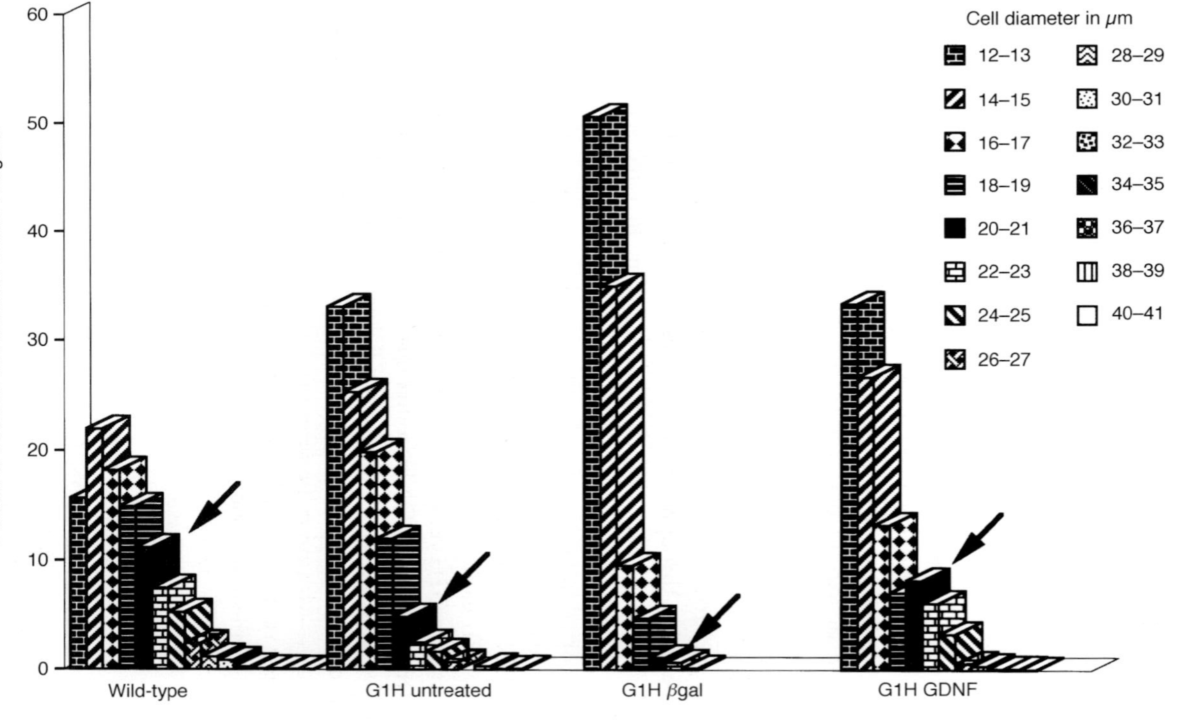

FIG. 4.   Morphometric analysis of the size distribution of motoneuron (MN) somal diameters expressed as a percent of FG-labelled MNs counted. At 18 weeks of age and 12 weeks after the beginning of treatment, the percentage of large MN innervating the GDNF-treated muscles in G1H mice is greater than that in control groups of G1H mice. The total number of FG-positive cells larger than 12 μm in diameter innervating the MG and LG muscle was set as 100%. The percentage of MNs with a defined diameter (given in the figure key, from 12–41 μm) is plotted as the function of genotype and treatment of mice. Note the shift of MN size toward smaller diameters in all G1H groups compared to wild-type mice. Note also that GDNF-treated G1H mice have a larger percentage of large MNs when compared to other control G1H mice (see arrows indicating 20–21 μm). (Reproduced with permission from Mohajeri et al 1999.)

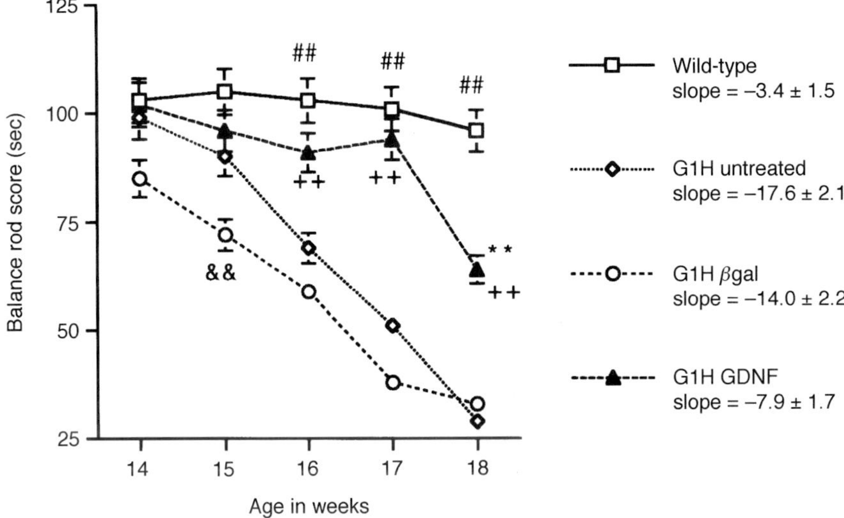

FIG. 5. Performance of mice in the balance rod test. At 14 weeks, no statistically significant difference was observed among experimental groups. Over the next 4 weeks, performance of untreated and β-galactosidase (βgal, control vector) treated mice deteriorated significantly, whereas the performance of GDNF-treated mice did not show a significant difference from that in wild-type mice until 18 weeks of age (**, $P \leqslant 0.01$ for GDNF vs wild-type; ##, $P \leqslant 0.01$ for wild-type vs. βgal and untreated; &&, $P \leqslant 0.01$ for βgal vs. GDNF and wild-type; ++, $P \leqslant 0.01$ for GDNF vs. βgal and untreated). (Reproduced with permission from Mohajeri et al 1999.)

GDNF promotes the survival and function of DA neurons whether the vector is injected prior to or subsequent to a 6-OHDA lesion. However, differential effects are observed depending on the site of vector injection relative to the DA terminals and soma, and the timing of vector injection relative to the degenerative signal. These studies provide a foundation for exploring the application of GDNF gene therapy in humans afflicted with ALS or PD. It is of utmost importance to develop means for safe, effective, and regulatable delivery of the GDNF gene to the human CNS. As a first approach, testing of novel vector systems in the non-human primate CNS is critical to identify an ideal gene transfer vector. Another potentially valuable direction will be to test other gene candidates for their ability to interfere directly with apoptotic pathways in animal models of neurodegenerative diseases.

References

Aebischer P, Pochon NA, Heyd B et al 1996a Gene therapy for amyotrophic lateral sclerosis (ALS) using a polymer encapsulated xenogenic cell line engineered to secrete hCNTF. Hum Gene Ther 7:851–860

Aebischer P, Scluep M, Déglon N et al 1996b Intrathecal delivery of CNTF using encapsulated genetically modified xenogeneic cells in amyotrophic lateral sclerosis patients. Nat Med 2:696–699 (erratum: 1996 Nat Med 2:1041)

Akerud P, Alberch J, Eketjäll S, Wagner J, Arenas E 1999 Differential effects of glial cell line-derived neurotrophic factor and neurturin on developing and adult substantia nigra dopaminergic neurons. J Neurochem 73:70–78

Baumgartner BJ, Shine HD 1997 Targeted transduction of CNS neurons with adenoviral vectors carrying neurotrophic factor genes confers neuroprotection that exceeds the transduced population. J Neurosci 17:6504–6511

Baumgartner BJ, Shine HD 1998a Neuroprotection of spinal motoneurons following targeted transduction with an adenoviral vector carrying the gene for glial cell line-derived neurotrophic factor. Exp Neurol 153:102–112

Baumgartner BJ, Shine HD 1998b Permanent rescue of lesioned neonatal motoneurons and enhanced axonal regeneration by adenovirus-mediated expression of glial cell line-derived neurotrophic factor. J Neurosci Res 54:766–777

Bennett J, Zeng Y, Bajwa R, Klatt L, Li Y, Maguire AM 1998 Adenovirus-mediated delivery of rhodopsin-promoted bcl-2 results in a delay in photoreceptor cell death in rd/rd mouse. Gene Ther 5:1156–1164

Betz AL, Yang G-Y, Davidson BL 1995 Attenuation of stroke size in rats using an adenoviral vector to induce overexpression of interleukin-1 receptor antagonist in brain. J Cereb Blood Flow Metab 15:547–551

Bilang-Bleuel A, Revah F, Colin P et al 1997 Intrastriatal injection of an adenoviral vector expressing glial-cell-line-derived neurotrophic factor prevents dopaminergic neuron degeneration and behavioral impairment in a rat model of Parkinson disease. Proc Natl Acad Sci USA 94:8818–8823

Blesch A, Tuszynski MH 1997 Robust growth of chronically injured spinal cord axons induced by grafts of genetically modified NGF-secreting cells. Exp Neurol 148:444–452

Bohn MC, Choi-Lundberg DL 1998 Gene therapies for Parkinson's disease. In: Chiocca EA, Breakefield XO (eds) Gene therapy for neurological disorders and brain tumors. Humana Press, Towata, NJ, p 377–395

Boulis NM, Bhatia V, Brindle TI et al 1999 Adenoviral nerve growth factor and beta-galactosidase transfer to spinal cord: a behavioral and histological analysis. J Neurosurg (suppl) 90:99–108

Castel-Barthe MN, Jazat-Poindessous F, Barneoud P et al 1996 Direct intracerebral nerve growth factor gene transfer using a recombinant adenovirus: effect on basal forebrain cholinergic neurons during aging. Neurobiol Disease 3:76–86

Cayouette M, Gravel C 1997 Adenovirus-mediated gene transfer of ciliary neurotrophic factor can prevent photoreceptor degeneration in the retinal degeneration (rd) mouse. Hum Gene Ther 8:423–430

Chen KS, Gage FH 1995 Somatic gene transfer of NGF to the aged brain: behavioral and morphological amelioration. J Neurosci 15:2819–2825

Chiu AY, Zhai P, Dal Canto MC et al 1995 Age-dependent penetrance of disease in a transgenic mouse model of familial amyotrophic lateral sclerosis. Mol Cell Neurosci 6:349–362

Choi-Lundberg DL, Lin Q, Chang YN et al 1997 Dopaminergic neurons protected from degeneration by GDNF gene therapy. Science 275:838–841

Choi-Lundberg DL, Lin Q, Schallert T et al 1998 Behavioral and cellular protection of rat dopaminergic neurons by an adenoviral vector encoding glial cell line-derived neurotrophic factor. Exp Neurol 154:261–275

Connor B, Kozlowski DA, Schallert T, Tillerson JL, Davidson BL, Bohn MC 1999 Differential effects of glial cell line-derived neurotrophic factor (GDNF) in the striatum and substantia nigra of the aged Parkinsonian rat. Gene Ther 6:1936–1951

Cunningham LA, Hansen JT, Short MP, Bohn MC 1991 The use of genetically altered astrocytes to provide nerve growth factor to adrenal chromaffin cells grafted into the striatum. Brain Res 561:192–202

Cunningham LA, Short MP, Breakfield XO, Bohn MC 1994 Nerve growth factor released by transgenic astrocytes enhances the function of adrenal chromaffin cell grafts in a rat model of Parkinson's disease. Brain Res 658:219–231

Dal Canto MC, Gurney ME 1994 The development of central nervous system pathology in a murine transgenic model of human amyotrophic lateral sclerosis. Am J Pathol 145:1271–1279

Date I, Ohmoto T, Imaoka T, Shingo T, Emerich DF 1996 Chromaffin cell survival from both young and old donors is enhanced by co-grafts of polymer-encapsulated human NGF-secreting cells. Neuroreport 7:1813–1818

Déglon N, Heyd B, Tan SA, Joseph JM, Zurn AD, Aebischer P 1996 Central nervous system delivery of recombinant ciliary neurotrophic factor by polymer encapsulated differentiated C2C12 myoblasts. Hum Gene Ther 7:2135–2146

Dekker AJ, Fagan AM, Gage FH, Thal LJ 1994 Effects of brain-derived neurotrophic factor and nerve growth factor on remaining neurons in the lesioned nucleus basalis magnocellularis. Brain Res 639:149–155

Deng HX, Hentati A, Rainer JA et al 1993 Amyotrophic lateral sclerosis and structural defects in Cu, Zn superoxide dismutase. Science 261:1047–1051

Emerich DF, Hammang JP, Baetge EE, Winn SR 1994a Implantation of polymer-encapsulated human nerve growth factor-secreting fibroblasts attenuates the behavioral and neuropathological consequences of quinolinic acid injections into rodent striatum. Exp Neurol 130:141–150

Emerich DF, Winn SR, Harper J, Hammang JP, Baetge EE, Kordower JH 1994b Implants of polymer-encapsulated human NGF-secreting cells in the nonhuman primate: rescue and sprouting of degenerating cholinergic basal forebrain neurons. J Comp Neurol 349:148–164

Emerich DF, Cain CK, Greco C et al 1997a Cellular delivery of human CNTF prevents motor and cognitive dysfunction in a rodent model of Huntington's disease. Cell Transplant 6:249–266

Emerich DF, Winn SR, Hantraye PM et al 1997b Protective effect of encapsulated cells producing neurotrophic factor CNTF in a monkey model of Huntington's disease. Nature 386:395–399

Emerich DF, Bruhn S, Chu Y, Kordower JH 1998 Cellular delivery of CNTF but not NT-4/5 prevents degeneration of striatal neurons in a rodent model of Huntington's disease. Cell Transplant 7:213–225

Federoff HJ, Geschwind MD, Geller AI, Kessler JA 1992 Expression of nerve growth factor *in vivo* from a defective herpes simplex virus 1 vector prevents effects of axotomy on sympathetic ganglia. Proc Natl Acad Sci USA 89:1636–1640

Frim DM, Short MP, Rosenberg WS, Simpson J, Breakefield XO, Isacson O 1993a Local protective effects of nerve growth factor-secreting fibroblasts against excitotoxic lesions in the rat striatum. J Neurosurg 78:267–273

Frim DM, Simpson J, Uhler TA et al 1993b Striatal degeneration induced by mitochondrial blockade is prevented by biologically delivered NGF. J Neurosci Res 35:452–458

Frim DM, Uhler TA, Galpern WR, Beal MF, Breakefield XO, Isacson O 1994 Implanted fibroblasts genetically engineered to produce brain-derived neurotrophic factor prevent 1-methyl-4-phenylpyridinium toxicity to dopaminergic neurons in the rat. Proc Natl Acad Sci USA 91:5104–5108

Galpern WR, Frim DM, Tatter SB, Altar CA, Beal MF, Isacson O 1996 Cell-mediated delivery of brain-derived neurotrophic factor enhances dopamine levels in an MPP+ rat model of substantia nigra degeneration. Cell Transplant 5:225–232

Geschwind MD, Hartnick CJ, Liu W, Amat J, Vandewater TR, Federoff HJ 1996 Defective HSV-1 vector expressing BDNF in auditory ganglia neurite ougrowth: model for treatment of neuron loss following cochlear degeneration. Hum Gene Ther 7:173–182

Giménez y Ribotta M, Revah F, Pradier L, Loquet I, Mallet J, Privat A 1997 Prevention of motorneuron death by adenovirus-mediated neurotrophic factors. J Neurosci Res 48:281–285

Gravel C, Götz R, Lorrain A, Sendtner M 1997 Adenoviral gene transfer of ciliary neurotrophic factor and brain-derived neurotrophic factor leads to long-term survival of axotomized motor neurons. Nat Med 3:765–770

Gurney ME, Pu H, Chiu AY et al 1994 Motor neuron degeneration in mice that express a human Cu,Zn superoxide dismutase mutation. Science 264:1772–1775 (erratum: 1995 Science 269:149)

Haase G, Kennel P, Pettmann B et al 1997 Gene therapy of murine motor neuron disease using adenoviral vectors for neurotrophic factors. Nat Med 3:429–436

Haase G, Pettmann B, Vigne E, Castelnau-Ptakhine L, Schmalbruch H, Kahn A 1998 Adenovirus-mediated transfer of the neurotrophin-3 gene into skeletal muscle of pmm mice: therapeutic effects and mechanisms of action. J Neurol Sci (suppl) 160:S97–S105

Haase G, Pettmann B, Bordet T et al 1999 Therapeutic benefit of ciliary neurotrophic factor in progressive motor neuronopathy depends on the route of delivery. Ann Neurol 45:296–304

Henderson CE, Phillips HS, Pollock RA et al 1994 GDNF: a potent survival factor for motoneurons present in peripheral nerve and muscle. Science 266:1062–1064 (erratum: 1995 Science 267:777)

Hoffman D, Breakefield XO, Short MP, Aebischer P 1993 Transplantation of a polymer-encapsulated cell line genetically engineered to release NGF. Exp Neurol 122:100–103

Iijichi A, Noel F, Sakuma S, Weil MM, Tofilon PJ 1996 *Ex vivo* gene delivery of platelet-derived growth factor increases 0-2A progenitors in adult rat spinal cord. Gene Ther 3:389–395

Isenmann S, Klöcker N, Gravel C, Bahr M 1998 Short communication: protection of axotomized retinal ganglion cells by adenovirally delivered BDNF *in vivo*. Eur J Neurosci 10:2751–2756

Kawaja MD, Rosenberg MB, Yoshida K, Gage FH 1992 Somatic gene transfer of nerve growth factor promotes the survival of axotomized septal neurons and the regeneration of their axons in adult rats. J Neurosci 12:2849–2864

Kim DH, Gutin PH, Noble LJ, Nathan D, Yu JS, Nockels RP 1996 Treatment with genetically engineered fibroblasts producing NGF or BDNF can accelerate recovery from traumatic spinal cord injury in the adult rat. Neuroreport 7:2221–2225

Klein RL, Muir D, King MA et al 1999 Long-term actions of vector-derived nerve growth factor or brain-derived neurotrophic factor on choline acetyltransferase and Trk receptor levels in the adult rat basal forebrain. Neuroscience 90:815–821

Kojima H, Abiru Y, Sakajiri K et al 1997 Adenovirus-mediated transduction with human glial cell line-derived neurotrophic factor gene prevents 1-methyl-4-phenyl-1,2,3,6-tetrahydropyridine-induced dopamine depletion in striatum of mouse brain. Biochem Biophys Res Comm 238:569–573

Kozlowski DA, Connor B, Tillerson JL, Schallert T, Bohn MC 2000 Delivery of a GDNF gene into the substantia nigra after a progressive 6-OHDA lesion maintains functional nigrostriatal connections. Exp Neurol, in press

Labandeira-Garcia JL, Rozas G, Lopez-Martin E, Liste I, Guerra MJ 1996 Time course of striatal changes induced by 6-hydroxydopamine lesion of the nigrostriatal pathway, as studied by combined evaluation of rotational behaviour and striatal Fos expression. Exp Brain Res 108:69–84

Lapchak P, Araujo D, Hilt D, Sheng J, Jiao S 1997 Adenoviral vector-mediated GDNF gene therapy in a rodent lesion model of late stage Parkinson's disease. Brain Res 777:153–160

Lawrence MS, McLaughlin JR, Sun GH et al 1997 Herpes simplex viral vectors expressing Bcl-2 are neuroprotective when delivered after a stroke. J Cereb Blood Flow Metab 17:740–744

Levivier M, Przedborski S, Bencsics C, Kang UJ 1995 Intrastriatal implantation of fibroblasts genetically engineered to produce brain-derived neurotrophic factor prevents degeneration of dopaminergic neurons in a rat model of Parkinson's disease. J Neurosci 15:7810–7820

Lin L-FH, Doherty DH, Lile JD, Bektesh S, Collins F 1993 GDNF: a glial cell line-derived neurotrophic factor for midbrain dopaminergic neurons. Science 260:1130–1132

Lindner MD, Winn SR, Baetge EE et al 1995 Implantation of encapsulated catecholamine and GDNF-producing cells in rats with unilateral dopamine deletions and parkinsonian symptoms. Exp Neurol 132:62–76

Linnik MD, Zahos P, Geschwind MD, Federoff HJ 1995 Expression of bcl-2 from a defective herpes simplex virus-1 vector limits neuronal death in focal cerebral ischemia. Stroke 26:1670–1674

Lucidi-Phillipi CA, Gage FH, Shults CW, Jones KR, Reichardt LF, Kang UJ 1995 Brain-derived neurotrophic factor-transduced fibroblasts: production of BDNF and effects of grafting to the adult rat brain. J Comp Neurol 354:361–376

Mandel RJ, Spratt SK, Snyder RO, Leff SE 1997 Midbrain injection of recombinant adeno-associated virus encoding rat glial cell line-derived neurotrophic factor protects nigral neurons in a progressive 6-hydroxydopamine-induced degeneration model of Parkinson's disease in rats. Proc Natl Acad Sci USA 94:14083–14088

Martínez-Serrano A, Fischer W, Björklund A 1995a Reversal of age-dependent cognitive impairments and cholinergic neuron atrophy by NGF-secreting neural progenitors grafted to the basal forebrain. Neuron 15:473–484

Martínez-Serrano A, Lundberg C, Horellou P et al 1995b CNS-derived neural progenitor cells for gene transfer of nerve growth factor to the adult rat brain: complete rescue of axotomized cholinergic neurons after transplantation into the septum. J Neurosci 15:5668–5680

Martínez-Serrano A, Fischer W, Söderström S, Ebendal T, Björklund A 1996 Long-term functional recovery from age-induced spatial memory impairments by nerve growth factor gene transfer to the rat basal forebrain. Proc Natl Acad Sci USA 93:6355–6360

Mohajeri MH, Figlewicz DA, Bohn MC 1998 Selective loss of alpha motoneurons innervating the medial gastrocnemius muscle in a mouse model of amyotrophic lateral sclerosis. Exp Neurol 150:329–336

Mohajeri MH, Figlewicz DA, Bohn MC 1999 Intramuscular grafts of myoblasts genetically modified to secrete glial cell line-derived neurotrophic factor prevent motoneuron loss and disease progression in a mouse model of familial amyotrophic lateral sclerosis (FALS). Hum Gene Ther 10:1853–1866

Morgan JI, Curran T 1991 Simulus-transcription coupling in the nervous system: involvement of the inducible proto-oncogenes fos and jun. Annu Rev Neurosci 14:421–451

Mourelatos Z, Gonatas NK, Stieber A, Gurney ME, Dal Canto MC 1996 The Golgi apparatus of spinal cord motor neurons in transgenic mice expressing mutant Cu,Zn superoxide dismutase becomes fragmented in early preclinical stages of the disease. Proc Natl Acad Sci USA 93:5472–5477

Mulder DW, Kurland LT, Offord KP, Beard CM 1986 Familial adult motor neuron disease: amyotrophic lateral sclerosis. Neurology 36:511–517

Nakahara Y, Gage FH, Tuszynski MH 1996 Grafts of fibroblasts genetically modified to secrete NGF, BDNF, NT-3 or basic FGF elicit differential responses in the adult spinal cord. Cell Transplant 5:191–204

Niijima K, Chalmers GR, Peterson DA, Fisher LJ, Patterson PH, Gage FH 1995 Enhanced survival and neuronal differentiation of adrenal chromaffin cells cografted into the striatum with NGF-producing fibroblasts. J Neurosci 15:1180–1194

Rosen DR, Siddique T, Patterson D et al 1993 Mutations in Cu/Zn superoxide dismutase gene are associated with familial amyotrophic lateral sclerosis. Nature 362:59–62 (erratum: 1993 Nature 364:362)

Rosenberg MB, Friedmann T, Robertson RC et al 1988 Grafting genetically modified cells to the damaged brain: restorative effects of NGF expression. Science 242:1575–1578

Rosenblad C, Martínez-Serrano A, Björklund A 1998 Intrastriatal glial cell line-derived neurotrophic factor promotes sprouting of spared nigrostriatal dopaminergic afferents and induces recovery of function in a rat model of Parkinson's disease. Neuroscience 82:129–137

Sagot Y, Tan SA, Baetge E, Schmalbruch II, Kato AC, Aebischer P 1995 Polymer encapsulated cell lines genetically engineered to release ciliary neurotrophic factor can slow down progressive motor neuronopathy in mouse. Eur J Neurosci 7:1313–1322

Sagot Y, Tan SA, Hammang JP, Aebischer P, Kato AC 1996 GDNF slows loss of motorneurons but not axonal degeneration or premature death of pmm/pmm mice. J Neurosci 16:2335–2341

Sanchez-Capelo A, Corti O, Mallet J 1999 Adenovirus-mediated over-expression of TGF-beta1 in the striatum decreases dopaminergic cell survival in embryonic nigral grafts. Neuroreport 10:2169–2173

Sauer H, Oertel WH 1994 Progressive degeneration of nigrostriatal dopamine neurons following intrastriatal terminal lesions with 6-hydroxydopamine: a combined retrograde tracing and immunocytochemical study in the rat. Neuroscience 59:401–415

Schumacher JM, Short MP, Hyman BT, Breakefield XO, Isacson O 1991 Intracerebral implantation of nerve growth factor-producing fibroblasts protects striatum against neurotoxic levels of excitatory amino acids. Neuroscience 45:561–570

Shults CW, Kimber T, Martin D 1996 Intrastriatal injection of GDNF attenuates the effects of 6-hydroxydopamine. Neuroreport 7:627–631

Siddique T, Pericak-Vance MA, Brooks BR et al 1989 Linkage analysis in familial amyotrophic lateral sclerosis. Neurology 39:919–925

Siddique T, Figlewicz DA, Pericak-Vance MA et al 1991 Linkage of a gene causing familial amyotrophic lateral sclerosis to chromosome 21 and evidence of genetic-locus heterogeneity. N Engl J Med 324:1381–1384 (errata: 1991 N Engl J Med 325:71, 325:524)

Staecker H, Gabaizadeh R, Federoff H, Van De Water TR 1998 Brain-derived neurotrophic factor gene therapy prevents spiral ganglion degeneration after hair cell loss. Otolaryngol Head Neck Surg 119:7–13

Takahashi K, Schwarz E, Ljubetic C, Murray M, Tessler A, Saavedra RA 1999 DNA plasmid that codes for human Bcl-2 gene preserves axotomized Clarke's nucleus neurons and reduces atrophy after spinal cord hemisection in adult rats. J Comp Neurol 404:159–171

Tan SA, Deglon N, Zurn AD et al 1996 Rescue of motorneurons from axotomy-induced cell death by polymer encapsulated cells genetically engineered to release CNTF. Cell Transplant 5:577–587

Trupp M, Arenas E, Fainzilber M et al 1996 Functional receptor for GDNF encoded by the c-ret proto-oncogene. Nature 381:785–788

Tseng JL, Baetge EE, Zurn AD, Aebischer P 1997 GDNF reduces drug-induced rotational behavior after medial forebrain bundle transection by a mechanism not involving striatal dopamine. J Neurosci 17:325–333

Tseng JL, Bruhn SL, Zurn AD, Aebischer P 1998 Neurturin protects dopaminergic neurons following medial forebrain bundle axotomy. Neuroreport 9:1817–1822

Tuszynski MH, Peterson DA, Ray J, Baird A, Nakahara Y, Gage FH 1994 Fibroblasts genetically modified to produce nerve growth factor induce robust neuritic ingrowth after grafting to the spinal cord. Exp Neurol 126:1–14

Tuszynski MH, Roberts J, Senut MC, U HS, Gage FH 1996a Gene therapy in the adult primate brain: intraparenchymal grafts of cells genetically modified to produce nerve growth factor prevent cholinergic neuronal degeneration. Gene Ther 3:305–314

Tuszynski MH, Gabriel K, Gage FH, Suhr S, Meyer S, Risetti A 1996b Nerve growth factor delivery by gene transfer induces differential outgrowth of sensory, motor, and noradrenergic neurites after adult spinal cord injury. Exp Neurol 137:157–173

Tuszynski MH, Murai K, Blesch A, Grill R, Miller I 1997 Functional characterization of NGF-secreting cell grafts to the acutely injured spinal cord. Cell Transplant 6:361–368

Winkler C, Sauer H, Lee CS, Björklund A 1996 Short-term GDNF treatment provides long-term rescue of lesioned nigral dopaminergic neurons in a rat model of Parkinson's disease. J Neurochem 16:7206–7215

Winn SR, Hammang JP, Emerich DF, Lee A, Palmiter RD, Baetge EE 1994 Polymer-encapsulated cells genetically modified to secrete human nerve growth factor promote the survival of axotomized septal cholinergic neurons. Proc Natl Acad Sci USA 91:2324–2328

Winn SR, Lindner MD, Lee A, Haggett G, Francis JM, Emerich DF 1996 Polymer-encapsulated genetically modified cells continue to secrete human nerve growth factor for over one year in rat ventricles: behavioral and anatomical consequences. Exp Neurol 140:126–138

Wong PC, Pardo CA, Borchelt DR et al 1995 An adverse property of a familial ALS-linked SOD1 mutation causes motor neuron disease characterized by vacuolar degeneration of mitochondria. Neuron 14:1105–1116

Yamada M, Oligino T, Mata M, Goss JR, Glorioso JC, Fink DJ 1999 Herpes simplex virus vector-mediated expression of Bcl-2 prevents 6-hydroxydopamine-induced degeneration of neurons in the substantia nigra *in vivo*. Proc Natl Acad Sci USA 96:4078–4083

Yang GY, Zhao YJ, Davidson BL, Betz AL 1997 Overexpression of interleukin-1 receptor anatagonist in the mouse brain reduces ischemic brain injury. Brain Res 751:181–188

Yang GY, Liu XH, Kadoya C et al 1998 Attenuation of ischemic inflammatory response in mouse brain using an adenoviral vector to induce overexpression of interleukin-1 receptor antagonist. J Cereb Blood Flow Metabol 18:840–847

Yenari MA, Fink SL, Sun GH et al 1998 Gene therapy with HSP72 is neuroprotective in rat models of stroke and epilepsy. Ann Neurol 44:584–591

Yoshimoto Y, Lin Q, Collier TJ, Frim DM, Breakefield XO, Bohn MC 1995 Astrocytes retrovirally transduced with BDNF elicit behavioral improvement in a rat model of Parkinson's disease. Brain Res 691:25–36

Zhang Y, Dijkhuizen PA, Anderson PN, Lieberman AR, Verhaagen J 1998 NT-3 delivered by a adenoviral vector induced injured dorsal root axons to regenerate into the spinal cord of adult rats. J Neurosci Res 54:554–562

Zigmond MJ, Abercrombie ED, Berger TW, Grace AA, Stricker EM 1993 Compensatory responses to partial loss of dopaminergic neurons: studies with 6-hydroxydopamine. In: Schneider J, Gupta M (eds) Current concepts in Parkinson's disease research. Hogrefe & Huber, Gottingen, p 99–140

DISCUSSION

Olson: We are now discussing the delivery of large protein molecules to the brain. Have you looked at how GDNF distributes in a dopamine-innervated versus a dopamine-denervated striatum? Is it taken up and transported away from a dopamine-denervated area, for example?

Bohn: We haven't examined that in a rigorous way. However, you raise an interesting point, because we have some evidence that lesions cause up-regulation of GDNF receptors. If you're studying the effects of a growth factor, you also have to worry about your model and how it is responding to that growth factor.

Olson: How far does GDNF travel from where you deposit your vector?

Bohn: When we use an infusion pump, 2 μl of vector covers about 3 mm in the rat; in the monkey, we can cover about 12–16 mm with a 20 μl injection. When we were first trying out vectors we did a study in which we put in a βgal vector and counted neurons. It seemed to have a stable expression, but then in our experiments with the 6-OHDA lesion we had a decline in the number of βgal-expressing cells as well as a decline in GDNF expression. This decline was greater when we put the vector near the substantia nigra than it was in the striatum. In the substantia nigra, both GDNF protein and GDNF mRNA levels declined, whereas GDNF vector DNA remained constant. We thought it might be a brain region effect, or it could be that if the vector is put into a region where there is a lot of cell death, this may result in down-regulation of the promoter.

Price: There are other interpretations of the effect that you showed on the size distribution of the MNs when you label from muscle. It is conceivable that you could be filling different sized populations with greater or lesser efficiency, through some effect on axonal transport or uptake. This is what GDNF could be affecting. Did you say that the total of number of cells labelled was the same in all conditions?

Bohn: I showed the MN data expressed two ways. First, I showed total counts of FG-labelled MNs broken down into large ($\geqslant 20$ μm) and small (12–19 μm) neurons. These data showed that in all groups, there was little difference in the total number of small MNs projecting to the treated muscles from that in wild-type mice. In contrast, there was a large deficit in large MNs in the transgenic mice compared to wild-type mice, and this deficit was partially compensated for by GDNF. The second way I showed the MN data was by size distribution in which the percentage of total MNs for each diameter of neuron in 2 μm increments was plotted. These data showed that GDNF shifted the size distribution towards larger motoneurons, but that in all groups of transgenic mice, there was a significant increase in smaller diameters compared with wild-type mice. The data demonstrate that one can get a high number of neurons labelled via retrograde transport of FG even at the late stages of neurodegeneration in these mice. Although these mice have been reported to have bundles or neurofilaments and inclusions in their axons, and could have compromised retrograde transport, it seems that this does not interfere significantly with retrograde labelling. The data suggest rather that there is a shrinkage of motoneurons in the transgenic mice which is ameliorated by GDNF. We do not have data on MN populations that served other muscles.

Price: There are many other nerves that project from the muscle apart from the primary MNs. It is conceivable that you're affecting the uptake of your marker into those.

Perry: There are several problems with using GDNF for any chronic degenerative disease. Firstly, MNs are not a homogeneous population of cells. Recent work shows that different MN groups require different growth factors (Henderson et al 1998). You will have to deliver your agent to different muscle groups in the appropriate way, and this will involve multiple injections of the virus. Of course, adenovirus has already a poor history in therapy, and it's not really clear how one is going to get round the immunological problems. All gene therapies delivered for chronic degenerative diseases are going to have to confront the immunological problems.

Bohn: That is absolutely the crucial issue for applying gene therapy in humans. We are conducting a large study in monkeys with Gene Redmond at Yale to compare systematically different types of viral vectors. In the mouse studies we didn't use an adenovirus. In that mouse strain we could never get infection of muscle after the mice were older than two weeks old. These experiments instead involved transplanting myoblasts transfected with a retrovirus.

Perry: Presumably the muscle cell will then express retroviral proteins, which is another potential problem. Many laboratory studies have been done in clean animals that have not been exposed to infections. If you deliberately give animals related infections to the viral vector that you might use as a delivery tool, you get a completely different immunological responses from what happens if you use a specific-pathogen free (SPF) animal. Immunological priming is a real problem out there in the dirty world that we live in.

Price: I presume that you use replication-incompetent retroviral vectors which don't express retroviral protein. You won't therefore in that system get any retroviral gene products expressed.

Bohn: If you're going to implant cells to provide a neurotrophic factor to treat ALS, the real problem is how to get the factor to all the motoneurons. Do you do 50 or 60 injections to the muscles, or do you wait until you have some kind of mesenchymal stem cell that can be injected peripherally that will home to the muscles and deliver the gene?

Aebischer: I'm not sure that the injection needs to be in the periphery. It was shown that if you deliver it in the cerebrospinal fluid (CSF) there is retrograde transport. We should look at the CSF in ALS treatment because buy doing this it may be possible to affect the entire spinal axis.

On a separate issue, aren't you a bit concerned about the results in the SOD transgenic mouse? There have been five or six reports going from Bcl-2 to vitamin C, all showing an effect of around 10%, both in life expectancy and in onset of disease. This is not a lot. I think ALS is going to be a more complex disease and trophic factors are not the whole solution.

Perry: I would have thought that developmental dependency for growth factors wouldn't suddenly disappear.

Peschanski: My view is that trophic factors are not protective in the adult in the same discrete manner they are protective during development. Ciliary neurotrophic factor (CNTF) would not be as extensively used, for example, if this were not the case. There is a difference between the specificity of developmental stages and the kind of protection you can get with many trophic factors. This is true with the striatum and nerve growth factor (NGF): GABAergic medium spiny neurons are protected by NGF in the adult but not during development.

Perry: I only raised recent work from Henderson's laboratory because I thought it was relevant to the issue that, as Patrick Aebischer pointed out, most of these growth factor studies for ALS have been a failure. Is this because different cells require different growth factors?

Gage: In situations where we are looking at the effects of growth factors and getting a read out, in very few cases have we identified the mechanism by which that growth factor is having an effect. We make assumptions that the growth factor is working on this cell, but there are often many other cell types that have receptors that that growth factor can respond to. For example, with the NGF effects on the striatum, its not clear that the effects are direct, or whether they stimulate an interaction with other cells. Growth factors can make astrocytes do lots of things, or there could be an inflammatory response which could result in trophic factor release. Until we can tease out the exact effect of the growth factor on the adult population and can define what cell type it is actually acting on to give a survival effect, we can't make a comparison between the adult and the developmental system. In development the experiments were done with defined populations of cells where you know the effect is on that cell: these experiments haven't been done in the adult and all we have is a read-out of survival.

Bohn: In all the studies on lesions of motoneurons in adult rats and mice at different levels, GDNF has been able to protect them. Even though a cocktail of growth factors may work better, different populations of MNs don't appear to lose the ability to respond to GDNF.

Peschanski: The same can be said for brain-derived neurotrophic factor and CNTF.

Gray: From all that, what's the take-home message about the likelihood that the kind of results Martha Bohn has been talking about will deliver a clinically effective strategy with reasonably robust results within the foreseeable future?

Bohn: Our results represent a proof of principle. If we could get the gene in the right place for a prolonged time in humans, it has the potential of slowing neurodegeneration.

A ebischer: There is also the question of the disease. ALS is very complicated, and therapy will require more than just delivering the trophic factor closely. We have a good model for ALS with the SOD mouse, and in this model nothing really works. In comparison, in Parkinson's disease GDNF works rather well in all kinds of models that have been studied. Studies we have done show that if you co-transplant grafts with GDNF-producing cells this has a major effect on the survival of transplanted neurons. This can be correlated with behaviour. In terms of the clinical probability of using trophic factors, we have to think about what is the best way to proceed. I do not think that ALS is the best candidate: Parkinson's or Huntington's disease are better candidates than MNs.

Gray: If you are going to use delivery of growth factors as a way of aiding a transplant, isn't it going to be more efficient to transfect the gene into the cells you are going to transplant rather than do it through a separate route?

A ebischer: It's a question of the feasibility of the approach. With all the problems of transplant procurement, it is tricky to keep the cells alive while you transfect them. An *ex vivo* gene therapy approach is probably the way to start.

Gray: I was thinking of putting together the growth factor approach with the engineered cell line approach, as distinct from primary fetal grafts. You could transfect the gene for delivery of GDNF into that cell population, or you could have two cell populations, one with GDNF, one without. Wouldn't that be a more effective way of doing it?

Bohn: There are other factors to consider. It might be good to have a growth factor gene in the brain prior to the graft, because you are likely to need immediate nurturing of those neurons.

Reference

Henderson CE, Yamamoto Y, Livet J, Arce V, Garces A, de Lapeyrière O 1998 Role of neurotrophic factors in motoneuron development. J Physiol Paris 92:279–281

Repair of corticospinal axons by transplantation of olfactory ensheathing cells

Geoff Raisman

Division of Neurobiology, National Institute for Medical Research, The Ridgeway, Mill Hill, London NW7 1AA, UK

Abstract. This paper examines the possibility of repairing cut central connections by transplantation of glial cells which modify the glial pathways and take advantage of the inherent growth capacity in adult neurons. We found that transplants of cultured olfactory ensheathing cells into lesions of the adult rat corticospinal tract induced long growth of cut axons across the lesion. Acquisition of a directed forepaw reaching function was restored on the operated side.

2000 Neural transplantation in neurodegenerative disease. Wiley, Chichester (Novartis Foundation Symposium 231) p 94–109

One of the peculiarities of the nervous system is that virtually no neurons are made in the adult. So far at this meeting we have been talking about the replacement of nerve cells in conditions in which nerve cells are lost. But there is another peculiarity: nerve cells are not like any other cells morphologically. They have a long process, the axon, which can be very long. Consequently, in the case of the nervous system we find a unique kind of injury, which is the cutting of axons while sparing the nerve cell bodies, but disconnecting them from their normal targets and therefore destroying their function. One of the challenges facing us is whether it is possible to reconnect cut axons to their original targets. The nerve cells are still alive and we assume that if we could reconnect them, it seems likely that some lost functions could be restored.

We got into this field looking at lesions of central nervous pathways many years ago. Our starting point was our observation that new synaptic connections form in the adult CNS after injury. Then, following the methodology that Anders Björklund had pioneered of putting embryonic tissue into adults, we showed (Zhou et al 1990), as others have done, that if you put different types of embryonic tissue into adult hippocampus, you get a pattern of connections that reproduces the normal differential patterns of connections which the various types of donor tissues normally form in the hippocampus. From this, we made the assumption that new connections do form in the damaged adult CNS, they can be induced to form by transplants, and at least in some cases, they will retain the correct specificity. The question is, how can we turn this ability to form new connections into a method for repair of injuries?

The model on which we based our project was a lesion of the peripheral nervous system (PNS). When a peripheral nerve is crushed, the cut axons sprout, explore the environment, find the distal stump and some grow through. It is not always a perfect repair, but some can repair and some function is restored. In the CNS, after lesions of the corticospinal tract, the cut fibres also sprout and explore the environment with exactly the same kind of growth cones as in the PNS. However, they do not advance along the pathway to reach their targets.

The pathway along which nerve fibres grow is highly organized. One of the organizing principles is that the glial cells are arranged in unicellular rows, evenly spaced throughout the tract. These rows comprise a number of different cell types. These include solitary astrocytes, contiguous oligodendrocytes, microglia and endothelial cells. Not only are the glial cells arranged in the rows, but they also generate long processes aligned along the axis of the pathway. The question is what can we do about this pathway to convert this resilient, non-permissive structure into a magic carpet which would allow axons to grow along it?

If we think of this problem in terms of development, we all knew how to grow nerve fibres when we were babies. Taking the rat fimbria as an example, the growing nerve fibres start at around the 15th day of embryonic life (E15), at which stage the pathway consists of radial glia which produce a palisade of radial fibres at right angles to the axis of the future tract. Around the time of birth, the progeny of dividing glial progenitor cells in the ependymal layer start to migrate into the body of the pathway. During the first week, the generative layer becomes depleted and the cells in the tract start to form longitudinal rows. This is the stage when axons are growing. It is only by the second month in the rat — and probably by the second year in humans — that the cells are arranged in the densely packed longitudinal rows typical of the adult. This is the stage when axons do not grow when they are cut.

The reason for this failure is not due simply to the adult maturational state of the pathway, because when we transplanted E15 rat hippocampal precursor cells (mainly neurons) into an adult fully myelinated fimbria, large numbers of axons consistently grew readily and rapidly out of the transplant and disseminated themselves through the pathway. By the second week they crossed to the opposite hippocampus. Thus, adult nerve fibre tracts will permit rapid, selective, aligned growth of embryonic axons. The embryonic neuron is still capable of doing that. More than that, if the nerve fibres from the embryonic graft have a choice between white matter and grey, they will selectively grow along the white.

Which is not surprising, because the white matter is where you normally find nerve fibres: if you give cars the chance between driving on fields or driving on roads, they will choose roads: that is where you find cars, that is where they go.

So, if embryonic nerve fibres can grow down adult pathways, what can we do to induce adult nerve fibres to do the same? The approach to this was described by Cajal (1928) in his book, and it was brought first into modern times by Aguayo (Vidal-Sanz et al 1987), who cut the optic nerve and bridged the cut ends with a transplant of a segment taken from the sciatic nerve, producing regeneration all the way to the optic tectum. The underlying idea is to take something from an environment in the PNS where regeneration can occur, and transplant it into the CNS where regeneration does not occur.

What is special about the PNS? It contains one unique cell type — the Schwann cell. If we transplant Schwann cells into the fimbria, after one day the cells start to migrate out of the graft, and after 10 days the grafts have massive cell division and cells are migrating along blood vessels. After about 10 days these Schwann cells stop growing, they leave the blood vessels and they migrate. By this approach, therefore, we have made a tissue which is a mixture of peripheral and central glia. We have woven another thread into the carpet. The Schwann cells have been accepted into a central pathway.

We can get the Schwann cells in, but can they make axons grow? Can we make them repair tract damage? We have looked at lesions of the corticospinal tract. Within the lesion we find cut nerve fibres with expanded endings that are sprouting (Li & Raisman 1995). If we didn't have sprouting persisting like this, we would have no basis for our repair. Our goal is to exploit this ability to sprout, but in addition to make these fibres do something useful. When we fill the lesion cavity by transplanting cultured peripheral nerve Schwann cells, we see a mass of nerve fibres growing in, with lots of pseudoterminal-type branching. We have indeed managed to induce the sprouts to grow, but the growth is still not enough: what we have not got is the re-entry of fibres into their original pathways.

With hindsight, we might not be too surprised because if you look at the normal distribution of Schwann cells they go along the dorsal roots as far as the spinal cord, as far as regeneration is concerned they are no good at mediating the re-entry of nerve fibres into the spinal cord. In fact, the only place in the adult body where we know that nerve cells are continuously replaced and nerve fibres continuously re-enter the CNS is in the olfactory system, where the fibres go into the olfactory bulb. At the entry point of the olfactory nerves there is a special, unique type of glial cell, which can be cultured, and has been called the olfactory ensheathing cell. After filling lesions of the corticospinal tract with these cells, we got something quite different from what we had ever seen before (Li et al 1998). There is massive movement of cells down through the lesion, and a long migration of cells down the adult host corticospinal tract, for about 15 mm. If we look at the cut ends of the nerve fibres, the ones in the region of the lesion are typically branched and not going anywhere, but the nerve fibres in contact with the transplanted olfactory ensheathing cells are long and unbranched with simple growing points. The regrowing fibres are intimately clothed by olfactory ensheathing cell processes and grow all the way down through the graft and on into the distal part of the corticospinal tract.

This is preliminary work. There is a lot to be done. We know that these fibres re-enter, but we have not yet any map of where they are going to. We don't even know the extent to which they make synapses. Then we made a shot in the dark: was there anything wrong with these animals that can be made better by the graft? We took something that Whishaw and Steve Dunnett have described — the acquisition of a directed paw reaching task (Dunnett et al 1987). We found that over the testing period of 50 trials a day for 10 days, the rats never used the hand of the completely lesioned side. In the case of the transplants, the paw reaching function was regained. At the moment, this is a straw in the wind, but it looks very encouraging. From this it will be a long way to the human goal, but we feel this is a strategy worth pursuing.

Acknowledgements

This project was supported by the Medical Research Council, the British Neurological Research Trust, the International Spinal Research Trust, the Barnwood House Trust, and Smith's Charities.

References

Cajal SR 1928 Degeneration and regeneration of the nervous system. Hafner, New York

Dunnett SB, Whishaw IQ, Rogers DC, Jones GH 1987 Dopamine-rich grafts ameliorate whole body motor asymmetry and sensory neglect but not independent limb use in rats with 6-hydroxydopamine lesions. Brain Res 415:63–78

Li Y, Raisman G 1995 Sprouts from cut corticospinal axons persist in the presence of astrocytic scarring in long-term lesions of the adult rat spinal cord. Exp Neurol 134:102–111

Li Y, Field PM, Raisman G 1998 Regeneration of adult rat corticospinal axons induced by transplanted olfactory ensheathing cells. J Neurosci 18:10514–10524

Vidal-Sanz M, Bray GM, Villegas-Pérez MP, Thanos S, Aguayo AJ 1987 Axonal regeneration and synapse formation in the superior colliculus by retinal ganglion cells in the adult rat. J Neurosci 7:2894–2909

Zhou CF, Li Y, Morris RJ, Raisman G 1990 Accurate reconstruction of three complementary laminar afferents to the adult hippocampus by embryonic neural grafts. Neurosci Res Suppl 13:S43–S53

DISCUSSION

Olson: In the experiment you described in which you grafted Schwann cells, where do those Schwann cells come from?

Raisman: We have used two kinds: we started off using neonate, but in fact adult sciatic nerve Schwann cells do better. However, neither of them give good evidence of re-entry.

Olson: But they do engraft and myelinate corticospinal axons?

Raisman: Yes.

Gage: What percentage of cells are fibroblasts in these grafts? Do you try to separate out the contributions of different cell types?

Raisman: You've gone straight to the jugular vein! There is a view, from Sue Barnett who has grown these much more that I, that the olfactory ensheathing cell population consists of two cell types: a Schwann-like cell and an astrocyte-like cell. She would not accept the word 'fibroblast'. I have the impression on the basis of electron micrographs, that that second cell type is a fibroblast. It may not be a regular dermal fibroblast, but it is more like a fibroblast than any other cell type. Numerically, about 50% of the cells are of this type. When you culture the cells they segregate. The fibroblast-like cell produces an enormous amount of intercellular junctions, and I suspect this cell type is very important in the repair process.

Blakemore: Robin Franklin believes that olfactory glia and Schwann cells are two different phenotypes. From his data, these two cells behave totally differently when you transplant them into our types of glial-free lesions. With Schwann cell cultures one never sees the multi-junctional cells that are a component of olfactory glia transplants. Also, one doesn't see the big glial fibrillary acidic protein (GFAP)-positive cells that tend to isolate glia.

Geoff Raisman, your results on the movement of Schwann cells are very different from the ones that we are getting. We are transplanting Schwann cells into normal white matter, and find no evidence for movement of these cells. Probably like you, we find after a period they actually disappear. It may therefore be important to know exactly what was the composition of your Schwann cell preparations, and have you driven them with growth factors?

Raisman: Part of the answer has to do also with the lesion. We make a big hole, so we're putting these cells into a lesion which has done a lot of damage. We are now using neuregulin to push them.

Gray: What age is the donor?

Raisman: Adult. We use the method of Jessen and Mirsky.

This work is preliminary. I am not convinced that we're all talking about the same cell types, or the same cell mixtures, because everyone is using slightly different sources and slightly different methods. We are trying hard to characterize the crucial cell in our mixture.

Björklund: In what ways are the Schwann-like cells different from Schwann cells?

Raisman: We have no way to distinguish the Schwann-like cell in this mixture from Schwann cells. The only way to distinguish them is their origin: one is taken from the olfactory bulb, and the other from sciatic nerves.

Gray: Can you separate the two into subpopulations?

Raisman: We haven't succeeded yet. We have got a fairly pure population of the Schwann-like cells, based on p75 FACS sorting, and it was very poor at repair.

It is important to mention in this context that if you simply make a lesion of a spinal cord and don't inject anything, it fills up with Schwann cells. As a consequence, I don't yet have definite evidence of all those Schwann-like cells are from the transplant, rather than from the host spinal cord.

Blakemore: It is important to bear in mind that Schwann cells can migrate. Therefore it is a question of who follows who. In the experiments in which you inject Schwann cells and don't have much damage, the key question concerns whether these cells migrate and survive. If they do migrate, they might attract the axons; if they don't then it means that they are actually following the axons. We know from the other experiments that you quoted that axons can grow within an intact adult nervous system, and so it does suggest that when you see Schwann cells with axons, they are actually followers not leaders, whereas in the case of the olfactory glia, they may be leaders not followers.

Raisman: That is not at all out of the question. We don't know which of the cell types is leading. The other interesting thing about the transplants is the re-entry. They are actually making a dorsal root-like entry situation in which one internode has Schwann cells and the next has oligodendrocytes.

Blakemore: Which would suggest that the axons are the pullers.

Raisman: They could well be.

Olson: To add a little bit to what Anders Björklund was asking about the differences between the olfactory ensheathing cells and the Schwann cells, we tried to look at the presence of neurotropic factors and receptors with *in situ* hybridization in the two populations. We could hardly find anything in olfactory ensheathing cells which makes them different from the Schwann cells, suggesting that what the olfactory ensheathing cells do is probably more related to molecules on their surfaces than releasable factors.

Gray: Isn't this the kind of issue that could be tackled by looking for gene expression in a whole bunch of Schwann cells and a bunch of olfactory ensheathing cells, using differential display?

Raisman: That is one way. Another is to see whether there are any other cells in the body that will have these properties. We've had great difficulty getting sufficient numbers of human olfactory glia.

Gray: Presumably, work first needs to be done working out the differences in gene expression between the Schwann-like cells and the Schwann cells, or the fibroblast-like cells and the Schwann cells.

Reier: If the axons have a problem re-entering the CNS with Schwann cells, why do you think this would be different with the olfactory epithelial cells? There is a basal lamina around these cells, as I recall. Are these ensheathing cells really entering the CNS? If there's basal lamina around the cell, it now becomes part of the non-CNS world. Are these cells really becoming indigenous to the CNS? If they are not, then the interface is a critical place to look irrespective of all the expressions, because there is something about ensheathing cells that changes the interface from an otherwise non-permissive PNS–CNS re-entry zone. This is very important.

Raisman: It's a bit semantic. In the olfactory system, how can you distinguish what is peripheral from what is central? The ensheathing cells are olfactory and they handshake with the astrocytes that allow their entry. The reason for going for it, was that we had re-entry in that system, and a specialized cellular interface.

Peschanski: It may not be a completely semantic question. When we look at the kainate lesion, which is a completely different model, we see Schwann cells in the area of neuronal loss, in the CNS. The problem is that over time these Schwann cells tend to attract a reaction of the astrocytes which then form a complete wall around them, and then the Schwann cells disappear. How long did you look for?

Raisman: We haven't gone beyond about six months so I don't know what will happen long term. I suspect they may be being gradually replaced by oligodendrocytes.

Blakemore: We know that some endogenous Schwann cell remyelination is stable for one or two years, but we have never followed Schwann cell grafts for a long time. What does seem to be important is that once a Schwann cell is actually on an axon there's no reason to believe that it should move, but Schwann cells that don't find an axon and find themselves within astrocyte territory don't like it, in either tissue culture or the animal.

Raisman: We've never seen excess Schwann cells apart from the ones that are myelinating.

Blakemore: Some of these astrocyte-like olfactory glia will form basal lamina and some don't. There seem perhaps to be three cells that can be generated from clonal lines generated from olfactory bulb. There is a cell that behaves like a Schwann cell, there's a cell that behaves like an astrocyte, and there's this other cell type. This third type can be GFAP-positive and behaves a little bit like an arachnoid cell, but it doesn't seem to induce basal lamina on astrocytes (Franklin et al 1996).

Gray: Is that third cell type what Geoff Raisman was calling the fibroblast-like cell?

Blakemore: Yes, and these cells are generated from clonal cell lines. They are cells that differentiate from a cell isolated from the olfactory bulb.

Raisman: Neural crest stem cells do the same kind of thing.

Price: There's some evidence that there are multiple sources of Schwann cells. Schwann cells classically come from the crest; there's no question about that. But there's been an argument in the literature for years about whether some of the peripheral Schwann cells actually migrate out from the tube along the ventral root. There were quite good studies in which the dorsal half of the neural tube was ablated—including the neural crest—and Schwann cells still migrated out along the ventral root, which implied that they were derived from the ventral half of the tube. Embryologically, there are therefore probably two sources of cells (Lunn et al 1987).

Raisman: The olfactory system develops from a placode, and the axons and the ensheathing cells migrate in to the CNS. I'm not sure whether those cells are completely distinguished from the rostral neural crest.

Olson: Geoff Raisman, you stated that axons prefer white matter to grey matter. This is surprising to me, because eventually they're all going to end up in grey matter. If they always prefer white matter, how are they going to get into grey matter? Would you like to comment on the work of Jerry Silver on sensory axons in microtransplants which grow longer distances in white matter (Davies et al 1999)?

Raisman: I'm happy that they grow longest in white matter. Wictorin, working in Anders Björklund's group, was the first to show that you can get embryonic tissue transplanted and it will grow up long axons in white matter. They select for it.

Olson: Do they select for it or are they entrapped?

Raisman: Whatever, but they travel in it. We have studied the question of how they get out, in the fimbria. As they go past the hippocampus which is their correct target, they give off branches at right angles which enter and break up into terminals. Our feeling is that the white matter pathways are encouraging the growth of long unbranched axons, and then some stimulus comes from the grey matter and collateral branches come off. The first clear demonstration of that was by O'Leary in the pontine nuclei looking at corticospinal tract growing down beside it (O'Leary et al 1990). He showed that only when and where the pontine nuclei developed did the collaterals come up. It is as though there are two types of axon guidance, one determining long distance growth and the other determining collaterization. In the corticospinal system particularly, this is played upon at different areas. The motor cortex retains the long branches to the corticospinal tract and the visual cortex starts off with them and then prunes them. It is a major decision point for the axons, whether to follow white matter tract or whether to go into grey. In every case I've seen that decision is marked anatomically by a rectangular T junction. I think this is saying something about the cytoskeleton.

Gage: It is one thing to say that axons can grow in white matter; it's another thing to say that they preferentially choose white matter over grey. Are you making the statement that given a choice, for example for fetal grafts at equal distance from the two areas, that they'll choose white matter over grey?

Raisman: Where we have a graft which is partly in the corticospinal tract and partly in the spinal grey, we see long axon growth down the white matter, and a cloud of terminal-type arborizations in the adjacent grey. What I should have said is that axons are responding differently to the white and to the grey.

Reier: These are obviously different circumstances because of the genetically modified fibroblast experiments in the cord where investigators resect an area of white matter and still preserve some grey. Corticospinal and other descending fibres seem not to grow through the modified cell implant. Instead, they tend to work around the graft using the grey matter.

Raisman: There's a big of divergence in the discussion of white and grey matter. There is a view that white matter is somehow inhibitory, and if you can prevent that inhibition fibres will grow. The basic evidence for that was actually showing fibres growing in grey matter. Why inhibit a white matter inhibitor to get them to grow in grey?

Björklund: In experiments with fetal human grafts, when we put the grafts in the spinal cord we also saw that kind of pattern of axon growth. The axons extending from these grafts were exposed to both grey and white matter. The fibres did grow into both grey and white matter, but elongation over long distances and maintenance of the direct growth was seen only in the white matter. At certain points we could see axons exiting from the white matter into the grey matter where they ramified. I think there may be two different mechanisms involved: those guiding the axons over longer distance and those recognizing the targets and making the axons ramify to make synaptic contacts.

Gray: This prompts the question: when the cell starts off by elongating its axon over a long distance, does it know where it is actually going to end up? It has to know in some sense or the brain would not make the kind of precise topographical connections that it does. How does it know when it starts growing which way to head off?

Björklund: Some years back, we did experiments with transplants of fetal human nigral or ganglionic eminence tissue, showing a remarkable directional specificity. When we put nigral grafts in the internal capsule, half-way between substantia nigra and striatum, we observed a preferential growth of the axons towards the striatum. When the axons reached the grey matter of the striatum we could see that the straight growth was changed into a ramifying network. Clearly, the axons did sense the direction towards the appropriate targets. Moreover, we saw ramification into varicose terminals only in those nuclei which normally receive dopamine innervation, such as the striatum, amygdala and nucleus accumbens. This suggests that the adult brain may possess a capacity to guide outgrowing axons to their appropriate targets and that these mechanisms may operate over quite long distances.

Price: Geoff Raisman, you referred obliquely to Martin Schwab's experiments (Kartje et al 1999). I'm confused how his findings, which I think are pretty robust, fit in with what you're saying. My understanding of his experiments is that, he's identified an inhibitory factor present in oligodendrocytes and myelin, NI 35/250. The observation there is that there is an inhibitory effect from myelin which can be overcome by a blocking antibody. I guess the difference between that and what you just described is that this work has to do with regeneration of adult corticospinal tract, whereas you're talking about embryonic axons preferring white matter to grey.

Raisman: The data I showed was with adult corticospinal lesions. There's no contradiction between the two. He will claim that there is an inhibitory molecule that's associated with myelinated cells. It is perfectly possible for the axons to grow without ever encountering myelin. They grow down a tract which has lost its fibres, where the myelin has degenerated. I showed them becoming remyelinated, but they obviously don't enter a myelin sheath: they grow first, and then they become myelinated. We can't say whether or not myelin would inhibit growth in our system.

Price: I guess the take-home message is whether or not you feel that they prefer grey or white, it would still be plausible that the white matter could be 'improved' by blocking NI 35/250.

Gage: Once again we have fetal donor tissue into adult white grey matter, and adult regeneration into white grey matter, which may or may not be demyelinated. Do we know what is preferential to axons? Do adult axons grow on non-demyelinated white matter?

Raisman: Simply to demyelinate is not enough to make them grow.

Gage: You were saying there was consistency between your results and Martin's results. I still find a slight mismatch.

Raisman: Martin is postulating that adult myelin is associated with a surface molecule which makes growth cones collapse. As soon as they see this molecule they won't grow through. You are asking why I get growth in a white matter tract. I'm saying that when we make a complete lesion of the corticospinal tract, axons degenerate, the myelin is removed—there are plenty of astrocytic membranes in there, it's perfectly possible that those axons could grow down there without encountering myelin.

Blakemore: They must encounter myelin. At the lesion point it may have disappeared, but when they cross the transection point they go straight into an area of Wallerian degeneration in the corticospinals, or ascending normally myelinated fibres. If they are going into the spinal cord, they cannot escape growing on myelin. The only difference would be if your olfactory glia grow first to form a sort of burrowing tube of cells that will then support axon growth.

Raisman: I'm just not convinced that anatomically we know what they're growing on at the growing end.

Reier: I don't know what the turnover or fate of Nogo is after myelin breakdown. If you look in the lesioned corticospinal tract distally, besides seeing a lot of astroglial reactivity, there are many macrophages with myelin debris which are present for a long time. If you look at this ultrastructurally there's no way, even in a chronic situation, that regrowing axons will escape myelin in some form. As far as whether it is myelin and/or reactive glia that inhibit regeneration, it still seems like a big puzzle, and we run into difficulty when we try to resolve this in absolute black-and-white terms. Recent work by Steve Davies and Jerry Silver (Davies et al 1997, 1999) throws yet another light on this consideration. Grafted dorsal root ganglion cells appear to be capable of growing in chronically degenerated CNS white matter.

Perry: With regard to the rate at which the debris disappears, Martin Schwab and colleagues have found in preliminary studies that Nogo disappears from a lesion rather slowly, like other myelin proteins (M. E. Schwab, personal communication).

Paul Reier's point is absolutely right: we are talking about a very small percentage of regenerating fibres. It is not as if 100% of the corticospinal tract suddenly rushed off down to the end of the spinal cord. This element of whether every neuron expresses the right number of receptors to make it susceptible to inhibition is an important part of it. Some fibres do make it: precisely how they make is at present unclear. If you were to add Nogo antibodies it may improve things dramatically.

Raisman: I tend to think that embryonic axons have the ability to grow through adult white matter tracts. Perhaps what these transplanted cells are doing is somehow converting the adult corticospinal axons into that form. Maybe they don't express the receptor for the inhibitory molecule.

Perry: That would be one suggestion with the dorsal root ganglion transplants, where one transplants the dorsal root ganglion that has been stripped of all its processes. These cells may have dedifferentiated completely and now no longer have the receptor, and that's why they grow so well in an adult tract.

Peschanski: I have always been interested in the 'mechanical' difference between the grey and white matter. When one injects a molecule into the grey matter the result is a small sphere. When one injects into the corpus callosum or the internal capsule, the injected material spreads. This is equally true with cells and with fluorescent beads. Many papers have mistakenly reported migration when cells are injected into the white matter just because of this purely physical phenomenon.

Perry: I think that's wrong. There are some excellent studies on diffusion in grey and white matter (see Nicholson & Syková 1998). Diffusion in fibre tracts is easier than in grey matter.

Peschanski: I was not talking about molecules; I was talking about cells.

Perry: That's what diffusion is; it is the same.

Peschanski: One thing that is quite striking is that when you implant a glioblastoma, a migrating cell, into the striatum and it goes up into the corpus callosum, within a week in the corpus callosum all the cells are gone. That is, they have spread into the corpus callosum while they only start to migrate along blood vessels into the grey matter at that time point. I was wondering whether this phenomenon was simply mechanical. People working on gliomas think that there may be specific cues for cells migrating along the blood vessel, but within the white matter they are wondering whether there is something or not.

Perry: Part of it must be geometry. Imagine a bag of peas, and you put a cell or a molecule in the middle of this bag. It will take a long time for it to get to the edge of the bag because it will have to go around a lot of peas. Alternatively, if you put it into a bag of spaghetti, which is all aligned, the distance is much shorter. The geometry makes a big difference. With regard to an actively migrating cell like a glioma cell, it may find the extracellular matrix of the grey matter and the white matter different.

Raisman: It also seems that the axon growth along the white matter is non-specific, because we get the same growth if we put hippocampal cells in the corticospinal tract: their axons grow down it. The white matter pathways don't have the same requirement for matching of axon type to pathway that the grey matter pathways do.

Gray: If that were true — that tracts didn't care about which axons entered them and axons didn't care about which tracts they entered — then you wouldn't get the topographic connections that wire the brain up in the rather reliable manner that they do.

Raisman: I see them as motorways: anyone can along the motorway as long as they have more than a 50 cc engine!

Gray: But you have to get on the right motorway. If you're going to Cambridge you don't get on the M40.

Price: You've got to distinguish between development and the situation in the adult.

Raisman: I think it is when you come off the motorway, then it is crucial to find the right junction to get to your target.

Gray: How close are we to the clinic with this?

Raisman: If we could get human cells in enough numbers I would be interested to see what would happen if we were to put them into lesions.

Gray: What would you see as a plausible first clinical target?

Raisman: It would have to be a nerve to start with: the optic nerve or dorsal root.

Peschanski: How long can you wait after the lesion before you treat to still get good results? These axons can't remain like that for a long time. After all, the neurosurgeons won't do something on a patient who just had a car accident, for example.

Gray: In your experiments it was quite a short delay was it?

Raisman: Yes; you'll never get out of the rat, with its 18 month lifespan, a model for a 10-year-old human spinal cord lesion.

Gray: The same question came up in relation to Helen Hodges' paper, and she answered that in the case of the hippocampal lesions it worked with a two week delay. It is worth adding in the context of this discussion that in our own work looking at lesions of the cholinergic nuclei that project to the forebrain, we have been able to wait six months after lesion prior to putting in a transplant of MHP36 cells, and we still saw complete recovery of function. There are many human conditions for which, after six months, you can be sure that a deficit will not show further rehabilitation.

Olson: In rats it has been shown that you can lesion them and wait a year and the corticospinal neurons and axons will still be present although they may have retracted a little, but they are fine electrophysiologically.

Reier: What type of lesion are you talking about treating, Geoff Raisman?

Raisman: I'd have to be guided by the neurosurgeons on what they want to do and are prepared to do.

Freeman: I disagree with many of my colleagues on these issues. I have seen too many trials driven by the neurosurgeon's opinion of what is practical and appropriate from the surgeon's perspective, even if the scientific basis for the trial is compromised or ignored. Instead, I think that clinical trial design has to follow the science.

Raisman: I think there are some criteria we have to think of in this, and they're very difficult to get out of the spinal cord. You have got to know that the condition you're treating will not get better without you doing something. You have to be fairly well assured that what you do won't make the patient worse.

Gray: I'm surprised: I thought that in the case of many spinal cord injuries one could be pretty sure they would not get better spontaneously.

Raisman: But you don't know this until nine months or so after the lesion.

Blakemore: Is there any evidence that intervention might be deleterious?

Raisman: It could well be. Think of a situation such as what we have heard about Christopher Reeve, where he's got as slight and somewhat variable recovery of breathing in a large lesion. How do we know where those fibres are which mediate that small return of function? Could you ensure that you could approach the spinal cord without damaging those?

Reier: This gets really tough. In the studies by Alstermark et al (1987) which deal with cat reaching, the bottom line is that you can lesion a tract and have a deficit in reaching, and then you can make sequential lesions in any tract which you think would normally mediate this reaching behaviour, and reaching behaviour is subserved by another pathway. Maybe there are aberrant fibres in other systems that we don't see on a routine anatomical basis. On the other hand, there may be ways that nature kicks in alternative pathways. My point is, there is a complicated background of potential plasticity, no matter how you deal with this. In that sense, if somebody talks to me about volunteering for something, my feeling is that in spite of their injury there is always some risk of losing something even though it's not overtly obvious.

Gage: One of the things we haven't talked about with respect to the regeneration of axons is the significance of the scar. We have talked about permissive molecules and environments, and their relationship to injury, and the message seems to be that all we need to do is provide the appropriate positive stimuli. Do people think that the axons will pass through the scar or around it?

Raisman: I can make one anatomical comment. In the picture I showed from Steve Davies', where he made a microlesion, the fibres turned back within four days: the non-permissive property was present four days after the lesion. If an astrocytic scar is going to occur, it will take weeks to form. Whether if you could get the axons started they would now prevent it, is something that is going to have to be explored. We have got our axons started with migrating cells. Whether they could bore their way through a scar or not needs investigating.

Gage: So your axons are growing within four days to the lesion site?

Raisman: We have had them work at five weeks, when there is quite a lot of astrocytic scarring.

Gage: In that case does it look different from the situations when you implant prior to scar formation?

Raisman: No, but that's not a very good test. We need to look at some solid scars to see whether we have to overcome them physically. All I'm saying is that we can't say that the scar is the cause of the failure, because the failure has occurred long before the scar has formed.

Gray: Supposing one had a patient with a lesion in cortical motor neurons, would there be something to be said for combining the various transplantation technologies — stem cells, primary fetal tissue or whatever — with olfactory ensheathing cells so that these cells might then provide a pathway for the transplanted cells to spread their axons? Is that a crazy idea?

Perry: There is an interesting observation by Martin Berry and colleagues on the optic nerve (Berry et al 1996). When they deliver growth factors by various routes to the retina, the scar in the crushed injured optic nerve disappears: the axons that are able to penetrate the scar and secrete molecules that are sufficient to degrade it. It does seem that if the neuron is given enough of a kick start to get going, the scar itself will dissipate in some way.

Gage: That's an important point because it's addressing the physical presence of the scar.

Olson: I think there is some key information here. If we translate this to spinal cord injury it suggests that we shouldn't focus too heavily on where the cut axon is: instead we should treat the cell body by adding trophic factors to the cell body level.

Gray: This was done by Benowitz et al (1999), who showed that application of the purine nucleoside, inosine, to the rat's sensorimotor cortex after transection of the corticospinal tract stimulated intact pyramidal cells to undergo extensive sprouting into the denervated spinal cord.

Perry: In the context of what we were discussing about the spinal cord injury, I can't imagine what the proximal end of a cut spinal cord or damaged spinal cord actually looks like.

Reier: There are two types of injury. A bullet wound, for example, would essentially be a physical transection, but the majority of cord injuries are the result of shearing or compression. In a compression lesion there is scarring around the injury site over time, but it is not the same type of fibroglial scarring seen in transections. Geoff Raisman is talking about a cut. In a contusion injury there are spared axons, which is one of the issues that we really need to address in spinal injury. There are spared but dysfunctional fibres. This may be because of demyelination, or there may be other reasons. If you are going to introduce something at the level of a contusion epicentre, you will have to deal with the scar. On the basis of Jerry Silver's work, if the scar is expressing chondroitin sulfate proteoglycans, this can be an inhibitory factor. However, if you can bypass that, these axons can apparently grow in what is now a denervated tract. In my personal experience, in both cat and rat with long-term cord injury I have never seen any hint of an axon growing through a three-dimensional scar. Years ago, we did the converse of the Aguayo experiments: we took an optic nerve scar and transplanted it into the periphery. The axons never grew through this. I still think that the scar is an important issue.

Freeman: I think the scar will be less of a problem than people hypothesize. There is a growing body of evidence in the neurosurgical literature that even if a patient has lost all motor function but has some preserved sensation after, for example, a subdural haematoma, decompression within 12 h can result in restoration of useful motor function. If a patient with no motor function but some sort of sensory preservation below the injury can gain useful motor function, this means that even a small number of surviving fibre tracts in the spine can be predictive of the return of useful function. It may just be a numbers game. There may just be a critical mass of neurons for useful function to come back. The scar may be an issue, but it may not present a formidable challenge.

Gage: Are you saying that the scar doesn't form in those cases?

Freeman: It may or may not, but the fact is a large percentage of people with complete motor deficit but sensory preservation whose injury is decompressed rapidly enough can develop useful motor function. So our hurdle may not be as high as we are predicting in some circumstances.

References

Alstermark B, Lundberg A, Petterson LG, Tantisira B, Walkowska M 1987 Motor recovery after serial spinal cord lesions of defined descending pathways in cats. Neurosci Res 5:68–73

Benowitz LI, Goldberg DE, Madsen JR, Soni D, Irwin N 1999 Inosine stimulates extensive axon collateral growth in the rat corticospinal tract after injury. Proc Natl Acad Sci USA 96:13486–13490

Berry M, Carlile J, Hunter A 1996 Peripheral nerve explants grafted into the vitreous body of the eye promote the regeneration of retinal ganglion cell axons severed in the optic nerve. J Neurocytol 25:147–170

Davies SJ, Fitch MT, Memberg SP, Hall AK, Raisman G, Silver J 1997 Regeneration of adult axons in white matter tracts of the central nervous system. Nature 390:680–683

Davies SJ, Goucher DR, Doller C, Silver J 1999 Robust regeneration of adult sensory axons in degenerating white matter of the adult rat spinal cord. J Neurosci 19:5810–5822

Franklin RJ, Gilson JM, Franceschini IA, Barnett SC 1996 Schwann cell-like myelination following transplantation of an olfactory bulb-ensheathing cell line into areas of demyelination in the adult CNS. Glia 17:217–224

Kartje GL, Schulz MK, Lopez-Yunez A, Schnell L, Schwab ME 1999 Corticostriatal plasticity is restricted by myelin-associated neurite growth inhibitors in the adult rat. Ann Neurol 45:778–786

Lunn ER, Scourfield J, Keynes RJ, Stern CD 1987 The neural tube origin of ventral root sheath cells in the chick embryo. Development 101:247–254

Nicholson C, Syková E 1998 Extracellular space structure revealed by diffusion analysis. Trends Neurosci 21:207–215

O'Leary DDM, Bicknesse AR, De Carlos JA et al 1990 Target selection by cortical axons: alternative mechanisms to establish axonal connections in the developing brain. Cold Spring Harb Symp Quant Biol 55:453–468

Neural transplantation in Parkinson's disease

Olle Lindvall

Section of Restorative Neurology, Wallenberg Neuroscience Center, University Hospital, SE-221 85 Lund, Sweden

Abstract. Transplanted human embryonic dopamine neurons reinnervate the striatum in patients with Parkinson's disease. The grafts can exhibit long-term survival without immunological rejection and despite an ongoing disease process and continuous antiparkinsonian drug treatment. Recent findings using positron emission tomography indicate that the grafts are functionally integrated in the patient's brain and release dopamine into the striatum. In the most successful cases, patients have been able to withdraw L-dopa treatment after transplantation and resume an independent life. About two-thirds of grafted patients have shown clinically useful, partial recovery of motor function: increased percentage of time in the 'on'-phase and reduced rigidity and hypokinesia during 'off'-phases, bilaterally but predominantly on the side contralateral to the graft. Gait, speed, balance and dyskinesias have not exhibited any major, consistent improvements. Current research aims at solving three main problems: (a) large amounts of human embryonic mesencephalic tissue are needed for therapeutic effects; (b) symptomatic relief is incomplete and varies between patients; and (c) patient selection and grafting procedure have not been optimized.

2000 Neural transplantation in neurodegenerative disease. Wiley, Chichester (Novartis Foundation Symposium 231) p 110–128

The basic principle underlying neural transplantation as a new therapeutic strategy is very simple, i.e. functional restoration in the diseased human brain should be achieved by replacement of dead neurons with implanted healthy neurons. There are three major reasons why this strategy is particularly suitable to explore in Parkinson's disease (PD). First, there is a definite need for new therapeutic approaches in PD. This disorder is characterized by tremor, rigidity, hypokinesia and postural instability. L-dopa treatment initially provides marked symptomatic relief, but within 5–10 years most patients exhibit a gradual loss of efficacy of L-dopa associated with diurnal oscillations in motor performance ('on–off' phenomena) and involuntary movements (dyskinesias). Although at this stage the patients often temporarily benefit from changes in medication, most patients become severely incapacitated. Second, the main pathology in PD is a rather

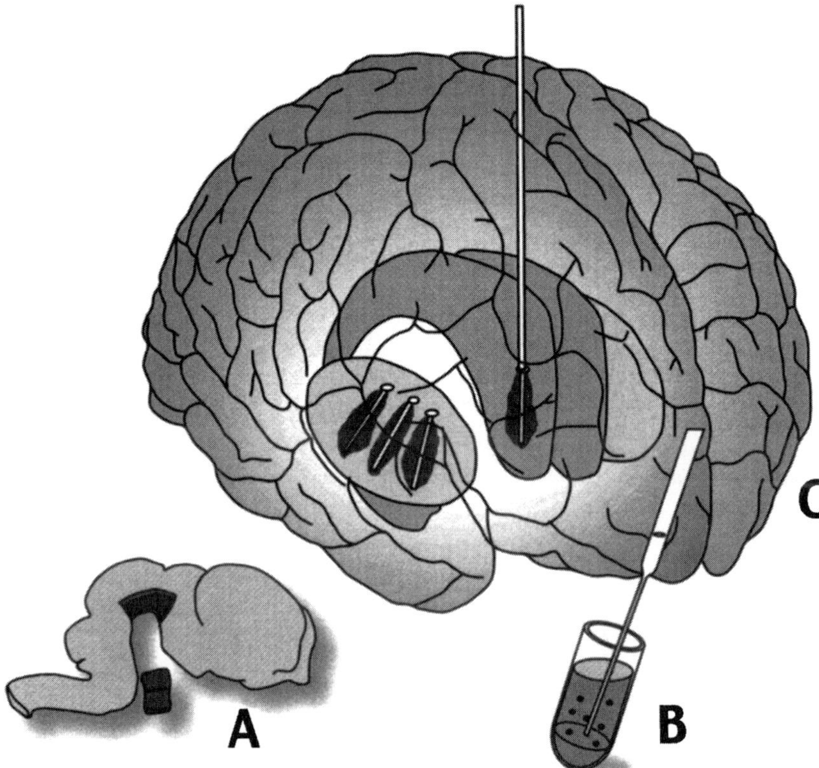

FIG. 1.   Schematic illustration of the most commonly used procedure for transplantation of human embryonic mesencephalic tissue into the striatum in patients with PD. Ventral mesencephalic DA-rich tissue (A) from human embryos aged 5.5–8 weeks postconception is dissociated (B) and then implanted unilaterally or bilaterally using stereotaxic surgery into the caudate nucleus or the putamen or both (C).

selective degeneration of the nigrostriatal dopamine (DA) system, i.e. of a specific neuronal population within a restricted area of the brain. This leads to a major reduction of DA levels in the striatum. The dopaminergic deficit in PD should be more easy to correct by transplantation as compared to, e.g. the more widespread loss of many different cell types in Alzheimer's disease. Third, studies in animal models of PD have shown that grafted embryonic DA neurons, taken from the ventral mesencephalon and implanted into the DA-denervated striatum in rodents and non-human primates, reinnervate the striatum, release DA and improve motor function, including the cardinal symptoms of human PD (Brundin et al 1994, Annett 1994).

So far, about 250 patients with PD have been grafted with embryonic tissue of human or porcine origin (Fig. 1). Here, I will argue that major scientific progress

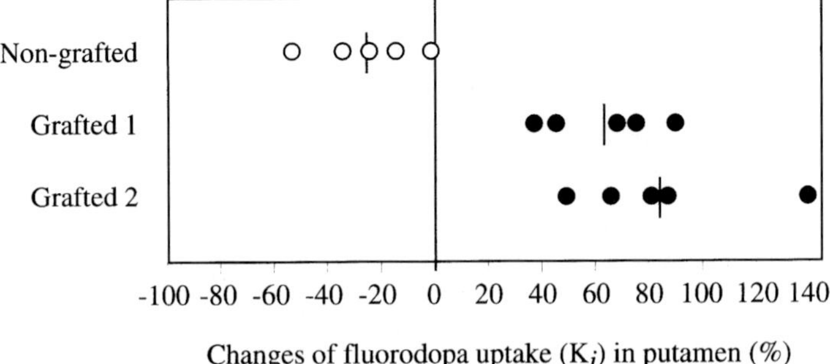

FIG. 2.   Survival of intrastriatal dopaminergic grafts after sequential implantation in the putamen in a group of five patients. Summary diagram showing the percent change of fluorodopa uptake (K_i-value) compared with preoperative value in the non-grafted putamen ('Non-grafted') and grafted putamen ('Grafted 1') at 8–12 months after the first transplantation, and at 12–18 months after the second transplantation in the recently grafted putamen ('Grafted 2'). Data from Wenning et al (1997) and Hagell et al (1999).

has been made in this field, clearly documenting that cell replacement can restore brain function for several years in humans. I will also underline some of the main problems that need to be solved for the further development of neural transplantation into a clinically useful therapeutic strategy for PD.

Experiences from clinical trials

Mesencephalic DA neurons from 5.5–9-week-old human embryos survive transplantation into the brain of PD patients. Significant increase of fluorodopa uptake in the grafted striatum has been shown using positron emission tomography (PET) in about 20 cases (Figs 2 and 3B) (Lindvall et al 1990, 1994, Sawle et al 1992, Widner et al 1992, Peschanski et al 1994, Remy et al 1995, Freeman et al 1995, Wenning et al 1997, Hagell et al 1999, Hauser et al 1999, Brundin et al 2000a). In one patient, the fluorodopa uptake in the putamen was normalized after transplantation (Fig. 3B) (Wenning et al 1997). Histopathological studies have confirmed the survival of the dopaminergic grafts

FIG. 3.   Illustration of the marked clinical improvement, correlated to normalization of [18F]dopa uptake, in a PD patient grafted unilaterally into the putamen with embryonic mesencephalic tissue from four human donors aged 6–8 weeks postconception. (A) Percentage of the day spent in the 'off' phase and motor examination score of the UPDRS in the practically defined 'off' phase at various time points after transplantation. Mean ±95% confidence interval. (B) [18F]dopa uptake in the grafted and in the non-grafted putamen in the same patient. Comparative data on [18F]dopa uptake in the putamen are given for a group of 16 healthy volunteers. Data from Wenning et al (1997) and Piccini et al (1999).

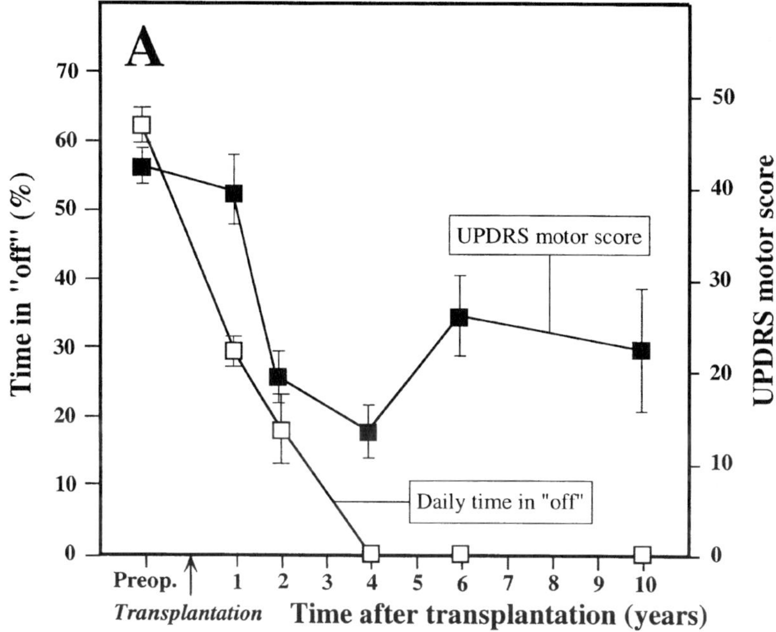
A
70
60
50
40
30
20
10
0
Time in "off" (%)
50
40
30
20
10
0
UPDRS motor score
UPDRS motor score
Daily time in "off"
Preop.
Transplantation
1 2 3 4 5 6 7 8 9 10
Time after transplantation (years)

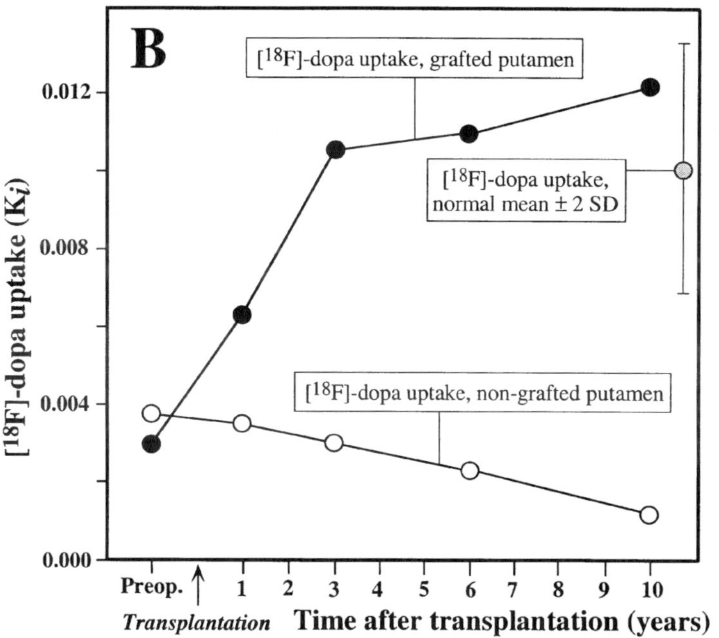
B
0.012
0.008
0.004
0.000
[18F]-dopa uptake (Ki)
[18F]-dopa uptake, grafted putamen
[18F]-dopa uptake,
normal mean ± 2 SD
[18F]-dopa uptake, non-grafted putamen
Preop.
Transplantation
1 2 3 4 5 6 7 8 9 10
Time after transplantation (years)

and demonstrated reinnervation of the striatum in two parkinsonian patients who died after transplantation (Kordower et al 1995, 1996, 1998). About 80 000–130 000 dopaminergic neurons had survived on each side (Kordower et al 1996). The neuritic outgrowth from the grafted neurons extended up to approximately 7 mm within the putamen (Kordower et al 1995). With six tracts, placed 5 mm apart, confluent reinnervation of 24–78% of the designated target area in the post-commissural putamen could be obtained, although in the patient with the densest reinnervation, the putamen was shrunken (Kordower et al 1998). The dopaminergic innervation occurred in a patch-matrix pattern and electron microscopy revealed synaptic connections between graft and host. There was no evidence that sprouting had occurred from the patient's own DA neurons.

Recently, it was demonstrated that synaptic DA release from embryonic mesencephalic grafts can be monitored *in vivo* in the striatum of a PD patient using [^{11}C]raclopride PET to measure DA D2 receptor occupancy by the endogenous transmitter (Piccini et al 1999). In a patient who had received a transplant in the right putamen 10 years earlier, D2 receptor binding was normal in the grafted putamen but was up-regulated in the non-grafted putamen. This indicates that the transplant continuously releases DA. Systemic amphetamine caused a substantial release of DA from the graft, of a magnitude similar to that observed from the intact nigrostriatal system in healthy controls.

Embryonic mesencephalic DA grafts can exhibit long-term survival despite an ongoing disease process and continuous antiparkinsonian drug treatment. In two patients who were transplanted unilaterally in the putamen, the fluorodopa uptake in the grafted structure was still high at 6 and 10 years after surgery (Fig. 3B) (Wenning et al 1997, Piccini et al 1999). In contrast, there had been a progressive fall of tracer uptake in non-grafted striatal regions, indicating degeneration of the patient's own DA neurons (Fig. 3B). Immunological rejection of the grafts has not been reported in any PD patient, even several years after withdrawal of immunosuppression. However, the presence of microglia, macrophages and T and B cells in the well-developed dopaminergic grafts in two patients subjected to autopsy (at 18 months after transplantation and 12 months after withdrawal of cyclosporin) suggests that there is a potential for immune reactions when immunosuppression is removed (Kordower et al 1997).

Several clinical research groups have demonstrated therapeutic improvement associated with graft survival in PD patients (Lindvall et al 1990, 1992, 1994, Pechanski et al 1994, Widner et al 1992, Remy et al 1995, Defer et al 1996, Wenning et al 1997, Freeman et al 1995, Hagell et al 1999, Hauser et al 1999, Brundin et al 2000a). In the most successful cases, patients have been able to withdraw L-dopa treatment after transplantation (Wenning et al 1997, Hagell et al 1999, Brundin et al 2000a). In our own series, three patients have managed without L-dopa for 2.5–4.5 years. About two-thirds of grafted patients have shown clinically useful, partial recovery of motor function: increased percent time in the 'on' phase and reduced rigidity and hypokinesia during 'off' phases (Lindvall et al 1990, 1992, 1994, Widner et al 1992, Pechanski et al 1994, Freeman et al 1995, Remy et al 1995, Defer et al 1996, Wenning et al 1997, Hagell et al 1999, Hauser et al 1999, Brundin et al 2000a). Some patients have demonstrated improved gait, speech and balance and fewer dyskinesias after transplantation (Widner et al 1992, Freeman et al 1995, Defer et al 1996), but in most cases these symptoms have not exhibited any major, consistent changes (Defer et al 1996, Wenning et al 1997, Hagell et al 1999).

Following unilateral grafts, the improvements are most pronounced in the contralateral limbs, but amelioration of parkinsonian symptoms on the ipsilateral side is also observed (Fig. 4). The most likely explanation for the symptomatic relief on both sides is that a major output from the striatum is, via the pallidum and thalamus, directed to the supplementary motor area (SMA), which has bilateral connections. The activation of the SMA and dorsolateral prefrontal cortex associated with movements is impaired in PD, which is believed to underlie parkinsonian hypokinesia. Piccini et al (2000) have recently shown using PET and rCBF measurements that intrastriatal grafts restored the activation of these frontal cortical areas, which was in agreement with the symptomatic relief in the patients. Unilateral dopaminergic grafts could, therefore, reduce motor symptoms bilaterally by restoring the functional integrity of the ipsilateral cortico-striato-thalamo-cortical loop and activating the SMA, which controls both sides of the body. In the study of Piccini et al (2000), the restoration of frontal cortical activation occurred in parallel to the clinical improvement but later than the increase of fluorodopa uptake, i.e. the striatal dopamine storage capacity. The temporal difference between these effects suggests that functional integration of the graft, with the establishment of afferent and efferent synaptic contacts with the host, is necessary for substantial symptomatic relief in PD patients.

Clinically valuable improvement and, in some cases, dramatic symptomatic relief allowing for withdrawal of L-dopa treatment can be induced by unilateral grafts (Fig. 3A) (Lindvall et al 1990, 1992, 1994, Wenning et al 1997). However, for maximum and long-lasting functional recovery, implants should be bilateral. This conclusion is based on two main observations. First, Hagell et al (1999) have reported from a series of patients transplanted sequentially on both sides that when a second intraputaminal graft was added contralateral to the first one, the functional effect was enhanced (Fig. 4). The magnitude of improvement induced by the second graft was less pronounced than that after the first implant. Second, after transplantation there is also a progressive degeneration of the patient's own DA neurons, which will lead to gradually increasing functional

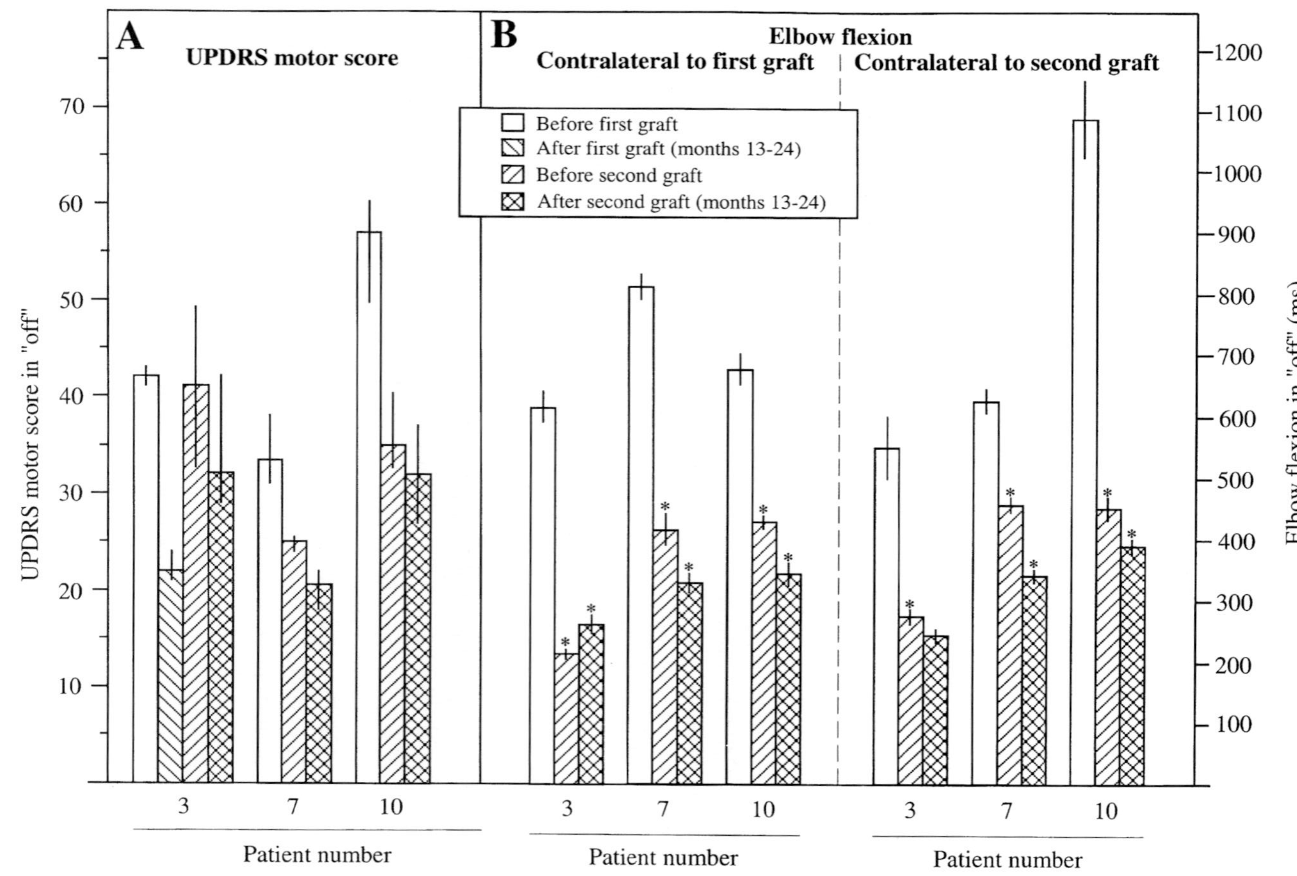

A
UPDRS motor score
B
Elbow flexion
Contralateral to first graft
Contralateral to second graft
Before first graft
After first graft (months 13-24)
Before second graft
After second graft (months 13-24)
70
60
50
40
30
20
10
UPDRS motor score in "off"
1200
1100
1000
900
800
700
600
500
400
300
200
100
Elbow flexion in "off" (ms)
3
7
10
Patient number
3
7
10
Patient number
3
7
10
Patient number

impairment predominantly on the side of the body contralateral to the non-grafted striatum (Lindvall et al 1994, Wenning et al 1997).

Current research problems and future directions

The demonstration that grafted DA neurons can survive and improve motor function in patients represents an important step towards a transplantation therapy in PD. Research should now aim at solving the scientific problems which, on basis of the clinical experience, can be clearly defined.

(1) Large amounts of human embryonic mesencephalic tissue are needed for therapeutic effects

Each substantia nigra in the human brain contains 550 000 dopaminergic neurons (Pakkenberg et al 1991). About 250 000 of these neurons have been estimated to innervate the putamen and a similar number to project to the caudate nucleus. Transplantation of dissociated human embryonic mesencephalic tissue into immunosuppressed parkinsonian rats results in about 40 000 surviving DA neurons from each donor (aged 6–8 weeks postconception) (Frodl et al 1994). Thus, less than 4% of human DA neurons survive grafting into rats and similar findings (5–10% survival) have been reported after transplantation to patients (Kordower et al 1995, 1996, 1998). The low yield of surviving DA neurons after transplantation, which is also observed with animal tissue, is a major obstacle for the application of this procedure in a large number of patients. Using currently available procedures, mesencephalic tissue from at least 3–4 human embryos (giving rise to about 100 000–150 000 surviving grafted DA neurons) probably needs to be implanted per side in each patient in order to induce a substantial clinical improvement and consistent significant increase of fluorodopa uptake.

FIG. 4.   Illustration that (i) unilateral grafts have bilateral but predominantly contralateral effects, (ii) a second, contralateral graft implanted 10–56 months after the first one gives rise to additional symptomatic relief, and (iii) the magnitude of improvement induced by the second graft in these patients is less pronounced than that after the first implant. (A) Scores from the motor examination part of the UPDRS in the practically defined 'off' phase. Data are from assessments performed during the 6 months prior to each transplantation and during the second year following the second graft. Due to the long interval between the transplantations in patient 3 (56 months), data from the second postoperative year after the first graft are also included for this patient. Data are median ± 25th percentile. (B) Performance of elbow flexion contralateral to the first and second grafts, as assessed neurophysiologically. Data are mean ± SEM. Statistical comparisons were made between the measurements before the first and the second graft, and between measurements before and after the second graft. *$P < 0.05$; Student's *t*-test. Patient numbers refer to Lund–London series. Data from Hagell et al (1999).

Studies in animals indicate that the massive death of embryonic dopaminergic neurons occurs during the first week after grafting (for references, see Brundin et al 2000b). Brundin and co-workers (2000b) have distinguished four main events which cause DA neuronal death in transplantation: (1) hypoxic/hypoglycemic insult due to the removal of the embryo from its maternal blood supply; (2) axotomy and other damage during dissection and mechanical dissociation, and hypoxia before implantation; (3) implantation and the first 1–3 days thereafter in the new environment; and (4) lack of appropriate neurotrophic support at a later stage during maturation. Several improvements of basic transplantation methodology which increase DA neuron survival have been described (for references, see Brundin et al 2000b), including change of the medium for preparation, dissociation and storage of the tissue, less extensive dissociation of the tissue with implantation of a mixture of cell aggregates and single cells, and use of a microtransplantation technique to minimize the trauma at the implantation site in the host brain.

The survival of grafted dopaminergic neurons can also be improved by the administration of growth factors (Mayer et al 1993, Takayama et al 1995, Rosenblad et al 1996, Sinclair et al 1996, Zeng et al 1996, Sautter et al 1998, Sullivan et al 1998, Yurek 1998, Wilby et al 1999), and compounds which reduce oxidative stress (Nakao et al 1994, Björklund et al 1997, Othberg et al 1997) or inhibit caspases (Schierle et al 1999). Exposure of the graft to neurotrophic factors such as glial cell line-derived neurotrophic factor (GDNF) increases the survival of DA neurons at least twofold. Caspase inhibitors which block apoptosis can induce a greater than threefold increase of the number of surviving grafted DA neurons in rats. Whether these strategies increase graft survival also in PD patients is unknown. The only compound which has been tested clinically is the lazaroid, tirilazad mesylate, which inhibits lipid peroxidation. Administration of tirilazad mesylate supports a twofold increase of the number of surviving cultured rat mesencephalic DA neurons (Othberg et al 1997), and similar increases in the survival of rat DA neurons grafted to the anterior chamber of the eye (Björklund et al 1997). Furthermore, tirilazad mesylate significantly prolongs the time during which both rat and human embryonic mesencephalic cell suspensions displayed high viability when stored at room temperature (Othberg et al 1997). The clinical study of Brundin et al (2000a) provides evidence that tirilazad mesylate (administered to the graft tissue and intravenously to the patient) may improve survival of grafted DA neurons also in PD patients.

One way of obtaining large amounts of embryonic mesencephalic tissue could be to use xenografts. However, in the initial attempts with porcine xenografts in patients, survival of DA neurons has been poor and clinical benefits are as yet uncertain (Deacon et al 1997). A major concern with porcine xenografts, apart from immunological rejection and transfer of virus, is that if only 5–20% of DA neurons survive transplantation and the axonal growth capacity is less than that from human grafts, a large number of porcine donors and many implant sites may be needed to effectively reinnervate the human striatum.

Other sources of catecholamine-producing cells, such as adrenal medulla, sympathetic ganglia and carotid body, have also been considered potentially useful for transplantation in PD patients (Lindvall 1994, Espejo et al 1998). In clinical trials, adrenal medulla autotransplantation has only yielded modest symptomatic relief, probably due to poor graft survival. Two future strategies might be to implant genetically engineered L-dopa- or DA-producing cells, or dopaminergic neurons generated from mesencephalic precursor cells or stem cells. However, it has been difficult to demonstrate permanently high levels of tyrosine hydroxylase gene expression and DA synthesis and improvement of motor deficits resembling the symptoms in PD patients after transplantation of genetically engineered cells in animals (Fisher et al 1991, Anton et al 1994, Lundberg et al 1996), and these problems must be solved before clinical trials can be initiated. Recently, Studer and co-workers (1998) reported that precursor cells obtained from the embryonic rat mesencephalon could be expanded *in vitro* and differentiated into dopaminergic neurons, which ameliorated rotational asymmetry after transplantation in hemiparkinsonian rats. However, the overall yield of surviving DA neurons *in vivo* was quite low due to a major loss of cells (95–98%) in the grafting step. The data of Studer et al (1998) suggest that DA neurons, expanded from stem cells obtained from small quantities of early embryonic human tissue, might become useful for transplantation in patients with PD. In support of this idea, Wagner et al (1999) have provided the first evidence that dopaminergic neurons can be engineered from stem cells. Such cells derived from the mouse cerebellum were transfected with the Nurr1 gene, proliferated and exposed to a soluble signal secreted by type 1 astrocytes from the ventral mesencephalon. The stem cells then developed into neurons with a dopaminergic phenotype. These cells could be transplanted to the striatum and a small number of them survived for a few weeks.

(2) Symptomatic relief is incomplete and varies between patients

This problem may be partly due to that the ectopically placed, grafted nigral neurons lack some functional properties of intrinsic DA neurons, e.g. the appropriate synaptic input. Although some promising attempts of reconstructing the nigrostriatal pathway in rats have been reported (Brecknell et al 1996, Zhou et al 1996, Mendez et al 1996), clinical trials using such approaches seem distant. Another possibility is that the resistant symptoms are due to non-dopaminergic deficits which cannot be corrected for by mesencephalic grafts. Finally, and probably most importantly, the incomplete recovery may be explained by the fact that the graft-derived dopaminergic reinnervation has not reached all denervated areas, e.g. the ventral striatum. In the clinical studies, the magnitude of improvement of motor function has broadly corresponded to the degree of graft-derived reinnervation of the putamen, as revealed by the restoration of fluorodopa uptake (Remy et al 1995, Wenning et al 1997, Hagell et al 1999). The dopaminergic reinnervation of the putamen is incomplete with present transplantation procedures. To promote reinnervation, which most likely would lead to improved symptomatic relief, the number of implants has to be increased or the axonal outgrowth must be stimulated. Based on the findings of Kordower et al (1998) and our own experiences, we estimate that to cover most of the volume of the putamen with a dopaminergic innervation of significant density (25% or more of normal) requires tissue implanted along 6–7 tracts. Another approach to promote reinnervation is to stimulate axonal outgrowth by administration of a neurotrophic factor. For example, it has been shown that intrastriatal injections of GDNF (Rosenblad et al 1996) or implantation of polymer-encapsulated genetically modified GDNF-releasing cells (Sautter et al 1998) gives rise to increased DA fibre outgrowth from intrastriatal rat-to-rat grafts, suggesting strategies that might be useful also in PD patients.

(3) Patient selection and grafting procedure have not been optimized

On the basis of the idea that grafts act by replacing degenerated DA neurons, only patients with idiopathic PD, i.e. who have a relatively selective dopaminergic deficit should be grafted. The clinical data also indicate that patients with the following symptom profile should primarily be selected: fluctuations with good 'on' phases, severe hypokinesia and rigidity in 'off', and clear L-dopa response. Tremor should not be a dominant symptom. However, whether other symptoms, e.g. dyskinesias and axial symptoms, can be improved by grafts, and how this might be achieved remains to be determined. Knowledge about where a graft should be placed in order to reverse a particular symptom in a PD patient is currently poor. Studies in animals have shown that grafts placed in different subregions of the striatum compensate for specific features of the parkinsonian syndrome, and such a topography probably also exists in the human brain. A detailed preoperative PET scan with high resolution, to reveal the pattern of dopaminergic denervation in the individual PD patient, seems highly warranted both for patient selection and to determine the graft placements which will give rise to maximum improvements.

Conclusions

The clinical trials with neural transplantation in PD patients show, for the first time, that a cell replacement therapy can work in the human brain. At present, neural grafting is only one of several experimental procedures for the treatment of PD, including, for example, deep brain stimulation. The ongoing, placebo-controlled clinical trials will reveal the functional efficacy of the presently available transplantation procedures. It is conceivable, though, that in the future, scientific progress will lead to major improvements of the clinical usefulness of this approach in PD, firstly, by increasing the functional efficacy of the grafts and, secondly, by reducing the need for human embryonic tissue.

Acknowledgements

Our own work was supported by grants from the Swedish Medical Research Council, the Kock Foundation, the Wiberg Foundation, the King Gustav V and Queen Victoria Foundation and the Söderberg Foundation.

References

Annett L 1994 Functional studies of neural grafts in parkinsonian primates. In: Dunnett SB, Björklund A (eds) Functional neural transplantation. Raven Press, New York, p 71–102

Anton R, Kordower JH, Maidment NT et al 1994 Neural-targeted gene therapy for rodent and primate hemiparkinsonism. Exp Neurol 127:207–218

Björklund L, Spenger C, Strömberg I 1997 Tirilazad mesylate increases dopaminergic neuronal survival in the *in oculo* grafting model. Exp Neurol 148:324–333

Brecknell JE, Haque NSK, Du JS et al 1996 Functional and anatomical reconstruction of the 6-hydroxydopamine lesioned nigrostriatal system of the adult rat. Neuroscience 71:913–925

Brundin P, Duan W-M, Sauer H 1994 Functional effects of mesencephalic dopamine neurons and adrenal chromaffin cells grafted to the rodent striatum. In: Dunnett SB, Björklund A (eds) Functional neural transplantation. Raven Press, New York, p 9–46

Brundin P, Pogarell O, Hagell P et al 2000a Bilateral caudate and putamen grafts of embryonic mesencephalic tissue treated with lazaroids in Parkinson's disease. Brain 123:1380–1390

Brundin P, Karlsson J, Emgård M et al 2000b Improving the survival of grafted dopaminergic neurons: a review over current approaches. Cell Transplant 9:179–195

Deacon T, Schumacher J, Dinsmore J et al 1997 Histological evidence of fetal pig neural cell survival after transplantation into a patient with Parkinson's disease. Nat Med 3:350–353

Defer GL, Geny C, Ricolfi F et al 1996 Long-term outcome of unilaterally transplanted parkinsonian patients. I. Clinical approach. Brain 119:41–50

Espejo EF, Montoro RJ, Armengol JA, López-Barneo J 1998 Cellular and functional recovery of Parkinsonian rats after intrastriatal transplantation of carotid body aggregates. Neuron 20:197–206

Fisher LJ, Jinnah HA, Kale LC, Higgins GA, Gage FH 1991 Survival and function of intrastriatally grafted primary fibroblasts genetically modified to produce L-dopa. Neuron 6:371–380

Freeman TB, Olanow CW, Hauser RA et al 1995 Bilateral fetal nigral transplantation into the postcommissural putamen in Parkinson's disease. Ann Neurol 38:379–388

Frodl EM, Duan WM, Sauer H, Kupsch A, Brundin P 1994 Human embryonic dopamine neurons xenografted to the rat: effects of cryopreservation and varying regional source of donor cells on transplant survival, morphology and function. Brain Res 647:286–298

Hagell P, Schrag A, Piccini P et al 1999 Sequential bilateral transplantation in Parkinson's disease: effects of the second graft. Brain 122:1121–1132

Hauser RA, Freeman TB, Snow BJ et al 1999 Long-term evaluation of bilateral fetal nigral transplantation in Parkinson disease. Arch Neurol 56:179–187

Kordower JH, Freeman TB, Snow BJ et al 1995 Neuropathological evidence of graft survival and striatal reinnervation after the transplantation of fetal mesencephalic tissue in a patient with Parkinson's disease. N Engl J Med 332:1118–1124

Kordower JH, Rosenstein JM, Collier TJ et al 1996 Functional fetal nigral grafts in a patient with Parkinson's disease: chemoanatomic, ultrastructural, and metabolic studies. J Comp Neurol 370:203–230

Kordower JH, Styren S, Clarke M, DeKosky ST, Olanow CW, Freeman TB 1997 Fetal grafting for Parkinson's disease: expression of immune markers in two patients with functional fetal nigral implants. Cell Transplant 6:213–219

Kordower JH, Freeman TB, Chen EY et al 1998 Fetal nigral grafts survive and mediate clinical benefit in a patient with Parkinson's disease. Mov Disord 13:383–393

Lindvall O 1994 Neural transplantation in Parkinson's disease. In: Dunnett SB, Björklund A (eds) Functional neural transplantation. Raven Press, New York, p 103–137

Lindvall O, Brundin P, Widner H et al 1990 Grafts of fetal dopamine neurons survive and improve motor function in Parkinson's disease. Science 247:574–577

Lindvall O, Widner H, Rehncrona S et al 1992 Transplantation of fetal dopamine neurons in Parkinson's disease: one-year clinical and neurophysiological observations in two patients with putaminal implants. Ann Neurol 31:155–165

Lindvall O, Sawle G, Widner H et al 1994 Evidence for long-term survival and function of dopaminergic grafts in progressive Parkinson's disease. Ann Neurol 35:172–180

Lundberg C, Horellou P, Mallet J, Björklund A 1996 Generation of DOPA-producing astrocytes by retroviral transduction of the human tyrosine hydroxylase gene: *in vitro* characterization and *in vivo* effects in the rat Parkinson model. Exp Neurol 139:39–53

Mayer E, Dunnett SB, Fawcett JW 1993 Basic fibroblast growth factor promotes the survival of embryonic ventral mesencephalic dopaminergic neurons. II. Effects on nigral transplants *in vivo*. Neuroscience 56:389–398

Mendez I, Sadi D, Hong M 1996 Reconstruction of the nigrostriatal pathway by simultaneous intrastriatal and intranigral dopaminergic transplants. J Neurosci 16:7216–7227

Nakao N, Frodl EM, Duan WM, Widner H, Brundin P 1994 Lazaroids improve the survival of grafted rat embryonic dopamine neurons. Proc Natl Acad Sci USA 91:12408–12412

Othberg A, Keep M, Brundin P, Lindvall O 1997 Tirilazad mesylate improves survival of rat and human embryonic mesencephalic neurons *in vitro*. Exp Neurol 147:498–502

Pakkenberg B, Møller A, Gundersen HJG, Mouritzen Dam A, Pakkenberg H 1991 The absolute number of nerve cells in substantia nigra in normal subjects and in patients with Parkinson's disease estimated with an unbiased stereological method. J Neurol Neurosurg Psychiatry 54:30–33

Peschanski M, Defer G, N'Guyen JP et al 1994 Bilateral motor improvement and alteration of L-dopa effect in two patients with Parkinson's disease following intrastriatal transplantation of foetal ventral mesencephalon. Brain 117:487–499

Piccini P, Brooks DJ, Björklund A et al 1999 Dopamine release from nigral transplants visualized *in vivo* in a Parkinson's patient. Nat Neurosci 2:1137–1140

Piccini P, Lindvall O, Björklund A et al 2000 Delayed recovery of movement-related cortical function in Parkinson's disease following striatal dopaminergic grafts. Ann Neurol, in press

Remy P, Samson Y, Hantraye P et al 1995 Clinical correlates of [^{18}F]fluorodopa uptake in five grafted parkinsonian patients. Ann Neurol 38:580–588

Rosenblad C, Martínez-Serrano A, Björklund A 1996 Glial cell-line derived neurotrophic factor increases survival, growth and function of intrastriatal fetal nigral dopaminergic grafts. Neuroscience 75:979–985

Sautter J, Tseng JL, Braguglia D et al 1998 Implants of polymer-encapsulated genetically modified cells releasing glial cell line-derived neurotrophic factor improve survival, growth and function of fetal dopaminergic grafts. Exp Neurol 149:230–236

Sawle GV, Bloomfield PM, Björklund A et al 1992 Transplantation of fetal dopamine neurons in Parkinson's disease: PET [18F]6-L-fluorodopa studies in two patients with putaminal implants. Ann Neurol 31:166–173

Schierle GS, Hansson O, Leist M, Nicotera P, Widner H, Brundin P 1999 Caspase inhibition reduces apoptosis and increases survival of nigral transplants. Nat Med 5:97–100

Sinclair SR, Svendsen CN, Torres EM, Martin D, Fawcett JD, Dunnett SB 1996 GDNF enhances dopaminergic cell survival and fiber outgrowth in embryonic nigral grafts. Neuroreport 7:2547–2552

Studer L, Tabar V, McKay RDG 1998 Transplantation of expanded mesencephalic precursors leads to recovery in parkinsonian rats. Nat Neurosci 1:290–295

Sullivan AM, Pohl J, Blunt SB 1998 Growth/ differentiation factor 5 and glial cell line-derived neurotrophic factor enhance survival and function of dopaminergic grafts in a rat model of Parkinson's disease. Eur J Neurosci 10:3681–3688

Takayama H, Ray J, Raymon HK et al 1995 Basic fibroblast growth factor increases dopaminergic graft survival and function in a rat model of Parkinson's disease. Nat Med 1:53–58

Wagner J, Åkerud P, Castro DS et al 1999 Induction of a midbrain dopaminergic phenotype in Nurr1-overexpressing neural stem cells by type 1 astrocytes. Nat Biotechnol 17:653–659

Wenning GK, Odin P, Morrish P et al 1997 Short- and long-term survival and function of unilateral intrastriatal dopaminergic grafts in Parkinson's disease. Ann Neurol 42:95–107

Widner H, Tetrud J, Rehncrona S et al 1992 Bilateral fetal mesencephalic grafting in two patients with parkinsonism induced by 1-methyl-4-phenyl-1,2,3,6-tetrahydropyridine (MPTP). N Engl J Med 327:1556–1563

Wilby MJ, Sinclair SR, Muir EM et al 1999 A glial-cell line-derived neurotrophic factor-secreting clone of the Schwann cell line SCTM41 enhances survival and fiber outgrowth from embryonic nigral neurons grafted to the striatum and to the lesioned substantia nigra. J Neurosci 19:2301–2312

Yurek DM 1998 Glial cell line-derived neurotrophic factor improves survival of dopaminergic neurons in transplants of fetal ventral mesencephalic tissue. Exp Neurol 153:195–202

Zeng BY, Jenner P, Marsden CD 1996 Altered motor function and graft survival produced by basic fibroblast growth factor in rats with 6-OHDA lesions and fetal ventral mesencephalic grafts are associated with glial proliferation. Exp Neurol 139:214–226

Zhou FS, Chiang YH, Wang Y 1996 Constructing a new nigrostriatal pathway in the Parkinsonian model with bridged neural transplantation in substantia nigra. J Neurosci 16:6965–6974

DISCUSSION

Barker: Will the rescue strategies which you have outlined always rescue the same number of cells, or the same group of cells, or are they additive? For example, if you use the lazaroids, GDNF and the caspase inhibitors, will you achieve what you set out with a five- to tenfold increase in yield, or will you always get the same two- to threefold increase irrespective of which one of those strategies you employ?

Lindvall: This is a worry I have: that we may not reach 100% survival of DA neurons whatever we do. There are very few studies which try to combine these different approaches. I know that Patrik Brundin (Wallenberg Neuroscience Center, Lund, Sweden) is currently performing such studies. I believe that the most promising strategy will be to combine protective approaches with those generating more DA neurons from precursor cells taken from early embryonic tissue. For routine clinical use it would be acceptable if you could graft one patient with tissue from one donor.

Isacson: What are your views on how, in the future, we may select special DA neurons? When we looking at the surviving grafts we are looking at a fluorodopa scan from thousands of DA neurons. We don't know which of these are functionally relevant. Some of the transplanted non-dopaminergic neurons (90% of the fetal ventral mesencephalon) may not be doing much and may even be detrimental if they are not firing in the right place. Do you think this is an aspect that may enhance the clinical efficacy?

Lindvall: This is an important issue. We would like every case to be like patient number 4 in the Lund series, who has exhibited major clinical improvement. But the magnitude and pattern of symptomatic relief probably depend not only on the survival of grafted DA neurons, but also on other factors such as which areas of the striatum have been reinnervated, how efficiently the grafts are working in these areas, if the grafts are integrated into the host brain, and the preoperative denervation pattern in the patient. We have speculated about these issues for years and there are now imaging techniques which can help us. First, the resolution of the fluorodopa–PET method is much higher than previously, and we can now use it to look at the dopaminergic denervation and reinnervation patterns in different parts of the striatum. Second, we can measure DA release *in vivo* using [^{11}C]raclopride binding and PET. Third, the functional integration of the grafts can be explored using rCBF measurements with PET.

Isacson: Would you then use, for example, raclopride PET studies to determine DA receptor up-regulation prior to implantations?

Lindvall: Yes, we are doing that already.

Reier: In your studies, was lazaroid treatment limited to the graft preparation, or did you also administer it to the patient on a chronic basis?

Lindvall: In this series of patients we did both. The lazaroid tirilazad mesylate was present in the graft preparation. Then we gave tirilazad three times daily intravenously to the patient for three days. Whereas the first step has been supported by animal experimental data, the intravenous administration has not.

In the new patient series, we are not giving tirilazad mesylate systemically any more, because we had some side effects.

Aebischer: Why was patient 4 so special?

Lindvall: I could turn that question slightly around and ask whether there was anything special about the diagnosis of patient 4. I have now followed him for 12 years, and he has had Parkinson's disease for almost 20 years. The onset was according to the textbook, and there was nothing strange with the evolution of his disorder. However, he has behaved differently from the other grafted patients in two ways: first, he has exhibited the most pronounced clinical improvement, and second he is the only one who has had a complete restoration of fluorodopa uptake in the grafted putamen. This suggests that there might be something special with the graft in this patient.

Aebischer: How do your best patients compare with deep brain stimulation?

Lindvall: Stig Rehncrona, our neurosurgeon at the University Hospital in Lund, is responsible for transplanting the patients but is also putting electrodes into the subthalamic nucleus in other Parkinson patients. We are therefore in the fairly unique position of being able to compare the outcome of both procedures. According to Stig, without any detailed analysis, the outcome is presently about the same.

Gray: And what if you add to that comparison subthalamic surgery?

Lindvall: Subthalamic stimulation can give approximately the same outcome as fetal transplantation.

Gray: Can I clarify this: I thought there is a stimulation approach, and also an approach that involves the actual surgical removal of tissue.

Lindvall: We are not performing any lesions in the subthalamic nucleus.

Barker: I think Steve Gill in Bristol is actually moving towards subthalamo-tomy, as opposed to a subthalamic stimulator, because of the logistical problems with using stimulators and the number of patients requesting this treatment.

Annett: I heard Steve Gill talk recently about his subthalamic lesions in patients in Bristol, and his comment was that it is not a complete recovery, but 20–30% improvement.

Lindvall: I hesitate to make a comparison, because we have no hard facts.

Freeman: I have compared outcome results from our open-label transplant trial with published results from similar open-label trials of deep brain stimulation of the subthalamic nucleus. Such a comparison must be tempered by the fact that the trials are small, uncontrolled, performed in different centres and with unmatched groups of patients. However, there seems to be slightly more improvement with the deep brain stimulation, but the difference was 30–40% versus 50–60%. The numbers are too small to go beyond that generality.

But the real issue is that it doesn't matter. Direct comparison of surgical therapies is premature at this time. Deep brain stimulation is not clearly a viable therapy for large numbers of patients. Tony Lang had one neurologist working full time adjusting the deep brain stimulators for 200 patients. When you multiply the number of patients with Parkinson's disease by the number of stimulators, virtually every neurologist in the world would be adjusting these stimulators, or else you would have to train a huge number of nurses to be doing this. Of course, experience and technology changes may improve this problem. Second, the costs are incredible. Third, stimulators may not modify the disease process. Fourth, the surgical expertise required is tremendous, as opposed to targeting the putamen which is quite easy to reach reproducibly from a surgical perspective and for which the risks are more reasonable than going into the brainstem. What counts is not only the overall level of improvement, but the improvement in comparison with the ability to do the procedure, as well as the associated risks. Finally, there is tremendous potential to improve transplants in the future.

Peschanski: We have also compared deep brain stimulation with grafts. There are several differences that make deep brain stimulators more attractive to a number of people, both surgeons and patients. First, surgeons can just call the company, Medtronics, and get the stimulators. They don't have to liase with a biologist and an obstetrician to get the transplant done. The surgery can also be relatively fast (although implanting into the subthalamic nucleus can take up to 18 h when it is done in Grenoble). Technically, deep brain stimulation is much easier for the surgeon. At least in France, we have been unable to get a surgical group doing neural transplants, in addition to ours, even though results were good. Deep brain stimulation is now spreading to all the sterotactic neurosurgical departments in the country. Second, deep brain stimulation will give the patient immediate relief. After that it is necessary still to adapt the stimulation, but when it's well done a patient will actually be able to leave the hospital in a much better state.

Having said this, if there is a larger benefit for deep brain stimulation it is not major, and the results of this technique is just as heterogeneous as for the transplants. I disagree with your argument, in that I think that it is OK that one neurologist is working full time to adapt the stimulators in the groups which are doing a lot of deep brain stimulation. But if you begin to make calculations about the logistics of grafting all the patients with Parkinson's who will need some kind of surgical treatment, we would not be able to do it. These are just two different techniques that give partial recovery, and I don't think that a strict comparison should be carried out in this way.

Freeman: I think all of your points are exactly correct, and I think that's why surgeons are so enthusiastic about these interventions. Surgeons get paid for one and not the other, and that certainly has sparked an interest in pallidotomies, which are now performed in hundreds of centres. The same thing happened with adrenal transplants; surgeons charged for the procedures. Also, on the economic side, the neurologists gets paid very little for several hours of work adjusting the stimulator, so this factor will also come into play. I have heard this mentioned by several neurologists already.

In terms of fetal tissue being useful for hundreds of thousands of patients, unless one donor per patient is all that is needed, it may not be a useful therapy from a practical perspective. We have not established the optimal dose of cells yet. This is why we set up our dose-escalation trial, because we wanted to identify the absolute minimum number of cells necessary to induce meaningful benefit. But even if one donor per patient is adequate, there still are other considerations. It may not be reasonable to consider this a useful therapy for all patients worldwide until we have cell lines. It may be that what we are doing now is actually creating the roadmap for biotechnology trials, rather than creating the actual therapy.

Lindvall: I agree. It is unfair to compare these procedures at this early stage in neural transplantation. I think they should be developed in parallel. In my opinion, the use of several donors per patient on a routine basis is completely out of the question. We may end up using stem cells obtained from very small amounts of human embryonic tissue. We currently do not have a cell therapy with a potential for use in a large number of patients.

Olson: Perhaps one reason that we have had variable results is that the patients are genetically different. In some patients you have shown that the graft survives for 10 years, while the patients own DA system continues to degenerate. One reason for this might be some genetic defect that makes the endogenous DA neurons susceptible to whatever the disease process is, but not the grafted neurons because presumably they do not have this defect. Have you compared parkinsonian patients who have relatives with Parkinson's, to those cases who do not?

Lindvall: That is an interesting question, but we haven't looked at that. There are no familial cases among those we have grafted.

Gage: The finding that the graft survives in the context of the degenerating contralateral striatum answered a question that had been around for a long time: whether or not the host will continue to kill the transplant.

Sinden: The question about the heterogeneity of patients reminded me that the US blinded trials are on late stage PD patients only. Is it possible to compare the Swedish data with these US data?

Lindvall: There is one major difference between our patients and the US patients. The US team used tissue from two donors in the putamen in each side, and they cultured the tissue for four weeks. In the two patients who died 40 000 cells or fewer survived on each side. Our patients have received tissue from three to five donors in each putamen with an estimated number of 100 000–150 000 surviving DA neurons.

Sinden: I understand also that there was no immunosuppression.

Lindvall: They did not use immunosuppression. Whether this treatment is necessary or not we don't know. Several patients have withdrawn immunosuppression at 6 months to 3 years after grafting without any signs of rejection.

Transplantation of human fetal striatal tissue in Huntington's disease: rationale for clinical studies

Thomas B. Freeman*†‡, Robert A. Hauser†‡¶, Alison E. Willing*‡, Tanja Zigova*, Paul R. Sanberg*†‡ and Samuel Saporta*‡§

*Department of Neurosurgery, †Department of Pharmacology and Experimental Therapeutics, ‡The Neuroscience Program, ¶Department of Neurology, §Department of Anatomy, University of South Florida, 4 Columbia Drive, Suite 730, Tampa, FL 33606, USA

Abstract. Huntington's disease is a fatal neurological disorder characterized by chorea and deterioration in cognitive and neuropsychiatric function. Primary pathological changes are found in the striatum, where GABAergic neurons undergo degenerative changes. Local interneurons are relatively spared. Here, we describe the rationale for clinical trials of fetal striatal tissue transplantation for the treatment of Huntington's disease. Specifically, the reasons for utilizing tissue derived from the far lateral aspect of the lateral ventricular eminence as a source of striatal tissue will be discussed.

2000 Neural transplantation in neurodegenerative disease: current status and new directions. Wiley, Chichester (Novartis Found Symp 231) p 129–144

Huntington's disease (HD) is considered by some as a GABAergic deficiency (Peschanski et al 1995). However, pharmacological trials using GABA-related replacement therapies have failed to show objective or symptomatic relief for HD patients. This may be because many GABAergic neurons are serially connected within the brain, with only certain portions of this circuitry adversely affected by HD. This supports the need for local, appropriate reconstruction of the degenerating striatal circuitry in HD if a therapy with long-term benefit is to be developed.

Schmidt et al (1981) were the first to successfully implant fetal striatal tissue in an animal model of HD. Deckel et al (1983) subsequently reported behavioural improvement following striatal grafts in rodent models of HD. Fetal striatal grafts derived from rodents establish both afferent and efferent connections with the host brain in allograft models of HD (Pritzel et al 1986, Wictorin 1992, Dunnett & Svendsen 1993), and these connections are functionally integrated (Campbell et al 1993, 1995a,b, Sirinaibinghji et al 1993, Dunnett & Svendsen 1993,

Pakzaban et al 1993). In primate models of HD, Isacson and colleagues demonstrated improvement of drug-induced dyskinesia and hyperactivity following intrastriatal transplantation of striatal xenografts derived from rodent donors (Hantraye et al 1992). These grafts received afferent innervation from the host as well. Pig and human striatal grafts are capable of forming afferent and efferent connections with the brain via long axonal pathways (Wictorin 1992, Deacon et al 1994a). Human fetal striatal grafts similarly ameliorate some behavioural deficits in rodent models of HD (Sanberg et al 1997, Pundt et al 1996).

Development of a striatal graft capable of such connectivity has been a complex problem with an evolving understanding of non-striatal graft components. Striatal-like morphology has been demonstrated within grafts (Dunnett & Svendsen 1993). Initially, the 'patchy' appearance within grafts was interpreted as being reminiscent of striosome and matrix compartments seen in the normal striatum. However, a variety of other markers have subsequently been observed within 'striatal grafts' derived from the ganglionic eminence, including cortical and pallidal tissues, among others. At least 11 brain regions or fibre bundles develop within or adjacent to the ganglionic eminence, including the caudate nucleus, putamen, globus pallidus, nucleus accumbens, amygdaloid nuclei, pulvinar, piriform cortex, olfactory cortex, internal capsule, stria terminalis and the nucleus basalis (Graybiel & Ragsdale 1980, Candy et al 1985, Kostovic 1986, Pakzaban et al 1993, O'Rahilly & Müller 1994, Freeman et al 1995, de Carlos et al 1996, Anderson et al 1997). This accounts for the numerous cell types seen within grafts derived from non-selective dissection of the ganglionic eminence. For this reason, the ganglionic eminence has been recently characterized by O'Rahilly & Müller (1994) as the ventricular eminence, reflecting its morphological appearance rather than the specific progenitor cell types found within this developing brain region.

The striatal anlage that was dissected for early transplantation studies generally consisted of the combined medial and lateral ganglionic eminences (MGE and LGE) and in some cases included the body of the ganglionic eminence (see Wictorin 1992, Isacson et al 1987, Pakzaban et al 1993, Dunnett & Svendsen 1993). Subsequent studies demonstrated that only regions of the graft with striatal markers were anatomically and functionally integrated with the recipient brain (Wictorin 1992, Campbell et al 1993, 1995a,b, Pakzaban et al 1993, Deacon et al 1994a). Therefore Graybiel and colleagues named the graft regions with striatal markers 'P-zones', designating regions within grafts with patches of striatal-like tissue (Dunnett & Svendsen 1993). To distinguish between patch regions within grafts and 'patch-matrix' within the normal striatum, the term 'striosome' has been used instead of 'patch' when discussing the non-transplanted striatal region. Grafts themselves can have both matrix and striosome-like markers.

GABAergic projection neurons are found within the matrix component of both the normal striatum and striatal grafts (Wictorin 1992, Pakzaban et al 1993), so it was postulated by Pakzaban et al (1993) that increasing the proportion of these zones within grafts may be desirable. By elimination of the MGE and body of the ganglionic eminence from the dissection, they demonstrated that grafts contained P-zones consisting of up to 87% of the graft volume (Pakzaban et al 1993). These authors concluded that regions of grafts that did not label for striatal markers represented non-striatal regions that normally develop within or adjacent to the MGE or the body of the ganglionic eminence. Further clarification of this anatomic finding was provided by Deacon et al (1994a) and Olsson et al (1995). They found that GABAergic (DARPP-32-ir) neurons developed in the LGE, but not the adjacent MGE. They also demonstrated that only grafts derived from the LGE, but not the MGE integrated into the host striatum and innervated striatal efferent target sites within the host brain.

Connectivity between striatal grafts and the brain is important for several reasons. It has been suggested that there is a two-stage recovery following fetal striatal transplantation: a rapid neurotrophic or neurochemically mediated stage followed by a slower improvement secondary to afferent and efferent connectivity (Wictorin 1992, Peschanski et al 1995). However, if neural grafts are to be useful clinically for the treatment of HD, it is likely that anatomical connectivity will be crucial for long-term benefit (Freeman et al 1995, Peschanski et al 1995). Although primary pathological changes in HD and excitotoxin-lesioned rats are seen within the striatum, degeneration is also seen in multiple brain regions associated with either afferent or efferent striatal projections, including the globus pallidus, substantia nigra, subthalamic nucleus and cerebral cortex (Pritzel et al 1986, Töpper et al 1993, Wictorin 1992, Peschanski et al 1995, Hersch & Ferrante 1997). If this represents second-order degeneration, both afferent and efferent connectivity between graft and host may be necessary long-term if graft-derived trophic support is to arrest degeneration of these remote sites in HD (Pritzel et al 1986, Saji & Reis 1987, Sanberg et al 1993, Peschanski et al 1995).

Connectivity also plays an important role in graft-derived functional effects. Nakao et al (1996) demonstrated that behavioural improvement of paw reaching scores following rodent allografts correlated with the volume of the P-zones and the number of DARPP-32 positive neurons within the striatal grafts. Of importance, regression analysis demonstrated that significant behavioural improvement was observed when at least 25% of the graft volume was DARPP-32 positive, and behaviour improved to within one standard deviation of normal when 50% of the graft volume was DARPP-32 positive.

However, no investigator to date has demonstrated this volume of P-zones within human fetal striatal grafts transplanted into immunosuppressed rodents

(Pundt et al 1994, Sanberg et al 1994, 1997, Grasbon-Frodl et al 1996, Naimi et al 1996). Brundin and colleagues (1996) therefore concluded that the paucity of P-zones in human fetal striatal grafts did not favour the initiation of clinical trials of fetal tissue transplants for the treatment of HD.

Several explanations have been postulated for the species-specific differences encountered with human lateral ventricular eminence (LVE) grafts as compared to similar grafts derived from rodent or porcine donors (Deacon et al 1994b, Grasbon-Frodl et al 1996, 1997). Possible reasons for P-zone-poor grafts include prolonged ontogeny of human striatal neurons, loss of developmental cues in dissected tissues, the absence of species-specific trophic support, species-specific variability of GABAergic neuronal survival after transplantation, and incorrect donor age selection for grafts. We hypothesized that further regional dissection of the LVE is necessary with human fetal tissue in order to achieve optimal P-zones within human fetal striatal grafts. As the phylogenetic order is ascended, specific regions within the ventricular eminence assume greater volumetric representation. The percentage of the basal ganglia represented by pallidal tissue doubles as one ascends from non-human primate to humans (Harman & Carpenter 1950). Glial cells, seen commonly within the ventricular eminence, are more common in mammals with larger brains (Armstrong 1985) and can form an important component of striatal grafts (Deacon et al 1994b). Adjacent cortical tissue is frequently included in grafts (Dunnett & Svendsen 1993, Nakao et al 1996). Cortical brain regions have the most disproportionate growth across phylogenetic orders. There is increasing representation of the amygdaloid nuclei and nucleus basalis in the developing ventricular eminence in humans as compared to species of lower phylogenetic orders (Candy et al 1985, Kostovic 1986, O'Rahilly & Müller 1994, Chen et al 1996). This hypothesis is further supported by the fact that the non-P-zones within grafts have been found to have cells with primarily cortical and pallidal morphologies (Wictorin 1992, Dunnett & Svendsen 1993). Also, human and porcine striatal xenografts contain a high density of axons that remain within the graft (Wictorin 1992, Deacon et al 1994b). This is what would be expected if neurons that normally do not innervate the striatum are transplanted to this ectopic site (Schultzberg et al 1984).

The localization of the embryonic development of DARPP-32-positive striatal GABAergic neurons is quite similar across species, and it occurs within the LVE (Deacon et al 1994a, Naimi et al 1996). In humans, these neurons also develop in the LVE and anterior body of the ventricular eminence, anterior to the foramen of Monro (Freeman et al 1995, Naimi et al 1996). However, developing GABAergic neurons are displaced more laterally in the human LVE compared to other species, possibly due to the increased contribution of other developing regions within the human ventricular eminence.

We attempted to exclude developing regions of the nucleus basalis, amygdaloid nuclei, globus pallidus and cerebral cortex from human embryonic grafts by selectively dissecting the far lateral aspect of the human LVE (FLVE). We examined whether exclusion of non-striatal regions from human fetal grafts would increase the proportion of striatal P-zones within grafts to a level that has been predicted to be functionally relevant for therapeutic use in patients with HD (Brundin et al 1996).

Methods for tissue obtainment, storage, dissection and transplantation, as well as histological methods and results of transplant of FLVE grafts in a rodent model of HD have been described previously (Freeman et al 1999a). Briefly, the FLVE was dissected from human embryonic donors with a Carnegie Stage of 22–23. Solid grafts were transplanted stereotaxically into quinolinic acid-lesioned rodents that were immunosuppressed with cyclosporin. Tissue was evaluated histologically for neuronal phenotypes typical of the developing striatum.

All but one graft survived, and the largest graft size was $7.4\,mm^3$. Grafts contained patches with markers of both striatal projection (GABAergic) neurons as well as interneurons typically found in the striatum (ChAT- and NADPH-positive neurons). These patches of striatal tissue generally occupied greater than 30% of the graft volume, and in some cases involved over half of the graft volume. Ingrowth of host-derived tyrosine hydroxylase fibres was seen within the grafts. These fibres were generally localized within the periphery of grafts when examined at 8–12 weeks after transplantation, and in the medial aspects of grafts as well when evaluated 20–24 weeks after transplantation. Host-derived tyrosine hydroxylase fibres co-localized with markers of striatal tissue within grafts, suggesting targeted ingrowth of fibres into the patches of striatal tissue within the grafts. Graft-derived neuritic extensions into the host, visualized with an antibody to human neurofilament, were observed projecting to appropriate target regions including the globus pallidus, substantia nigra and the entopeduncular nucleus (see Freeman et al 1999a).

Therefore, grafts derived from the human fetal FLVE have been preliminarily demonstrated to survive in an animal model of HD, without evidence of graft overgrowth. Graft size has been similar to the size of grafts observed in human nigral transplants (Kordower et al 1995). The largest graft was $7.4\,mm^3$. The lack of graft overgrowth can be attributed to several factors. Only the FLVE was transplanted, as compared to other studies that transplanted other adjacent regions found within the ventricular eminence. Special care was taken not to 'button-hole' (cut completely through) the underlying donor cortex and arachnoid layer when performing the deep cut of the dissection in order to prevent potentially fatal graft overgrowth (Freeman et al 1999b). Due to problems inherent with long-term immunosuppression, it was not possible to evaluate graft growth potential after 24 weeks. It will therefore not be possible to delineate the final growth potential of FLVE grafts until such transplants are performed in patients with HD. However, graft size was markedly less than the size of the normal rat striatum ($25\,mm^3$), the human striatum ($11\,960\,mm^3$; Harman & Carpenter 1950), or the human striatum in advanced HD, which is about 60% smaller than the normal striatum (Lange et al 1976). Graft-derived neuritic extensions projected to regions within the host striatum that are typically innervated by striatal GABAergic projection neurons, including the globus pallidus, substantia nigra and entopeduncular nucleus. A similar pattern of projections from ganglionic eminence grafts was described by Wictorin (1992).

At least four groups to date have reported initial clinical results of fetal transplantation for the treatment of HD (Molina et al 1990, Sramka et al 1990, 1992, Madrazo et al 1991, 1993a,b, 1995, Kurth et al 1996, Philpott et al 1997, Kopyov et al 1998a,b). The first of these operations were performed collaboratively in Cuba and Poland in 1990 (Molina et al 1990, Sramka et al 1990). The groups from Cuba, Poland and Mexico all utilized tissue derived from the entire ventricular eminence. Kopyov et al (1998a,b) and Peschanski et al (1995, 1996) have argued that utilization of the LVE is appropriate for use in the initiation of clinical trials even though further basic research may be necessary. Kopyov and colleagues (1998a,b, Kurth et al 1996) have initiated their clinical transplant program using the LVE as the source of donor material.

However, most other investigators have been reluctant to initiate transplant programs for the treatment of HD, because (1) human embryonic grafts have not previously been demonstrated to survive reliably (Wictorin 1992, Brundin et al 1996, Grasbon-Frodl et al 1997), (2) uncontrolled graft growth can occur (with grafts measuring up to $4\times8\,mm$ in primates) (Hantraye et al 1992, Wictorin 1992, Pakzaban et al 1993, Freeman et al 1995, Brundin et al 1996, Grasbon-Frodl et al 1996, 1997) and (3) human fetal striatal grafts have not resulted in P-zone values that reproduced the rodent or porcine anatomical findings necessary for functional recovery (Naimi et al 1995, Peschanski et al 1995, Brundin et al 1996, Grasbon-Frodl et al 1997).

This last issue has been the most significant obstacle in proceeding with clinical trials. As discussed above, Brundin and colleagues have estimated that at least 25% of graft volume must contain P-zones to produce graft-induced behavioural recovery, and at least 50% of the graft should be P-zone-positive for the recovery to reach normal levels (Nakao et al 1996, Brundin et al 1996). In this respect, it is noteworthy that no long-term clinical improvement has been reported following trials performed in Cuba, Poland and Mexico, where dissections of the striatum utilized combined MVE, LVE and the body of the ventricular eminence. These grafts were unlikely to have an adequate volume of P-zones.

We demonstrated a higher percentage of zones containing striatal markers within human striatal xenografts than in comparison to all previous studies that utilized human fetal donors. All grafts evaluated after 12 weeks following transplantation had greater than 37% of volume occupied by striatal tissue. Over 50% of some grafts contained striatal-like markers. We also demonstrated that striatal regions within grafts received tyrosine hydroxylase terminals derived from the host brain. These findings are similar to what has been observed in functional rodent striatal allograft models (Wictorin 1992, Campbell et al 1993, Dunnett & Svendsen 1993, Sirinathsinghiji et al 1993).

It is our impression that the transplants derived from the FLVE have several advantages in comparison to grafts that include additional components of the ventricular eminence, as utilized in all previous studies. Patches of striatal-like tissue within the grafts occupy more of the graft volume than in all previous reports. Graft overgrowth is unlikely to occur. Numerous striatal neuronal phenotypes are found within FLVE grafts, including both typical striatal projection- and interneurons (including ChAT-ir neurons), which leaves open the possibility that a full complement of striatal neurons may be found within grafts derived from such a limited dissection. Finally, elimination of the MVE removes the graft-derived pallidum as an alternative preferential target region for transplanted GABAergic neurons (Olsson et al 1995).

We believe it is now appropriate to investigate the use of FLVE transplants in patients with HD. Such grafts meet the important requirement for P-zone volume proposed by Peschanski et al (1995) and Brundin et al (1996) for the initiation of clinical trials. Furthermore, graft survival in patients with HD is likely. Similar neural allografts survive in patients with Parkinson's disease (Kordower et al 1995). Transplanted fetal tissue does not contain the abnormal gene found in HD. Patients with HD develop the disease in later stages of life, and the disease is therefore less likely to adversely influence fetal tissue. Grafts demonstrate both afferent and efferent projections within the host brain, providing the possibility for connectivity and prevention of second order degeneration in areas remote from the transplant site. HD is a fatal neurological disorder for which therapies are primarily palliative. There is accumulating evidence that fetal transplantation into the striatum in patients with PD is safe. It is therefore our impression that the risks, both known and unknown, of transplantation of human fetal FLVE tissue into patients with HD are reasonable with respect to potential benefits in this fatal disease.

Results from our clinical transplant programme, as well as autopsy evidence of graft survival in a patient with HD will be reported subsequently.

References

Anderson SA, Eisenstat DD, Shi L, Rubenstein JLR 1997 Interneuron migration from basal forebrain to neocortex: dependence on *Dlx* genes. Science 278:474–476

Armstrong E 1985 Allometric considerations of the adult mammalian brain, with special emphasis on primates. In: Jungers WL (ed): Size and scaling in primate biology. Plenum Press, New York, p 115–146

Brundin P, Fricker RA, Nakao N 1996 Paucity of P-zones in striatal grafts prohibit commencement of clinical trials in Huntington's disease. Neuroscience 71:895–897

Campbell K, Kalén P, Wictorin K, Lundberg C, Mandel RJ, Björklund A 1993 Characterization of GABA release from intrastriatal striatal transplants: dependence on host-derived afferents. Neuroscience 53:403–415

Campbell K, Wictorin K, Björklund A 1995a Neurotransmitter-related gene expression in intrastriatal striatal transplants. I. Phenotypical characterization of striatal and non-striatal graft regions. Neuroscience 64:17–33

Campbell K, Wictorin K, Björklund A 1995b Neurotransmitter-related gene expression in intrastriatal striatal transplants. II. Characterization of efferent projecting graft neurons. Neuroscience 64:35–47

Candy JM, Perry EK, Perry RH et al 1985 Evidence for the early prenatal development of cortical cholinergic afferents from the nucleus of Meynert in the human foetus. Neurosci Lett 61:91–95

Chen EY, Mufson EJ, Kordower JH 1996 TRK and p75 neurotrophin receptor systems in the developing human brain. J Comp Neurol 369:591–618

Deacon TW, Pakzaban P, Isacson O 1994a The lateral ganglionic eminence is the origin of cells committed to striatal phenotypes: neural transplantation and developmental evidence. Brain Res 668:211–219

Deacon TW, Pakzaban P, Burns LH, Dinsmore J, Isacson O 1994b Cytoarchitectonic development, axon–glia relationships, and long distance axon growth of porcine striatal xenografts in rats. Exp Neurol 130:151–167

de Carlos JA, Lfipez-Mascaraque LL, Valverde F 1996 Dynamics of cell migration from the lateral ganglionic eminence in the rat. J Neurosci 16:6146–6156

Deckel AW, Robinson RG, Coyle JT, Sanberg PR 1983 Reversal of long-term locomotor abnormalities in the kainic acid model of Huntington's disease by day 18 fetal striatal implants. Eur J Pharmacol 93:287–288

Dunnett SB, Svendsen CV 1993 Huntington's disease: animal models and transplantation repair. Curr Opin Neurobiol 3:790–796

Freeman TB, Sanberg PR, Isacson O 1995 Development of the human striatum: implications for fetal striatal transplantation in the treatment of Huntington's disease. Cell Transplant 4:539–545

Freeman TB, Randall TS, Othberg AI et al 1999a Transplantation of human fetal striatal tissue derived from the far lateral ventricular eminence in a xenograft model of Huntington's disease: anatomical studies. Exp Neurol, submitted

Freeman TB, Hauser RA, Sanberg PR 1999b Fatal transplant cyst. J Neurosurg 90:1148–1150

Grasbon-Frodl EM, Nakao N, Lindvall O, Brundin P 1996 Phenotypic development of the human embryonic striatal primordium: a study of cultured and grafted neurons from the lateral and medial ganglionic eminences. Neuroscience 73:171–183

Grasbon-Frodl EM, Nakao N, Lindvall O, Brundin P 1997 Developmental features of human striatal tissue transplanted in a rat model of Huntington's disease. Neurobiol Dis 3:299–311

Graybiel AM, Ragsdale CW Jr 1980 Clumping of acetylcholinesterase activity in the developing striatum of the human fetus and young infant. Proc Natl Acad Sci USA 77:1214–1218

Hantraye P, Riche D, Maziere M, Isacson O 1992 Intrastriatal transplantation of cross-species fetal striatal cells reduces abnormal movements in a primate model of Huntington's disease. Proc Natl Acad Sci USA 89:4187–4191

Harman PJ, Carpenter MB 1950 Volumetric comparisons of the basal ganglia of various primates including man. J Comp Neurol 93:125–137

Hersch SM, Ferrante RJ 1997 Neuropathology and pathophysiology of Huntington's disease. In: Watts RL, Koller WC (eds) Movement disorders: neurologic principles and practice. McGraw-Hill, New York, p 503–518

Isacson O, Dawbarn B, Brundin P, Gage FH, Emson PC, Björklund A 1987 Neural grafting in a rat model of Huntington's disease: striosomal-like organization of striatal grafts as revealed by acetylcholinesterase histochemistry and receptor autoradiography. Neuroscience 22:481–497

Kopyov OV, Jacques S, Kurth M et al 1998a Fetal transplantation in Huntington's disease; clinical studies. In: Freeman TB, Widner H (eds) Cell transplantation for neurological disorders: toward reconstruction of the human central nervous system. Humana Press, Totowa, NJ, p 95–134

Kopyov OV, Jacques S, Lieberman A, Duma CM, Eagle KS 1998b Safety of intrastriatal neurotransplantation for Huntington's disease patients. Exp Neurol 149:97–108

Kordower JH, Freeman TB, Snow BJ et al 1995 Neuropathologic evidence of graft survival and striatal reinnervation after the transplantation of fetal mesencephalic tissue in a patient with Parkinson's disease. N Engl J Med 332:1118–1124

Kostovic I 1986 Prenatal development of nucleus basalis complex and related fiber systems in man: a histochemical study. Neuroscience 17:1047–1077

Kurth MC, Kopyov O, Jacques DB 1996 Six month follow-up of motor function after fetal transplantation in a patient with Huntington's disease. Movement Disord 11:250

Lange H, Thörner G, Hopf A, Schröder KF 1976 Morphometric studies of the neuropathological changes in choreatic diseases. J Neurol Sci 28:401–425

Madrazo I, Franco-Bourland RE, Cuevas C et al 1991 Fetal neural grafting for the treatment of Huntington's disease (HD) — report of the first case. Soc Neurosci Abst 17: 902

Madrazo I, Cuevas C, Castrejon H et al 1993a The first homotopic fetal homograft of the striatum in the treatment of Huntington's disease. Gac Med Mex 129:109–117

Madrazo I, Franco-Bourland RE, Castrejon H et al 1993b Fetal striatal brain homografting in two patients with Huntington's disease. Soc Neurosci Abstr 19:864

Madrazo I, Franco-Bourland RE, Castrejon H, Cuevas C, Ostrosky-Solis F 1995 Fetal striatal homotransplantation for Huntington's disease: first two case reports. Neurol Res 17:312–315

Molina H, Sramka M, Alvarez L et al 1990 Neurotransplantation in Huntington's chorea. 9th Congress of the European Society for Stereotactic and Functional Neurosurgery, Marbella, Spain, Sept 1990, p 54–56 (abstr)

Naimi S, Jeny R, Hantraye P, Peschanski M, Riche D 1996 Ontogeny of human striatal DARPP-32 neurons in fetuses and following xenografting to the adult rat brain. Exp Neurol 137:15–25

Nakao N, Grasbon-Frodl EM, Widner H, Brundin P 1996 DARPP-32-rich zones in grafts of lateral ganglionic eminence govern the extent of functional recovery in skilled paw reaching in an animal model of Huntington's disease. Neuroscience 74:959–970

O'Rahilly R, Müller F 1994 The embryonic human brain: an atlas of developmental stages. Wiley-Liss, New York

Olsson M, Campbell K, Wictorin K, Björklund A 1995 Projection neurons in fetal striatal transplants are predominantly derived from the lateral ganglionic eminence. Neuroscience 69:1169–1182

Pakzaban P, Deacon TW, Burns LH, Isacson O 1993 Increased proportion of acetylcholinesterase-rich zones and improved morphological integration in host striatum of fetal grafts derived from the lateral but not the medial ganglionic eminence. Exp Brain Res 97:13–22

Peschanski M, Césaro P, Hantraye P 1995 Rationale for intrastriatal grafting of striatal neuroblasts in patients with Huntington's disease. Neuroscience 68:273–285

Peschanski M, Césaro P, Hantraye P 1996 What is needed versus what would be interesting to know before undertaking neural transplantation in patients with Huntington's disease. Neuroscience 71:899–900

Philpott LM, Kopyov OV, Lee A J et al 1997 Neuropsychological functioning following fetal striatal transplantation in Huntington's chorea: three case presentations. Cell Transplant 6:203–212

Pritzel M, Isacson O, Brundin P, Wiklund L, Björklund A 1986 Afferent and efferent connections of striatal grafts implanted into the ibotenic acid lesioned neostriatum in adult rats. Exp Brain Res 65:112–126

Pundt L, Kondoh T, Low WC 1994 Transplantation of human fetal striatal brain tissue from spontaneous abortuses into a rodent model of Huntington's disease. Cell Transplant 3:212

Pundt LL, Kondoh T, Conrad JA, Low WC 1996 Transplantation of human fetal striatum into a rodent model of Huntington's disease ameliorates locomotor deficits. Neurosci Res 24:415–420

Saji M, Reis D J 1987 Delayed transneuronal death of substantia nigra neurons prevented by gamma-aminobutyric acid agonist. Science 235:66–69

Sanberg RR, Koutouzis TK, Freeman TB, Cahill DW, Norman AB 1993 Behavioural effects of fetal neural transplants: relavence to Huntington's disease. Brain Res Bull 32:493–496

Sanberg RR, Borlongon CV, Freeman TB et al 1994 Transplantation of striatal human fetal tissue in excitotoxin model of Huntington's disease: neuroanatomical and behavioral effects. Soc Neurosci Abstr 20:470

Sanberg PR, Borlongan CV, Koutouzis TK, Norgren RB Jr, Cahill DW, Freeman TB 1997 Human fetal striatal transplantation in an excitotoxic lesioned model of Huntington's disease. Ann NY Acad Sci 831:452–460

Schmidt RH, Björklund A, Stenevi U 1981 Intracerebral grafting of dissociated CNS tissue suspensions: a new approach for neuronal transplantation to deep brain sites. Brain Res 218:347–356

Schultzberg M, Dunnett SB, Björklund A et al 1984 Dopamine and cholecystokinin immunoreactive neurons in mesencephalic grafts reinnervating the neostriatum: evidence for selective growth regulation. Neuroscience 12:17–32

Sirinaibinghji DJS, Heavens RP, Torres EM, Dunnett SB 1993 Cholecystokinin-dependent regulation of host dopamine inputs to striatal grafts. Neuroscience 53:651–663

Sramka M, Rattaj M, Vojtassak J, Rusnak I, Belan V, Ruzicky E 1990 Transplantation of embryonal tissue in treatment of Parkinson disease and Huntington's chorea. International Congress of Bioenergetical and Biological Medicine, SSPKN, Bratislava, p 39–40

Sramka M, Rattaj M, Molina H, Vojtassak J, Belan V, Ruzicky E 1992 Stereotactic technique and pathophysiological mechanisms of neurotransplantation in Huntington's chorea. Stereatact Funct Neurosurg 58:79–83

Töpper R, Gehrmann J, Schwarz M, Block F, Noth J, Kreutzberg GW 1993 Remote microglial activation in the quinolinic acid model of Huntington's disease. Exp Neurol 123:271–283

Wictorin K 1992 Anatomy and connectivity of intrastriatal striatal transplants. Prog Neurobiol 38:611–639

DISCUSSION

Price: An embryological question: I was slightly surprised that you had to go so lateral in the piece of tissue you take. My understanding is that what you have taken is the precursor of the amygdala.

Freeman: The amygdaloid nuclei almost entirely arise from the MGE (O'Rahilly & Müller 1994). We take just the lateral aspect of the LVE.

Price: The current embryological thinking is that this lateral bit of the ventricular zone are the cells that give rise to the amygdala. It is sort of an intermediate region: it isn't truly ganglionic eminence (Fernandez et al 1998).

Freeman: I agree that a minority of the precursors of the four amygdaloid nuclei are located in the medial eminence. I don't think it's going to be possible to select precisely a pure GABAergic cell line with any particular dissection. With the mesencephalic dissection, for example, the dopamine neurons are only 10% of a particular dissection on average. The bigger the dissection, the more non-specific the dissection is with the ventricular eminence, and so our goal was to make it as selective as possible. The regions that develop adjacent to the striatum in the LVE push the developing GABAergic neurons more laterally in the developing human brain than in the rodent brain. We tried a number of different variables to increase the P-zone percentage in human striatal grafts, and this is the one variable that seemed to help the most. Also, in serial sections from our autopsy study following striatal transportation in a patient with HD, areas where there were no P-zones contained primarily cells that stained for glial fibrillary acidic protein (GFAP). I think the dissection is therefore about as free of non-striatal cell types as is possible in our hands.

Isacson: Let me clarify a couple of issues in the autopsy work that we did on this case that Tom Freeman described. With regard to the dissection procedure, we find that in the pig and human, the embryonic LGE does contain all the striatal markers, including cholinergic ones.

The GFAP staining in the surviving grafts in human cases that you showed is actually normal in the developing cluster on neurons. What appears as high staining in the other regions, is actually developing striatum—more of the immature kind—and there are plenty of neurons in those regions too. We see exactly the same thing in developing pig tissue. In the patient, even at this 18 month time point, I believe that this striatum is still developing. What we are watching here is a dynamic process in which the implanted cells are still growing and integration is taking place with the host brain.

Dunnett: I think you need to be careful about emphasizing the *proportion* of P-zone: it might instead be the *amount* of P-zone or striatal tissue that is important. In our experience, when we dissect just LGE rather than whole ganglionic eminence, we get a higher proportion of P-zone but smaller grafts, and so there is less striatal tissue when estimated as total amount. Ultimately, we are probably going to have to address this as an empirical issue. I'm sure several groups here have been being looking at functional consequences of different dissections. In our experience it's not straightforward. We have done quite a number of experiments in which whole ganglionic eminence has been compared with just lateral (we haven't looked at far lateral), and on balance we get more consistent and extensive recovery with the whole ganglionic eminence than we do with LGE. This suggests that it is the total amount of P-zone tissue rather than the proportion that is important for mediating functional recovery.

Isacson: Might there not be a simple explanation for that? When we do co-grafting of LGE and substantia nigra in the Parkinson model, we get more dopamine tissue and better innervation because we provide a trophic support to trophic neurons via the target LGE tissue. When you use LGE and MGE, you get larger grafts, as you are actually transplanting a trophically dependent system rather than just a striatum. Regarding behavioural recovery, we know from previous work that co-grafting into the substantia nigra may also be better in the Parkinson model. I think we need to separate — even if is just for transient scientific purposes — the embryological developmental questions from the functional mechanisms at work in the HD models.

Dunnett: I don't think the two are directly comparable. When you co-graft a nigra and striatum in the nigral graft model, the target striatum tends to attract dopamine ingrowth and you may get less functional recovery than if you have a nigral graft alone. The issue which we are only beginning to address is whether cells in the MGE are influencing differentiation and the development of the LGE cells. It is clear that the majority of the medium spiny neurons are developing in the LGE. It also seems clear that if you co-graft LGE with MGE pieces, you get more striatal cells surviving in the co-graft. It looks like the medial parts that would normally develop adjacent actually are influencing the development of the LGE. Therefore I don't think we can assume that we will get the optimal functional recovery just by concentrating on the lateral dissection.

Freeman: We don't have any answers, but we have a lot of hypotheses. One of the working hypotheses before we started our clinical programme was that we were seeing evidence of ChAT-positive neurons in the FLVE grafts. This was one of our major concerns. Therefore, we felt it was reasonable to use a selective dissection, in that we would have a full complement of at least the important cholinergic interneurons within the striatum. Secondly, we wanted to avoid using the medial ventrivular eminence (MVE). Because the developing pallidum is found in the MVE, we did not want to provide an alternative target for the developing GABAergic neurons. We felt that the neurons would have preferential growth towards a developing pallidum as opposed to a diseased pallidum. Finally, even if greater benefit may occur with a non-selective dissection, we were not concerned as our primary goal with the immediate benefit of the graft. Our main aim was to obtain neuritic outgrowth in order to provide the opportunity to prevent second-order degeneration of regions that connect with the striatum. The disease progresses in such a clear-cut and fatal fashion, if we can't stop second-order degeneration, any benefit gained would only be transient.

Peschanski: We have also transplanted a series of five HD patients bilaterally (Bachoud-Lévi et al 2000) and we have used whole ganglionic eminence. This was a historical choice: when the first patient was going to be grafted in 1996, we decided that there was a lot of data with whole ganglionic eminence, and even though we knew that the neurons to give P-zones were in the LGE, we were unsure of the consequence of eliminating the MGE which had been used in hundreds of experiments before in animals. I'm not completely sure that this issue is solved. You have very nice anatomical data, but you don't have very nice physiological data yet. The experimental work still has to provide the real answer as to whether we need it or not.

There is one problem: we are not dealing any longer with fetuses of 6 or 7 weeks post-conception, but instead 8 or 9 weeks. When it comes to transplantation, this means that the striatum, as opposed to the ventral mesencephalon that we are using in Parkinson's, is very large. When you get the whole ganglionic eminence and try to stick it into the brain of the patient, if you have one 8-week-old fetus, it is possible. However, if you have two fetuses, you cannot transplant the entire thing. It is a matter of knowing whether it would be better to graft more striatal neurons, and then we would have to turn to the LGE because we cannot increase the number of striatal neurons if we don't do this.

Björklund: In the rat there is evidence from Kenny Campbell's work that MGE normally contributes interneurons to the striatum during development. It is possible, therefore, that the full complement of neurons in the striatal grafts may require both LGE and MGE tissue. An important issue is whether or not the effective part of the graft is just the projection neurons or if it is the collective output of a machinery that includes also the interneurons.

Freeman: What is your impression of the cholinergic neurons that we saw in both our xenografts and allografts?

Björklund: At the fetal age when you take your LGE tissue the precursors of the cholinergic interneurons may already have migrated from the MGE into the LGE.

I agree with Steve Dunnett that the best interpretation of the animal data is that it is the total size of the P-zones rather than the proportion of P-zone that is important for a functional effect. The combined LGE and MGE grafts seem to generate larger P-zones.

Do you have any idea of the total volume of your grafts in cubic millimetres?

Freeman: We haven't looked at each graft, but the one I demonstrated was about 7×2 mm.

Björklund: The normal human pallidum is about 4000 mm^3. What you say suggests that relative to the normal total number of P-zone cells, your grafts represent a small percentage.

Freeman: Likewise, with nigral grafts, the grafts present a very small percentage of the overall striatal volume. It is the connectivity issue which we have to count on, unless we're trying to reproduce an entire striatum in terms of volume. One of the big fears is graft overgrowth: the French group has started with a very small volume to prevent that problem from occurring. If one looks at the striatal grafts from the Los Angeles group, they are huge. Is the goal to re-create an entire striatum, or is it to make a small centres of striatal-like tissue with the appropriate outgrowth?

Björklund: Are they big enough to be seen with magnetic resonance imaging?

Freeman: In one or two of the patients we could see the grafts a year out.

Isacson: Let's clarify this question. About 1% of striatal neurons are cholinergic interneurons. We find in our grafts, like you do, there is about that number of cholinergic neurons in the LVE or LGE. If we look in the basal part of the MGE we find more cholinergic neurons there than in the normal caudate putamen. Consequently, Campbell's paper shows a huge increase in the cholinergic markers of LGE grafts when MGE is included (Olsson et al 1998). I don't think it is an appropriate interpretation to say that therefore cholinergic neurons from the striatum are in the MGE, since the MGE could also include extra-striatal cholinergic neurons (Pakzaban et al 1993, Deacon et al 1994).

Bjorklund: The cholinergic neurons appear to be generated in the MGE and then migrate into the LGE. The exact stage when the LGE tissue is taken may therefore be important: if the LGE tissue is taken after the precursors have entered LGE, the grafts may indeed contain a normal complement of cholinergic neurons.

Isacson: Secondly, the overgrowth, or rather the amount of tissue that grows from this HD patient's graft that we studied seems to fill 25% of the putamen. It looks from a structural point of view as being quite appropriate.

Freeman: We did a pilot experiment where we looked at the entire LGE versus the FLVE, and we labelled it with p75, which is a marker of the developing nucleus basalis. In the LGE grafts we saw a lot of p75 marker, whereas in the FLVE grafts we did not. It may be that nucleus basalis cholinergic neurons are some of the cholinergic phenotypes observed in grafts derived from either the LGE or the entire ganglionic eminence.

Perry: I wanted to ask about the secondary degeneration, which is clearly very marked in these patients. There is an old and rather unfashionable literature on transneuronal degenerative phenomena: the removal of a target leads to the loss of neurons synapses. This happens and is dramatic in primates and humans, but does not happen in rodents to the same extent. I was wondering whether in the transgenics with HD, anyone had studied the secondary degenerative phenomena there?

Dunnett: The cell loss in the R6/2 transgenic mouse strain (which is the only one that has been characterized at all, to my knowledge) is very little and very late. So this is not a good model of the human disease. Inclusion formation is a predominant feature of the pathology in the mouse, but there is very little cell loss until late on.

Freeman: But you are talking about primary cell loss there, not secondary.

Dunnett: That is looking throughout the brain, so it is not even primary cell loss.

Finsen: I would like to address the immunological issues. I was a bit concerned about the MHC class 2 expression you saw. I know MHC class 2 is not the only molecule required for a cell to present antigen to a naïve T cell. Have you tried to look with other markers, such as dendritic leukocytic markers?

Freeman: That is what we have looked with so far. With the human nigral transplants we have almost identical up-regulation of the HLA-DR marker, but the grafts were viable 18 months after transplantation without immuno-suppression for the last year. I showed the worst of the grafts: others had less marker expressed. There is clearly some up-regulation, but it is an aberrant immune rejection process if there is rejection in that these grafts—both nigral and striatal—still look very viable.

Perry: That is a good point, because you said that there was the same numbers of CD4 and CD8 T cells in the surrounding tissue as in the graft, whereas in the normal brain there are essentially no CD4 or CD8 T cells.

Freeman: These markers were seen in the penumbra around the graft, but not in areas remote from the graft.

Finsen: The simultaneous presence of HLA-DR-positive cells and CD4 and CD8 cells indicates that there is a fine balance in between graft survival and graft rejection. As these grafts do not undergo rejection, the infiltrating T cells could be immunosuppressive but they could also be looking for foreign antigen.

What is known about the number of amoeboid microglial cells in the human donor tissue? This is a situation where antigen presentation may have taken place, and this could be mediated by graft antigen-presenting cells which have escaped from the graft immediately after grafting. Does anyone know the composition of amoeboid microglia and macrophages in immature human brain tissue?

Peschanski: We have looked at that (Geny et al 1995). When you do a xenotransplantation to the rat, the proportion of macrophage-like cells (i.e. cells you can label with macrophage markers from human) is very small at first, and decreases all the time. The human graft in a rat host is invaded by microglial cells from the host that come into the graft, and there differentiate into ramified microglia. The human-like macrophage cells tend to disappear over time. The same is true with the endothelial cells. These tend to integrate into the vascular supply that essentially comes from the host (Geny et al 1994).

I don't think that the macrophages are going to be a problem in this kind of set-up. Fetal tissue does not contain the entire set of macrophages and microglia that are found later on in development. In the fetal tissues that we take, I think these cells are essentially perivascular cells and not microglia.

References

Bachoud-Lévi A-C, Bourdet C, Brugières P et al 2000 Safety and tolerability assessment of intrastriatal neural allografts in five patients with Huntington's disease. Exp Neurol 161:194–202

Deacon TW, Pakzaban P, Isacson O 1994 The lateral ganglionic eminence is the origin of cells committed to striatal phenotypes: neural transplantation and developmental evidence. Brain Res 668:211–219

Fernandez AS, Pieau C, Repérant J, Boncinelli E, Wassef M 1998 Expression of the *Emx-1* and *Dlx-1* homeobox genes defines three molecularly distinct domains in the telencephalon of mouse, chick, turtle and frog embryos: implications for the evolution of telencephalic subdivisions in amniotes. Development 125:2099–2111

Geny C, Naimi-Sadaoui S, Jeny R, Belkadi AM, Juliano SL, Peschanski M 1994 Long-term delayed vascularization of human neural transplants to the rat brain. J Neurosci 14:7553–7562

Geny C, Naimi-Sadaoui S, Belkadi AE, Jeny R, Kammoun M, Peschanski M 1995 Microglial chimaerism in human xenografts to the rat brain. Brain Res Bull 38:383–391

Olsson M, Björklund A, Campbell K 1998 Early specification of striatal projection neurons and interneuronal subtypes in the lateral and medial ganglionic eminence. Neuroscience 84:867–876

O'Rahilly R, Müller F 1994 The embryonic human brain: an atlas of developmental stages. Wiley-Liss, New York

Pakzaban P, Deacon TW, Burns LH, Isacson O 1993 Increased proportion of acetylcholinesterase-rich zones and improved morphological integration in host striatum of fetal grafts derived from the lateral but not the medial ganglionic eminence. Exp Brain Res 97:13–22

General discussion I

Prospects for fetal transplants

Gray: Tom Freeman earlier made a very provocative statement. His view is that the clinical work of applying fetal transplants from a fresh donor into a patient's brain is an important stepping stone or road map towards one or other of the novel techniques that we are also discussing at this meeting, but that it has no future on its own. Do we believe this? Have I expressed your view properly, Tom?

Freeman: Fetal transplants are certainly serving as a road map for future trials of novel cellular therapies. It may be too extreme to say that they have no potential, but I believe they only have limited potential.

Dunnett: It is worth clarifying that there is a strong and a weak form of Tom's hypothesis. The strong form, that I think everyone would agree with, is that we will need several fetuses per site for transplantation, which is the current situation. In this case, because of practical constraints, it is never going to be widely available. However, if improvements are made so that one donor will then be sufficient for one patient, I'm not so sure that fetal transplantation is automatically ruled out as a practical therapy, at least for the immediate future, in particular if it turns out to be more effective than any of the alternatives.

Peschanski: I agree. We also have to keep in mind that the major constraint is actually social. Potentially, there is a huge number of fetuses that could be available. In France there was a report stating that there were 220 000 elective abortions per year. Considering that there are 80 000 Parkinson's patients, out of whom some 20 000 would benefit from surgery, then within one year there would be sufficient fetuses to transplant these patients. The problem is that we lack the social organization to achieve this. Whether this problem is completely intractable or not, I don't know. Thinking about the situation with heart transplants, there is a logistic that is one or two orders of magnitude worse than that needed for fetal transplants. Despite this, heart transplants are done routinely. I think it is more a social problem than a scientific one.

If, however, we are talking about long-term prospects, I agree that fetal transplants are not the best hope. However, the best long-term prospect is not surgery or neural transplants or stem cells, it is preventive treatment: how can we stop people developing Parkinson's disease and Huntington's disease. With

Huntington's disease, we know exactly which patients will develop it in advance, so there are several decades during which we could make an intervention.

Isacson: The view that surgery will disappear altogether is incorrect. I don't think it is realistic to protect all the world's Parkinson's patients prior to signs of disease. Therefore cell transplantation of some form will likely be needed. Let us look at Huntington's disease. Even though we have neuroprotection data in our own experiments, I doubt whether one will be able to prevent Huntington's disease from occurring in all cases. If we delay the disease by 15 years, for example, we will still have a large number of patients who will need some form of repair. From this perspective, my guess is that we will still need cell transplantation in some form.

The work by Olle Lindvall and colleagues in Parkinson's patients shows what can be done currently with a non-optimal procedure. Even so, their positive results can be improved. In this regard, when we saw the first car being compared with the bicycle, many people wanted to stick with the bicycle, because it seemed safer and more reliable. Most of us in the field believe that there is a significant potential for development of transplantation science and technology. Stem cells directed to become specific transplantation cell types would allow better procedures and combined with improved surgical cell placements will permit a more complete repair.

Blakemore: For remyelination, where we are interested in transplanting just one particular cell, our history has been very similar to the experiences in neural transplantation. First we used bits of brain, but it has now become clear that we need large numbers of committed progenitors and the only way to get these is either from fetuses or by manipulating primary tissue. However, I am now sure that simply implanting stem cells is the way forward in our particular disease and I suspect it may be in neural transplantation also. One therefore has to go back and do the science that will allow us to commit cells to the required lineage and hope and pray that you only need one cell type to achieve repair.

Freeman: From the biotechnology point of view, very few companies are willing to take a position in any product that is based on human fetal tissue as the primary source. Few large pharma companies (as opposed to small biotech start-ups) will risk subjecting their entire product line to the ethics debates and financial exposure that would be associated with a fetal-based technology of a comparatively minor US$20 million product. Historically, small companies that have produced biologics that are based on human fetal technology never found large corporate collaborators. From this point of view I think that human fetal tissue transplants are a dead end.

Besides the procurement difficulties, regardless of the number of donors, the next problem is related to issues surrounding good manufacturing practices

(GMPs). There have been two autopsy cases where dissection methods were based on inexperience, and two patients have died due to graft overgrowth. There are certainly contamination issues which are a major problem, particularly once hundreds of centres become involved. Most neurosurgeons do not have GMPs available to them, nor do they want to learn what they are. From all these points of view, fetal tissue is fraught with problems.

Neurotransplantation in neurodegenerative disease: a survey of relevant issues in developmental neurobiology

Jack Price, Dafe Uwangho*, Scott Peters*, Diane Galloway* and Karen Mellodew*

*Institute of Psychiatry, De Crespigny Park, Denmark Hill, London SE5 8AF and *ReNeuron Limited, Europoint Centre, 5–11 Lavington Street, London SE1 0NZ, UK*

Abstract. Neural development and transplantation therapies in neurodegenerative disease share a particular feature. In both cases, undifferentiated neural precursor cells are required to differentiate into a range of neural cell types in a tissue-specific fashion. This similarity opens the possibility that the mechanisms that drive neural development play a similar role in CNS repair. In this chapter, two aspects of neural development are considered in terms of their relevance to CNS repair: the diversity of neural precursor cells and positional specification. We present evidence to suggest that neural stem cells have a degree of diversity that is beyond what might have been expected a priori. We also show that neural stem cells express genes that might encode a positional specification for these cells, and consider a number of hypotheses about the role of positional specification in CNS repair.

2000 Neural transplantation in neurodegenerative disease. Wiley, Chichester (Novartis Foundation Symposium 231) p 148–165

There is a sense in which neurotransplantation as a therapy for neurodegeneration is an attempt to recapitulate development. In both cases, undifferentiated neural precursor cells are required to generate neurons and glia appropriate to a particular brain region. They must do this by activating their own developmental potential in response to a set of particular cues in the tissue environment, and thereby arrive at an appropriate complement of neural cells. Of course, there are also profound differences between repair and development. The scale and cellular composition of the embryonic and adult brains are quite dissimilar. Development is a precisely orchestrated series of events, the outcome of one process setting the stage for the next. Brain damage is unpredictable and variable, and complicated by degeneration and inflammation. The developmental processes of migration, axon pathfinding, synaptogenesis follow specific cues and guides. These will have long disappeared from the adult brain to be replaced by a maze of tracts and processes.

So there are similarities and differences, but the similarities between the two processes are worth consideration for at least two reasons. First, we understand development better than we understand repair. Development is better studied. It also proceeds as a matter of course, whereas repair is difficult to engineer and is less predictable in its outcome. If development and repair have any processes in common, we may find the mechanisms already described for us by neuro-embryologists. Second, embryonic cells are plentiful and have some capacity to repair. Indeed, what little proof-of-concept there is in this area has mostly come from studies with embryonic cells. So if we are to understand how repair works, embryonic precursor cells are a reasonable place to start.

We could profitably examine a range of developmental processes, but in this chapter we will concentrate on two. First, what do we know about sub-populations of precursor cells that might be relevant to our study of neural stem cells? Second, is the issue of positional specification relevant to the process of repair?

Neural precursor cell subpopulations

All embryonic neural precursor cells are not the same. One way they differ is in their positional specification. We will return to this issue later, but suffice it to say that cortical precursor cells generate pyramidal cells; cerebellar precursor cells generate Purkinje cells. A second way in which precursor cells differ is their degree of specification. Some neural precursor cells appear to be determined to give rise to a single cell type. For example, cells can be identified late during retinal development that give rise only to rod photoreceptors. Others appear to be multipotential; that is able to give rise to the range of cell types that make up the brain (Turner & Cepko 1987). Multipotential precursor cells have been identified in the retina, cerebrum, tectum and a number of other structures (Turner & Cepko 1987, Grove et al 1993, Price & Thurlow 1988, Galileo et al 1990). Yet others seem to have a potential somewhere between the two. There is a precursor cell type in the embryonic cortex that generates just neurons and oligodendrocytes (Williams et al 1991). In the optic nerve, the precursor that generates oligodendrocytes can also generate astrocytes in culture, although it is unclear whether it ever does this *in vivo* (Raff 1989). Most of these designations are tentative because it is very difficult to be sure one has observed the full potential of a cell, and that it does not have other tricks up its sleeve. Moreover, very few convincing markers have been derived that distinguish these different precursor populations, which means that the only way to discover what a cell can do is by getting it to do it. This automatically means that the experiment cannot be repeated under different conditions to see if the cell would do anything different. Consequently, there is always uncertainty whether the cell that generates cell A in the first experiment is the 'same cell' that generates cell B in the second experiment.

These two parameters: positional specification and degree of determination must be linked, because the degree of determination varies between populations of precursor cells from different parts of the CNS. For example, multipotential precursor cells are relatively rare in the rodent cerebral cortex from about the midpoint of neurogenesis. Precise estimates differ — in our own studies about 5% of precursor cells appeared to be multipotential (Williams & Price 1995) — but apparently most cortical precursor cells become committed to the production of a single cell type. In the retina, most precursor cells seem to retain their multipotency right through the period of neurogenesis (Turner & Cepko 1987), but this does not mean that all retinal precursor cells are the same. Subpopulations can be isolated that differ from each other in the precise combination of retinal cell types they generate (Alexiades & Cepko 1997). The pattern of subpopulations was found to be complex and to change with developmental time but one population, for example, generates mostly horizontal cells and amacrine cells. Thus the potential of these precursor cells is restricted, but not to the generation of a single cell type, as is the case with the determined precursor cells considered above. Why retinal precursor cells should have evolved in this (to our eyes) strange fashion is unclear. There is presumably some advantage, but it must lie in some aspect of histogenesis that we do not currently understand.

The lesson that we learn from these studies of development is an important one for studies of transplantation. It is axiomatic in the field that multipotential precursor cells are what is required for repair, which is not to say that other approaches are not currently extant. But could there not be different populations of multipotential cells, some that repair and some that do not? In fact, our own studies support precisely this conclusion. We have studied a number of conditionally-immortalized neuroepithelial stem cell lines that were derived from the 'immortomouse' (Jat et al 1991). This transgenic mouse line carries a temperature-sensitive allele of the SV40 large T immortalizing oncogene (the tsA58 allele). Since the oncogene is inactive at normal body temperature (the non-permissive temperature), the mouse is viable and apparently normal. If cells are taken from immortomouse embryonic CNS, however, and grown at 33 °C (the permissive temperature), lines emerge that can be shown to be multipotential and retain this property for at least 60 passages. A range of such lines has been generated. In particular the 'MHP' lines were generated from a single preparation of embryonic day (E)14 hippocampus (Sinden et al 1997). One of these, MHP36, has attracted particular attention since it has the capacity to repair CNS damage. This has been demonstrated in a number of animal different models of disease (see Gray et al 2000, Hodges et al 2000, this volume.)

What of the other MHP lines? Two other lines have been studied in some detail, MHP15 and MHP3. In addition we have looked at a line, SVE10, which also came from the immortomouse, but from E10 telencephalon. All four lines are essentially indistinguishable if grown at permissive temperature. The cells are all nestin-positive. They have roughly the same morphology, growth characteristics and growth factor dependence (a requirement for fibroblast growth factor [FGF]2 and little else). They all appear to be multipotential. MHP36, MHP15 and SVE10 certainly are; the data on MHP3 are not yet complete. This can be shown in a number of ways, but the simplest is to plate them onto dissociated cultures of (normal) embryonic mouse cortex. The MHP cells differentiate to give neurons, astrocytes and oligodendrocytes.

None the less, these immortomouse lines are not identical. First, their patterns of gene expression are not the same. If the genes expressed by the four lines are visualized by differential display (DD), it is clear that no pair of lines is identical, but MHP3 and MHP36 are very similar and MHP15 and SVE10 are very similar (Fig. 1). The two pairs are, however, markedly different from each other. So while it is relatively difficult to identify a DD band differentially expressed between, say, MHP36 and MHP3, many bands distinguish MHP36 and MHP15. We find this a very surprising difference. That two apparently identical, multipotential cell lines, both isolated from the same tissue at the same stage, should have such wildly differing patterns of expression, is quite remarkable.

Clearly, we would like to know what this expression difference means for the cells. We are characterizing the genes that distinguish the pairs of lines, and we currently have eight that we have confirmed to be differentially expressed according to the pattern we have described. These sequences are under investigation. A more fundamental observation, however, is that there is a very strong correlation between the two expression patterns and the capacity to repair. MHP36 cells can repair CNS damage (Sinden et al 1997), and MHP3 cells share this capacity for the four-vessel occlusion (4VO) model of hippocampal damage, the only model in which this line has been tested. MHP15 cells do not have this capacity to repair 4VO damage, though they may have other capacities to repair that we have yet to discover. SVE10 cells have not yet been tested. So for the three lines tested there is a correlation: MHP36 and MHP3 are alike and repair; MHP15 is different and does not. It is tempting to conclude that we have discovered the molecular basis for the capacity to repair the hippocampus, but needless to say the numbers are small and the study is not yet complete.

Positional specification

A further difference between MHP lines emerged when we began to study homeobox genes. In order to set this into a developmental context let us first

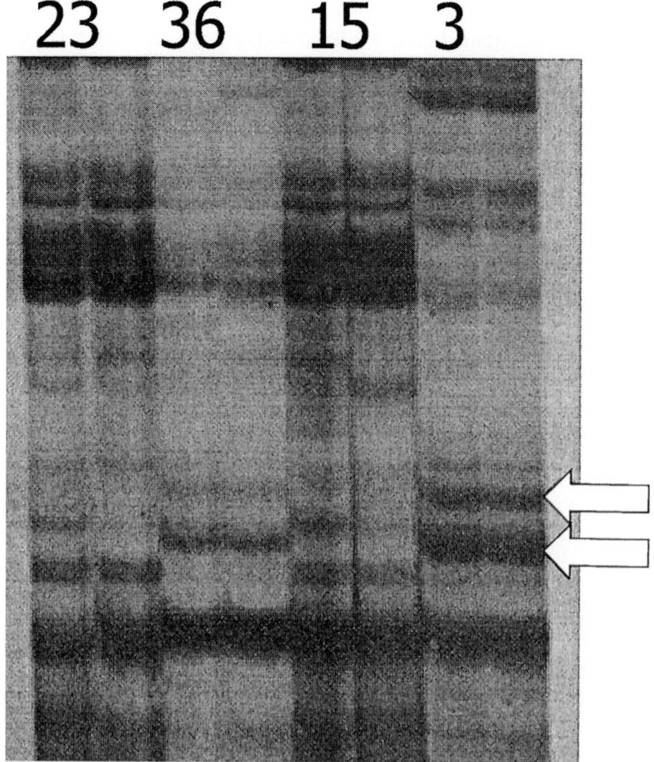

FIG. 1.   Part of a differential display gel comparing the genes expressed by three cell lines (SVE10 clone 23, MHP36, MHP15 and MHP3). The banding pattern of MHP36 and MHP3 are similar, as are those of SVE10 and MHP15, while the two pairs of lines differ from each other more markedly. Two bands indicated with arrows indicate bands shared by MHP36 and MHP3 that are not expressed by the other two lines.

consider the molecular basis of positional specification. There is now good evidence that a cell's positional specification is dictated by the pattern of homeobox genes (and other transcription factors) expressed by itself and its neighbours. By positional specification, we mean the tendency of a cell, or population of cells, to take on behaviours appropriate to their position in the embryo. Our understanding of how this works is by no means complete, but the involvement of homeobox genes is now unequivocal. Somehow, the members of this extended family of transcription factors drive the expression of downstream genes so that the cells behave in a fashion that results in histogenesis and differentiation appropriate to the cells' position.

Our best understanding of how this specification works is not in the forebrain (which is where the MHP lines come from), but in the hindbrain (Lumsden &

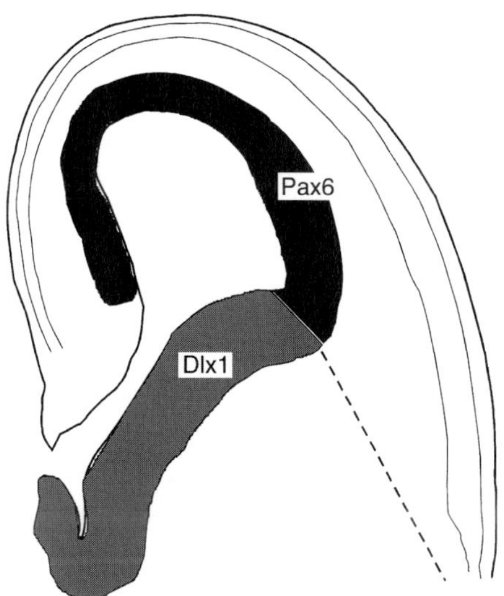

FIG. 2. Schematic of a coronal section through one cerebral hemisphere of an E15 mouse embryo. The shaded regions are the germinal areas (ventricular zones) of cortex (dark shading) and the ganglionic eminences (light shading). They are characterized by the expression of *Pax6* and *Dlx1*, respectively.

Krumlauf 1996) and the spinal cord (Lee & Jessell 1999). None the less, we now have some grasp of telencephalic positional specification (Rubenstein & Beachy 1998). The two genes that we need to concern ourselves with most for this discussion are *Pax6* and *Dlx1*, and their distribution is shown in Fig. 2. *Dlx1* is expressed in the ventral telencephalic anlage, the ganglionic eminences (Bulfone et al 1993). We know now that the pattern of migration of cells from this germinal region is complex and less restricted that was once thought (Pearlman et al 1998). None the less, essentially this is the piece of tissue that will give rise to the neurons and glia of the basal ganglia. Conversely, *Pax6* is expressed by the dorsal telencephalic anlage, the region that will generate the cerebral cortex (Stoykova & Gruss 1994). Both genes are expressed primarily by the cells of the ventricular zone (VZ), the germinal cells for each region. The expression patterns are reciprocal: cells one side of the boundary express one gene, while cells the other side express the other. Moreover, we have good reason to believe that these two genes are instrumental in establishing the character of the two tissue blocks; that is they are part of the mechanism that specifies position. In mice that carry null mutations in one or the other of these genes, the development of the appropriate part of the brain is compromised (Stoykova et al 1996, Anderson et al 1997). In *Pax6* mutants, the cortex is severely dysplasic. The pattern of cortical lamination is severely disrupted, and corticogenesis is massively disrupted. In *Dlx1* mutants,

TABLE 1   The expression pattern of three genes, *Pax6*, *Dlx1* and *Emx2*, in three cell lines grown at permissive temperature in the presence of FGF2

	MHP36	*MHP15*	*SVE10*
Pax6	−	+	+
Dlx1	+	+	+
Emx2	+	+	+

Expression was detected using reverse transcriptase PCR.

there is considerable disruption of the development of the striatal subventricular zone and in the differentiation of the striatal matrix neurons. Of course, these are not the only genes involved in the development of either of these two regions, and the interpretation of the mutants is complicated by the roles played by other genes. For example, there is a second gene, *Dlx2*, which is expressed similarly to *Dlx1* and can compensate for its loss of function (Anderson et al 1997). The important point, though, is that each gene is expressed in a particular domain, and is required for the normal positional specification of the tissue that is derived from that domain.

We have looked at the expression of homeobox genes in our MHP lines, and an interesting set of observations emerges (Table 1). First, the pattern of expression is generally what would be expected for hippocampal cells. Most of this data is not shown, but *Emx2* is given as an example in Table 1. During development, this gene is expressed by precursor cells across the cortical mantle (Gulisano et al 1996), and is indeed expressed by the three lines that we have tested, MHP36, MHP15, and SVE10. None the less, the pattern of expression in these lines of *Pax6* and *Dlx1* is not typical for hippocampus. The phenotype we expected is $Pax6^+Dlx^-$, but none of the lines express this pattern. Surprisingly, all the lines express *Dlx1*, which is not typical of hippocampus. The one gene with variable expression is *Pax6*. The line that repairs, MHP36, does not express *Pax6*, while those that do not repair do express this gene. We do not yet have the data for the other repairing line, MHP3.

How do these odd phenotypes arise? First we have to take seriously the possibility that the lines might not be truly hippocampal, but have arisen from some contaminating source of tissue. MHP36, for example, could be considered striatal with its $Pax6^-Dlx1^+$ phenotype, but the *Emx2* expression does not fit with that. The problem with this explanation is that the predominant phenotype $Pax6^+Dlx1^+$ is not typical for any recognized embryological region. We are currently studying the derivation of these phenotypes. The starting material— the primary hippocampal cells—is $Pax6^+$ and $Dlx1^-$ as would be expected, although we have not shown that every precursor cell is $Pax6^+$, and indeed we would not expect that to be the case. Our current hypothesis is that the atypical phenotypes arise as clones of immortalized stem cells emerge.

What might be the significance of positional specification genes for neural stem cells? The replacement of nerve cells lost as a consequence of disease poses an interesting problem for positional specification. As we have seen, embryonic precursor cells carry a positional specification. The data presented above indicate that neural stem cells express the genes that encode a positional specification, albeit that they express phenotypes not typical for embryological cells. How do the cells interpret that information during the process of repair? There appear to be three possibilities, each of which is supported to some extent by the data. The first is that neural stem cells do indeed carry a positional specification like that carried by embryonic precursor cells. This hypothesis predicts that each stem cell population can only generate the neural cell types appropriate to its specification. This may still leave a broad range of possible lineages open to a given stem cell population. None the less, it implies a restriction on the range of differentiated progeny that a particular line can generate, and therefore a restriction in the range of damage to which it could appropriately respond.

The second hypothesis is that neural stem cells carry a positional specification, but that it is plastic and can change in response to the tissue environment in which the cells find themselves. Thus any neural stem cell could respond to any CNS damage by changing its phenotype to fit the requirements. We know of no direct evidence to support this hypothesis, but it is consistent with two pieces of information. First, some lines—MHP lines and others—can repair damage in multiple sites of the CNS (Gray et al 1999). Second, some embryonic precursor cells show plasticity despite carrying a positional specification. There are several examples of this. Forebrain precursor cells can be respecified as hindbrain under certain circumstances (Martinez et al 1991). Dorsal telencephalic precursor cells can be respecified as ventral telencephalic precursors (Fishell 1997). The unresolved question is whether the pattern of expression of positional specification genes is changed following transplantation into an 'inappropriate' area of the brain.

A third hypothesis is that neural stem cells do not carry a positional specification at all. Rather these cells have the capacity to generate 'generic' neurons, which they do in response to any CNS damage. This hypothesis suggests that the positional gene expression observed in the MHP lines is irrelevant to their fate in the positional sense, and that might be thought unlikely. It is, however, supported by one piece of evidence. Gage and his colleagues transplanted a hippocampal stem cell line into embryonic retina and discovered that the cells integrated into the retinal tissue and differentiated appropriately as judged by morphological criteria (Takahashi et al 1998). None the less, the retinal cells they generated were lacking expression of key markers of retinal cell identity. A particularly pertinent example was the lack of opsin expression in the putative phtoreceptors. So although they looked the part, they were not functionally specialized retinal cells.

This appears to be an example of cells managing to make cells with neuronal properties — 'generic' neurons, if you will — but being unable to adopt the range of specialized properties required. Although a rod without rhodopsin is probably not much use, it is easy to imagine situations where a generic neuron might be better than nothing.

These three hypotheses are all currently open, but they are all testable. This seems to be an area that we need to pursue if we are to proceed with neural stem cell transplantation therapy.

Acknowledgement

This work was supported financially by the European Commission.

References

Alexiades MR, Cepko CL 1997 Subsets of retinal progenitors display temporally regulated and distinct biases in the fates of their progeny. Development 124:1119–1131

Anderson SA, Qiu M, Bulfone A et al 1997 Mutations of the homeobox genes *Dlx-1* and *Dlx-2* disrupt the striatal subventricular zone and differentiation of late born striatal neurons. Neuron 19:27–37

Bulfone A, Puelles L, Porteus MH, Frohman MA, Martin GR, Rubenstein JL 1993 Spatially restricted expression of *Dlx-1*, *Dlx-2 (Tes-1)*, *Gbx-2*, and *Wnt-3* in the embryonic day 12.5 mouse forebrain defines potential transverse and longitudinal segmental boundaries. J Neurosci 13:3155–3172

Fishell G 1997 Regionalization in the mammalian telencephalon. Curr Opin Neurobiol 7:62–69

Galileo DS, Gray GE, Owens GC, Majors J, Sanes JR 1990 Neurons and glia arise from a common progenitor in chicken optic tectum: demonstration with two retroviruses and cell type-specific antibodies. Proc Natl Acad Sci USA 87:458–462

Gray JA, Grigoryan G, Virley D, Patel S, Sinden JD, Hodges H 2000 Conditionally immortalized, multipotential and multifunctional neural stem cell lines as an approach to clinical transplantation. Cell Transplant 9:153–168

Grove EA, Williams BP, Li DQ, Hajihosseini M, Friedrich A, Price J 1993 Multiple restricted lineages in the embryonic rat cerebral cortex. Development 117:553–561

Gulisano M, Broccoli V, Pardini C, Boncinelli E 1996 *Emx1* and *Emx2* show different patterns of expression during proliferation and differentiation of the developing cerebral cortex in the mouse. Eur J Neurosci 8:1037–1050

Hodges H, Sowinski P, Virley D et al 2000 Functional reconstruction of the hippocampus: fetal versus conditionally immortal neuroepithelial stem cell grafts. In: Neural transplantation in neurodegenerative disease. Wiley, Chichester (Novartis Found Symp 231) p 53–69

Jat PS, Noble MD, Ataliotis P et al 1991 Direct derivation of conditionally immortal cell lines from an H-2K^b-tsA58 transgenic mouse. Proc Natl Acad Sci USA 88:5096–5100

Lee KJ, Jessell TM 1999 The specification of dorsal cell fates in the vertebrate central nervous system. Annu Rev Neurosci 22:261–294

Lumsden A, Krumlauf R 1996 Patterning the vertebrate neuraxis. Science 274:1109–1115

Martinez S, Wassef M, Alvarado-Mallart RM 1991 Induction of a mesencephalic phenotype in the 2-day-old chick prosencephalon is preceded by the early expression of the homeobox gene *en*. Neuron 6:971–981

Pearlman AL, Faust PL, Hatten ME, Brunstrom JE 1998 New directions for neuronal migration. Curr Opin Neurobiol 8:45–54
Price J, Thurlow L 1988 Cell lineage in the rat cerebral cortex: a study using retroviral-mediated gene transfer. Development 104:473–482
Raff MC 1989 Glial cell diversification in the rat optic nerve. Science 243:1450–1455
Rubenstein JL, Beachy PA 1998 Patterning of the embryonic forebrain. Curr Opin Neurobiol 8:18–26
Sinden JD, Rashid-Doubell F, Kershaw TR et al 1997 Recovery of spatial learning by grafts of a conditionally immortalized hippocampal neuroepithelial cell line into the ischaemia-lesioned hippocampus. Neuroscience 81:599–608
Stoykova A, Gruss P 1994 Roles of *Pax* genes in developing and adult brain as suggested by expression patterns. J Neurosci 14:1395–1412
Stoykova A, Fritsch R, Walther C, Gruss P 1996 Forebrain patterning defects in *Small eye* mutant mice. Development 122:3453–3465
Takahashi M, Palmer TD, Takahashi J, Gage FH 1998 Widespread integration and survival of adult-derived neural progenitor cells in the developing optic retina. Mol Cell Neurosci 12:340–348
Turner DL, Cepko CL 1987 A common progenitor for neurons and glia persists in rat retina late in development. Nature 328:131–136
Williams BP, Price J 1995 Evidence for multiple precursor cell types in the embryonic rat cerebral cortex. Neuron 14:1181–1188
Williams BP, Read J, Price J 1991 The generation of neurons and oligodendrocytes from a common precursor cell. Neuron 7:685–693

DISCUSSION

Bohn: The real question concerns whether the derivatives, such as the glial fibrillary acidic protein (GFAP)-expressing astrocytes or the neurofilament-expressing neurons, are composed of subpopulations that show differential display of genes themselves. It is possible that a precursor cell is not giving rise to two identical cells, even if both express a single marker gene. You are possibly giving rise to cells that would give a differential gene display pattern.

Price: So you are asking whether astrocytes, for example, from MHP36 are the same as the astrocytes from MHP15. I haven't looked at that, although it is a good experiment. I would be even more surprised if they were different. All we have looked at is the parent cells. What I can tell you is that the pattern of gene expression for the different lines is the same whether you grow at permissive or non-permissive temperatures, so it is not some artefact of the oncogene.

Blakemore: How did you do your differentiation assay, and can you alter the proportions of the different cells?

Price: We simply plate out a cortical or striatal culture. We can do this both with dissociated cultures or slice cultures. We then plate on the MHP line, and leave it for 10–14 days until we get terminal differentiation. Then we do conventional immunohistochemistry. We find that the results are very reproducible in terms of the proportion of each cell type in any given culture. They are also reproducibly different between different lines. The proportions for any particular line vary depending on the type of co-culture you use. If you plate MHP36 cells onto neonatal cortex rather than embryonic cortex, for example, you get more oligodendrocytes.

Blakemore: Can you induce it to flip totally towards one cell type?

Price: Not in these co-cultures, but we can treat cells on their own in a certain way to achieve this. We can get them to turn into exclusively oligodendrocytes, for instance, just by growing them at very low density.

Smith: The idea that you might have two different classes of progenitor cell is attractive. But it surely has to be equally possible that one or even both of these cell lines is just an *in vitro* artefact, not representing anything real.

Price: What do you mean by an *in vitro* artefact? That doesn't help me very much. I agree that this has arisen in a culture dish, but we still have to explain this distinction.

Smith: You are growing these cells out in culture, and you want to be clear that they are the same as cells *in vivo*.

Price: Hang on, I haven't made that leap.

Smith: You are arguing on the basis of marker expression that they could be representative of distinct progenitor cells *in vivo*.

Price: I put that forward as a hypothesis on the basis of the *Pax6* expression, but it is no more than a hypothesis.

Gray: How might that evidence be obtained?

Price: The hypothesis is that *Pax6* expression is the key: there are two populations to start with, and they expand to give the two types of cell line. Currently we are doing the experiment of separating the *Pax6*-positive cells from the negatives using a cell sorter. We can take these populations and do differential display or gain-of-function experiments, to extrapolate back to see if what I have suggested is indeed the case.

Smith: These are precisely the experiments that would be needed to show this. There are two different phenotypes in the cells that Jack Price islolates from these immortal lines. The question is, are they physiologically relevant? This is an important question if you then want to transplant these cells.

Price: I accept your point and we agree on the experiment that would need to be done to confirm my hypothesis. However, the important point is not whether these cells really are derived from two populations *in vivo*. For developmental biologists like us this may be of interest, but for this audience I would have thought that the importance is that there are two different stem cell phenotypes that apparently correlate with a capacity to repair. Whether we have generated these *de novo* in culture or not doesn't matter in this respect.

Smith: That depends on what is happening. You don't know what lesion might have happened to these cells in the process of establishing the culture. This is why the issue of the karyotype is so important.

Price: But remember these are still multipotential precursor cells that, both in culture and *in vivo*, differentiate to give neurons, astrocytes and oligodendrocytes. Even if they are a complete artefact and have lost a chromosome, for example, they would still be of interest with respect to what is the difference between them that correlates with their ability to repair.

Gage: I would agree that there is a distinction in terms of the value of the cells. One value would be as a transplantation tool, and the other is as a biological tool. We have no idea whether these cell lines represent an endogenous cell, because you haven't karyotyped the cells or mapped out any comparison between the cultured cells and the host cells. It is important to know this, because any information that you plan to learn about these cells as tools will be restricted to these cells if they are genetically different from an endogenous host cell. They may be viable for the clinical application, but the ability to extrapolate the information you gain from these cells to a general population would be limited. For this reason it will be important to determine through differential display just how different these cells are.

Price: It is difficult to prove that there is nothing wrong with something. We haven't done the karyotype, but these are cells that have been cultured extensively, so we could find that there are karyotypic differences between the lines. I wouldn't be surprised if that were the outcome. If one dismissed these cells as a consequence of that, to my mind that would be a mistake.

The more important experiment that we have to do is actually to generate more lines. We have currently only got the four that I described, and a few others in the freezer that we haven't studied yet. If it turns out that the vast majority of lines fall into one of these two categories, and let's say that it remains roughly a 50:50 split as we expand up to a dozen or so lines. This would argue that what we are describing here is real, in the sense that the lines are genuine. I would then be inclined to believe that it represented a stable viable phenotype, and not some oddity generated by the loss of a chromosome, for example.

Snyder: Karyotyping is obviously important, but it is also not the be-all and end-all. Rapidly dividing cells, even in the normal fetus, can transiently have abnormal karyotypes. For instance, in prenatal diagnosis with chorionic villus sampling it is well known that there are often karyotype abnormalities with no predictive value for the fetus. What Professor Gage is getting at, however, is crucial, and that is the definition of 'transformation' — i.e. at what point does a progenitor or stem cell become 'neoplastic'. It has been reported by us, now supported by multiple investigators, that human neural stem cells may be propagated by a variety of means (both epigenetic and genetic) that are equally safe and effective in yielding engraftable, migratory, responsive clones for multiple hosts. Genetically augmented expansion is not synonymous with 'transformation' as the term is rigorously used and defined by oncobiologists, nor is epigenetic manipulation or expansion of stem cells free from the concerns of becoming transformed. A short recitation of some of the criteria for proving that a cell is 'transformed'—or, more importantly, proving that it is *not* transformed by the absence of these criteria—are summarized on page 266.

Regarding phenotypic variations between ostensibly similar progenitor clones, do the expression pattern differences persist over time, or can these changes be dynamic? We have made the interesting observation that even with exactly the same clone, we can see differential expression of, for example, the spatial positional specifying genes *engrailed1* and *engrailed2*. Members of the same clone express *engrailed1* robustly while a sister cell expresses both 1 and 2, and this can fluctuate over time from passage to passage and still not predict or restrict the spatial integration of these cells following transplantation. Was what you were showing just a 'snapshot', so to speak, in the dynamic life of a given clone?

Price: We have only done one experiment related to that. We looked at passage 40 MHP36 cells compared with passage 60, and they gave the same expression pattern. However, these are both obviously quite late passage already. We haven't looked at really early passage and compared it with late passage.

Freeman: If one looks at a particular region in the subventricular zone over time, the same progenitor region produces numerous different cell types or nuclei. For example, the mesencephalic flexure produces the interpeduncular nucleus, nigral neurons and glial cells, depending on the timing. How closely have you looked at your temporal axis? Are these different gene expressions related to the time?

Price: All I can say is that one of those lines came from E10 material and the other three from E14. The E10 line fitted in with the other patterns, so it wasn't that the line from E10 had a different pattern to the ones that came from E14.

Gage: The other variable that might help with diversity would be using different conditions to amplify the cells initially. If you have used the same conditions to amplify the cells from the dissected tissue, there is some selection process there. Did you use FGF, epidermal growth factor or serum?

Sinden: None of the MHP cells saw serum, but the SV10 line did see a small amount at the beginning.

Gage: Was this an N2 medium with high FGF?

Sinden: 10 ng/ml FGF.

Gage: At one level you could say that the communality between the cells is not as surprising, given the fact that you might be using a condition that would select for a cell that would respond to this particular very defined medium. If you used different mitogens you might pull out a different population of cells with different characteristics.

Price: I accept that the selection procedure that we are using will have discriminated for certain populations and against others. However, the surprising thing about these cells is their difference, not their similarity.

Smith: But why is that surprising? T antigen can immortalize pretty much anything, and FGF is going to be a mitogen for pretty much anything.

Price: The reason I find it surprising is because as far as I can tell, these are all hippocampal precursors, and they are all multipotential. I would have expected them to be much more similar.

Gray: Is there a correlation between the ability of these cell lines to repair behavioural function and the extent to which they integrate into host brain tissue?

Price: I have addressed this as much as I can. We have a lot of data on the MHP36 cells: these clearly integrate, as Helen Hodges showed yesterday. We know much less about the other lines. The data we have on MHP15 suggest that there is a similar degree of integration in terms of cell survival and migration into the tissue.

Blakemore: It seems to me that it would be worth putting these cells back into embryos, because this would be a rapid assay to see whether you actually have different cells.

Price: Helen Hodges and I have discussed this and it is on our list of things to do. But if I think hard about that experiment, I ask myself what it will tell us.

Blakemore: It would only tell you something if the results are different.

Hodges: A follow up on what Jack Price was saying about making MHP36 cells *Pax*-positive Obviously, the first thing one would do would be to look to see whether they are still behaviourally effective. One could expect them to cease to repair behavioural deficits. A similar cross-over experiment could be done with the MHP15 cells. If they are made *Pax6*-negative they might become functionally effective.

Reier: I think some of this discussion raises considerations of what lessons have we learned from primary fetal tissue about carry over of developmental principles. If one reconstructs the life history of a graft, from anlage to the first hours and days after it is transplanted, then I think we would see a lot of carry over of developmental principles and mechanisms. In a simple-minded way it seems important to know what is going on in that situation, because the primary fetal grafts are an important template for the types of things we would hope to engineer ultimately by way of more defined cell populations. For example, we are looking at the floorplate and sonic hedgehog influences related to the maturation of fetal rat spinal cord transplants. Dr J. Velardo in my laboratory has shown that grafts of very basal E14 spinal cord have very different cytological features from those seen with transplants derived from extreme alar regions of fetal spinal cord (Velardo et al 1999). We can make a whole half of a spinal cord look like the superficial dorsal horn (substantia gelatinosa, myelin-free). It seems to me that there are some important principles we don't want to lose somewhere in all this.

Price: I'd make two points. First, the spinal cord results you have just cited are interesting. It goes without saying that those kinds of issues, about where signalling centres are (which is what the floorplate effectively is) need to be taken into consideration when one is thinking about grafting material. One of the problems is that we know much less about where those signalling centres are in relation to some of the material that is currently being grafted. There is evidence that sonic hedgehog can ventralize telencephalic structures (Kohtz et al 1998). If one takes material that is a source of these signalling molecules, they will have an effect on the host tissue.

Second, we will face a problem as we go from these undefined but none the less successful embryonic tissue grafts towards the kinds of cell lines I have described. We will have the advantage of using increasingly defined material, but we may discover that we have removed elements in the mixed cell population that contributed to our success.

Reier: I think there may be more to it than that. We have been transplanting E14 rat spinal cord tissue into various models of spinal cord injury. In an acute resection model, we found as part of an immunological study of transplantation that despite filling the cavity initially, only a vestige of the original graft could be found four days later, even where graft rejection was not an issue (Theele et al 1996). We looked more closely and found that there were little islands of immature neuroepithelial-like cells. I can't tell you their exact phenotype(s), because we are still examining this, but for all intents and purposes they are very germinal-looking. By E14 most of the ventral cord is developed, so what we are generating in the animal is a dorsal horn. We decided for other reasons that we would like to make these grafts more myelin-free, so on the basis of some work from Miller's laboratory (Warf et al 1991) we figured that we should take small areas of the cord near the floorplate region. When we did this we got a heavily myelinated graft, whereas if we take the extreme dorsal equivalent of that, you get essentially a substantia gelatinosa with very little myelin. In principle we have been transplanting the types of cells in an embryonic primary cell mixture that we talk about generating as an alternative to fetal tissue *per se*. As we look retrospectively at what we have been doing, there may be something in this whole thing that may have interesting molecular cues that tells us about what carries over developmentally and what is memorized by them. In lesion studies there are all kinds of things going on that you think would alter the program of these grafted cells, but obviously these programs are pretty well entrenched. Some of these cells are still on their way to making a dorsal horn, so they obviously have to be immature in that regard.

Dunnett: We have some direct evidence against that (Sinclair et al 1999). We have looked at dopamine cells in nigral grafts derived from E14 embryos. E14 is halfway through neurogenesis. A simple question to ask is: is it the cells that are already differentiated in the embryo that are surviving and contributing to the cell population that survives? Comparing a series of grafts where the donors were injected with BrdU prior to implantation, right up to 2 h prior to implantation, with separate animals that received standard grafts and then the host was labelled post-implantation, we saw that all the dopamine neurons surviving within the graft had differentiated prior to implantation. There were many neurons differentiating within the graft after implantation, but none of these exhibited a dopaminergic phenotype.

Gray: In Helen Hodges' paper she showed different features of the reconstitution of damaged tissue when she implanted fetal hippocampal tissue on the one hand, or the MHP36 cells on the other (Hodges et al 2000, this volume). This suggests that, although what Paul Reier has implied is true in some cases, it is not true in all.

Hodges: A lot must depend on the type of cell you take and your particular lesion model. For example, with 4VO ischaemia and loss of CA1 cells, we actually put in very late E18–19 fetal cells when they are already well differentiated, simply because of the need to dissect out the particular fields in the fetal hippocampus, which cannot be seen clearly before this age.

Björklund: Returning to the cell autonomous versus the extrinsic influences on cells after grafting: in the early transplantation work the ability of intact pieces of embryonic tissue to continue their normal development was thoroughly investigated. If the hippocampal primordium is taken at a stage when there is no dentate gyrus, and the pyramidal cells in the CA3/CA1 are starting to develop (i.e. E15/16 in the rat), and implanted into a cavity in the hippocampus, the tissue will continue to develop and forms a normal but smaller dentate with normal intrinsic connectivity. It looks a bit like an organotypic slice culture. When the architecture of the region is intact it can apparently continue its development and become quite complete with respect to internal organization and cell types. If the same tissue is dissociated and then injected into the hippocampus, the 3D organization is not retained and no dentate gyrus is formed. Interestingly, if the hippocampal tissue is taken out at an earlier stage, going back to E12/13, and grafted as a tissue piece in a well-organized hippocampus–dentate gyrus will not develop. The tissue will grow excessively and in a more disorganized manner. The take home message from these studies is that it is important to consider the stages that cells and neuronal subtypes go through during normal brain development. In critical stages of development, interactions between the cellular elements are probably very important. Mesencephalic dopamine neurons, for example, will develop and grow well after grafting if they are taken after the time point when they have irreversibly differentiated. These differentiated neuroblasts or young postmitotic neurons are then genuinely cell autonomous in what they do. If they are taken earlier, the interaction with other cells has not finished, and they may still need cross-talk with other cells in order to be able to progress through the later stages of differentiation. The earlier you take the primordial tissue, therefore, the more complex the interactions are likely to be. This is a challenge to any stem cell approach: the adult brain, as Jack Price pointed out, may lack at least some of the essential features of the embryonic environment, where extrinsic signalling and cell–cell interactions are both time- and position-dependent. We obviously need to learn more about these developmental mechanisms.

Isacson: The same also holds true for the striatum. E14 rat lateral ganglionic eminence when transplanted into the striatum region will develop into striatum in the same way as it will if you transplant it into the substantia nigra region. In response to what Paul Reier said, however, there is a point when you actually just see a string of surviving cells after one week post-transplantation. When you look at it fully developed, the cell commitment is very evident. We need also to think what trophic stage the cells are in, too. When you have an irreversible cell commitment, the growth and development of transplanted neurons seems to follow highly cell autonomous rules.

Sinden: Picking up on what Anders Björklund was saying, there is obviously a big difference between embryo and adult, but also we know very little about the damaged adult and what is going on there in terms of signalling.

For those of us making multipotential cells with extended self-renewal capacities (in other words, stem cells) for the purposes of transplantation, an important issue is whether or not we differentiate these cells prior to grafting. We put in undifferentiated cells after we have switched off the oncogene.

Olson: I also wanted to mention some experiments we did a long time ago in which we grafted tissues to the anterior chamber of the eye, and which addresses some of the issues raised in this discussion. The advantage with this experiment is that you can see the graft and follow its growth. After grafting a small piece of embryonic CNS tissue to the eye chamber, there is a small dip in volume before the graft becomes vascularized, but this is only a small dip. This suggests that growth is dependent on the survival of cells that came with grafting, rather than only on proliferation of stem cells.

Certain areas of the brain are highly dependent on contact with other areas for normal development to occur, others are not. For instance, if you transplant embryonic hippocampus or cerebellum, they have a built-in programme that will make them develop surprisingly normally even in the anterior chamber of the eye, in which the only part of the nervous system they see is the innervation of the host iris. There seems to be an intrinsic programme for their development. In contrast, if you transplant the cerebral cortex, it appears to be totally dependent on input for normal development. When it is placed alone in the eye chamber it doesn't do very well. However, if you transplant it to an eye that already carries another transplant from an area that normally provides input to cortex, it will do much better.

Gage: If we talk about committed cells being required, Steve Dunnett's experiment with dopaminergic neurons is very relevant. However, a necessary follow-up to that experiment would be to eliminate the proliferating cells, to show that the committed cells are not only necessary, but in themselves they are sufficient and that you don't need a background of proliferating cells that could act as a substrate or support cells. It may not be an either/or situation; the primitive uncommitted cells might give an important baseline. It would be interesting to see what would happen if you just grafted the pure committed population, having eliminated the proliferating cells.

Price: There are probably two different ways to repair. The observations presented here indicate that the immediately committed population is the element in the tissue grafts that is mediating repair. None the less, it is also evident that stem cells do work. It is probably the case that they are working in different ways.

References

Hodges H, Sowinski P, Virley D et al 2000 Functional reconstruction of the hippocampus: fetal versus conditionally immortal neuroepithelial stem cell grafts. In: Neural transplantation in neurodegenerative disease. Wiley, Chichester (Novartis Foundation Symposium 231) p 53–69

Kohtz JD, Baker DP, Corte G, Fishell G 1998 Regionalization within the mammalian telencephalon is mediated by changes in responsiveness to sonic hedgehog. Development 125:5079–5089

Sinclair SR, Fawcett JW, Dunnett SB 1999 Dopamine cells in nigral grafts differentiate prior to implantation. Eur J Neurosci 11:4341–4348

Theele DP, Schrimsher GW, Reier PJ 1996 Comparison of the growth and fate of fetal spinal iso- and allografts in the adult injured rat spinal cord. Exp Neurol 142:128–143

Velardo MJ, O'Steen BE, Reier PJ 1999 Regional differentiation of dorsal and ventral fetal spinal cord (FSC) transplants into adult rat spinal cord. Soc Neurosci Abstr 24

Warf BC, Fok-Seang J, Miller RH 1991 Evidence for the ventral origin of oligodendrocyte precursors in the rat spinal cord. J Neurosci 11:2477–2488

Molecular and cellular mechanisms in immune rejection of intracerebral neural transplants

Thomas Brevig*†, Erik Bo Pedersen* and Bente Finsen*[1]

*Department of Anatomy and Neurobiology, University of Southern Denmark–Odense University, and †Department of Clinical Immunology, Odense University Hospital, DK-5000 Odense C, Denmark

Abstract. Restorative transplantation of human embryonic nigral tissue for Parkinson's disease has given encouraging results with functional benefit and minimal signs of rejection in patients receiving standard immunosuppression. Due to the limited availability of human donor material and ethical concerns with its use, porcine tissue is considered an appropriate alternative. In animal studies, neural allo- and xenografts are usually rejected in the brain, emphasizing the necessity of understanding factors underlying survival and rejection of intracerebral neural transplants. Here, we review fundamental mechanisms of allo- and xenograft rejection, and discuss the privileged immune status of the brain, and how we may take advantage of this in order to improve and secure graft survival. Rejection of neural xenografts is expected to be of a cellular nature, like neural allograft rejection, but may also display unique features, and cannot be dealt with using conventional immunosuppressive therapies. The challenge therefore is to improve existing and design new strategies that allow permanent survival of histoincompatible neural grafts, taking advantage of the special immune status of adult CNS and immature donor brain tissue.

2000 Neural transplantation in neurodegenerative disease. Wiley, Chichester (Novartis Foundation Symposium 231) p 166–183

Clinical transplantation of embryonic human (Bachoud-Levi et al 2000, Freeman et al 1995a, Lindvall et al 1994, Peschanski et al 1994) or porcine (Friedrich 1999) neural tissue to patients suffering from neurodegenerative disorders highlight the question of how to secure long-term survival of allo- and xenogeneic neural tissue grafts in the brain. Preliminary results suggest that permanent survival and integration of allogeneic neural tissue may be achieved with temporary triple

---

[1]This chapter was presented at the symposium by Professor Finsen, to whom correspondence should be addressed.

immunosuppression, using cyclosporin, steroids and azathioprine (Lindvall et al 1994, Widner et al 1992, Pechanski et al 1994), and possibly with cyclosporin monotherapy (Freemann et al 1995a, Kopyov et al 1996, Spencer et al 1992). However, demonstration of T cell and macrophage infiltration and major histocompatibility complex (MHC) class II-antigen expression in well-established allografts in two patients in whom cyclosporin was withdrawn about 12 months prior to autopsy (Kordower et al 1997), and occurrence of graft regression in other patients who had cyclosporin withdrawn (Lopez-Lozano et al 1997), calls for caution. Such observations are consistent with animal studies, where histoincompatible neural transplants are prone to rejection in the CNS of immunocompetent recipients, although, quoting Barker & Billingham (1977), it usually happens in 'a delayed manner as compared to transplants of the same tissue placed in extracerebral, non-immune privileged sites'. Taken together with the observation that well-established intracerebral grafts are acutely rejected after peripheral sensitization (Lund et al 1988, Mason et al 1986), this suggests that the immune-privileged state of intracerebral transplants depends on inadequate presentation of donor antigens to the host immune system, and human allografts are therefore likely to be at continuous risk of being rejected. The immunology is far more complex in the case of porcine neural xenografts, which are rejected despite continuous cyclosporin treatment following transplantation into the human brain (Deacon et al 1997).

Principles of transplant rejection

The initial event in transplant rejection is the presentation of donor antigens to host T lymphocytes in peripheral lymphoid organs. Recognition of donor MHC antigens on donor antigen presenting cells (APCs) (direct pathway) or peptides from donor MHC or minor histocompatibility antigens presented by host dendritic cells (indirect pathway) leads to activation of naïve T cells (Fig. 1). Once activated, CD8 T cells lyse graft cells with MHC class I on their surface, either by secretion of perforin and granzyme B or through Fas-mediated induction of apoptosis. Activated CD4 T cells turn into helper cells, helping CD8 T cells in their activation, or inflammatory cells, activating macrophages in the graft to start a delayed-type hypersensitivity-like response, in which graft cells are thought to succumb to direct effects of toxic molecules such as tumour necrosis factor, nitric oxide, proteases and free radicals.

In allotransplantation and in most types of xenotransplantation, both direct and indirect recognition of antigen takes place (Fig. 1), but the relative contribution of indirect recognition increases the greater the species disparity (Auchincloss & Sachs 1998, Gill & Wolf 1995). The immune system is extremely efficient in mediating graft destruction, irrespective of the pathway of antigen recognition.

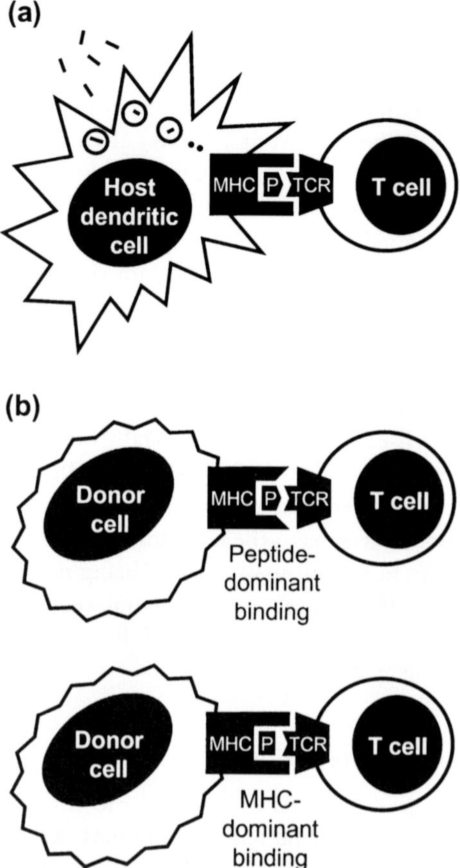

FIG. 1.   Indirect and direct pathways of antigen recognition by T cells. In the spleen and draining lymph nodes, antigens from intracerebral grafts are recognized via two distinct pathways or mechanisms: (a) an *indirect pathway* in which cell debris and shed molecules are endocytosed, processed and presented in the context of host MHC class I and II molecules by host dendritic cells (CD4 T cells recognize donor peptides bound to MHC class II, while CD8 T cells recognize donor peptides bound to MHC class I), and (b) a *direct pathway* in which donor MHC class I and II antigens on viable donor cells, e.g. microglia, are recognized by host CD8 and CD4 T cells, respectively. Direct recognition may come about in two ways, either with peptide or MHC contributing more to the strength of the binding. When both antigen (MHC and peptide) and co-stimulatory molecules, particularly CD40 and B7 (not shown), have been recognized, the T cell starts a proliferative response resulting in a clone of effector cells and memory cells (not shown). While direct antigen recognition only occurs following transplantation, indirect antigen recognition is the normal way in which invading microorganisms are recognized by the immune system. In xenotransplantation, the relative importance of indirect and direct antigen recognition by T cells depends on the phylogenetic disparity between host and donor species. MHC, major histocompatibility complex; P, peptide; TCR, T cell receptor.

On top of these cellular mechanisms, the humoral immune response may contribute to rejection by means of complement activation, opsonization of T cell antigens and antibody-dependent cellular cytotoxicity.

The α-galactosyl epitope (Galα1,3Galβ1,4GlcNAc-R), the major xenoantigen against which humans and other Old World primates have natural antibodies, is expressed by many cell types in the pig (Galili 1993), including microglia and endothelial cells in embryonic and adult brain (E. B. Pedersen & D. Møller, unpublished work, Sumitran et al 1999). In organ xenotransplantation, binding of host natural antibodies to graft endothelium activates the complement system, and since porcine complement regulatory proteins cannot efficiently inhibit human complement activation, the endothelial cells lyse or retract from one another, triggering platelet aggregation, microthrombi formation and graft rejection within minutes to hours (hyperacute rejection). Grafts derived from dissociated neural tissue contain only few donor endothelial cells and these are not, at least initially, arranged in vessels upon which the grafts depend to receive oxygen and nutrients. Consequently, these grafts do not undergo hyperacute rejection.

The immune privilege of the brain

CNS function depends on a stable microenvironment, which is secured by a highly specialized anatomical and histological organization. This also affords the CNS with a privileged immune status, which traditionally has been attributed to: (i) the lack of conventional lymphatics (Medawar 1948), (ii) the presence of a blood–brain barrier (BBB) (Björklund et al 1982), (iii) the lack of dendritic cells (Hart & Fabre 1981), and (iv) the fact that brain tissue in itself presents an immuno-suppressive environment (Bechmann et al 1999, Streilein 1993). Although devoid of conventional lymphatics, functional drainage routes from the CNS exist, enabling passage of cells and soluble antigens to regional lymph nodes and spleen (Broadwell et al 1994, Oehmichen et al 1979, Widner et al 1988).

The BBB excludes humoral immune factors and naïve, but not activated T cells from the brain parenchyma (Wekerle et al 1986). The BBB is broken at the time of grafting, and remains leaky for as long as infiltrating immune cells are present within the transplant (Finsen et al 1991). Consistent with the situation following grafting of syngeneic tissue, where the inflammatory response is of short duration and virtually without involvement of T cells, the BBB heals after a few days, provided that the host is efficiently immunosuppressed (Pedersen et al 1997a). This suggests that the BBB leakage observed in association with histo-incompatible neural transplants is the result rather than the cause of ongoing immune rejection, and emphazises the importance of avoiding antigen presentation and T cell infiltration.

Although the brain parenchyma has no dendritic cells (Hart & Fabre 1981), MHC class II-positive macrophages are abundant in the meninges, ependyma, choroid plexus (Matyszak et al 1992) and BBB-free circumventricular organs (Pedersen et al 1997b). These findings are consistent with those of Sloan et al (1990), that intraventricular transplants are rejected faster than intraparenchymal grafts, as well as with our finding that hippocampal xenografts survive longer after grafting into the striatum than into the hippocampal formation, in the latter location encroaching on the ventricles and/or the pial membrane (Pedersen 1997).

Mechanisms of neural graft rejection in the brain

Neural allograft rejection may be completed over a few weeks in rodents, or be delayed by weeks or even months, depending on the degree and type of histoincompatibility (Mason et al 1986, Sloan et al 1990). Incompatibility of several minor histocompatibility loci can elicit as strong rejection responses as disparity across MHC class I and/or II loci (Mason et al 1986). In immunocompetent rat hosts, murine xenografts are usually rejected within 5–8 weeks when grafted to the hippocampal formation (Finsen et al 1991). There has been no direct comparison of the relative contribution of T cells and macrophages to the cellular infiltrate in neural allo- and xenografts. Our studies have shown that the infiltrate in xenografts largely consists of macrophages and T cells, while B cells are present in very low numbers (Finsen et al 1991, Pedersen et al 1997a). Furthermore, it has been shown that host dendritic cells infiltrate intracerebral neural transplants during the course of rejection along with infiltrating macrophages and T cells (Lawrence et al 1990). As for allografts undergoing rejection, both CD8 and CD4 T cells are numerous (Nicholas et al 1987). Lymphocyte depletion studies have shown that CD4 T cells are necessary for rejection of neutral allografts (Nicholas et al 1990) and xenografts (Wood et al 1996).

Younger donor tissue does better when grafted into the CNS. This was first shown in mouse-to-rat xenotransplant studies (Zimmer et al 1988), and was later confirmed in human-to-rat studies (Freeman et al 1995b). One significant difference between very young embryonic and perinatal brain tissue is the low number or lack of microglial precursor cells in the young tissue (Dalmau et al 1997), thus attracting attention to this cell type as a potential APC. This hypothesis is supported by the ability of microglial precursor cells to express MHC antigens and co-stimulatory molecules in culture (De Simone et al 1995, Frei et al 1987), and the observation that the same type of microglia can stimulate naïve T cells (Frei et al 1987). Interestingly, similar observations have been made for porcine microglial precursor cells and human T cells (Brevig et al 1999). In combination with the existence of functional lymphatic drainage routes from the brain (Broadwell et al

1994, Oehmichen et al 1979, Widner et al 1988), these findings raise the possibility that the variable outcome in animal experiments, and possibly also in clinical neural transplantation, may be attributed to a variable content of microglial precursor cells in the donor tissue, most likely in combination with the effect of using different transplantation techniques and recipient sites.

The ability of neurons to express MHC class I antigens, and thereby be targets for cytotoxic T cells, is a matter of dispute. Although interferon (IFN)-γ-treated neurons can express MHC class I antigens *in vitro* (Neumann et al 1997), careful immunohistochemical analysis has not shown induction of MHC class I antigens on transplanted murine hippocampal neurons (Pedersen et al 1997a), although this type of graft is densely infiltrated with IFN-γ-expressing T cells (Pedersen 1997). These data are consistent not only with the xenograft studies by Zimmer et al (1988), but also with studies by Bartlett et al (1990), showing increased survival of allografts consisting of neuronal precursor cells selected on the basis of lack of MHC class I-antigen expression after culture with IFN-γ. Interestingly, Batten et al (1996) have shown that human IFN-γ does not work across the species barrier to pig, suggesting that neurons in pig-to-human neural xenografts are, in any case, not induced to express MHC class I antigens by T cell-derived IFN-γ.

Stability of intracerebral neural grafts

Like other types of grafts, neural allo- and xenografts are depleted of APCs over time, and repopulated with host APCs (Finsen et al 1997, Pedersen et al 1997a, Perry & Lund 1989). Donor antigens will, therefore, eventually be presented exclusively by the indirect pathway. In the normal CNS, the turnover of microglia is slow (Lawson et al 1992), and new microglial cells arise from proliferation of existing microglia *in situ*, or from bone marrow-derived cells entering the CNS from the circulation. In case of injury or other types of neurodegenerative phenomena, resting microglia become activated, proliferate and express MHC antigens and co-stimulatory molecules (Finsen et al 1996). Although never shown, it seems likely that some of these newly generated and strongly activated microglial cells might migrate to and present antigen in the draining lymph nodes. Interestingly, anterograde axonal and synaptic degeneration, which usually is considered a minor type of injury, has been shown to be sufficient to induce rejection of well-established neural xenografts (Lund et al 1988). The unpredictability of the outcome of neurodegenerative stimuli should, however, be emphasized. One of the earliest molecules to be induced in microglia along with MHC class I antigen is anti-inflammatory cytokine transforming growth factor β1, which remains expressed until the microglial cells return to their resting state days to weeks after the injury (Finsen et al 1996, Lehrmann et al 1998). The possibility, therefore, exists that different types of injury and degenerative changes may induce different levels of microglial activation and capacity to present antigen to T cells in the draining lymph nodes or already present in the graft (Kordower et al 1997).

Strategies to overcome neural xenograft rejection

In pig-to-human neural xenotransplantation, the role of antibodies, complement and natural killer cells is largely unknown, and T cells are generally thought to be sufficient for graft destruction. It is, therefore, of immense importance that non-T cell-mediated responses are investigated and that strategies to overcome the T cell response are developed. Cyclosporin, which effectively inhibits T cell alloreactivity, has been shown to be insufficient in xenotransplantation. In rats, cyclosporin monotherapy cannot maintain neural xenografts (Pedersen et al 1997a). A post-mortem histological analysis of a Parkinson patient that had received porcine embryonic neural grafts about 8 months earlier and been continuously immunosuppressed with cyclosporin since, showed low T cell reactivity in direct proximity to grafts of poor survival (Deacon et al 1997). The presence of T cells, even in small numbers, suggests that porcine embryonic neural tissue induces a T cell response also in patients treated with cyclosporin. In the clinical setting, the immunosuppression must therefore be more aggressive, which may lead to serious side effects, or supplemented with other strategies inhibiting or preventing the host T cell response. A non-exhaustive list of

TABLE 1   Strategies to overcome cellular immune rejection of porcine neural xenografts in humans

---

Donor manipulations

Pure-breeding of low-immunogenic strain

Genetical manipulation
    Transgenics
    Knockouts

Pretreatment of donor tissue
    Cell-subset depletion
    Antigen masking
    Encapsulation
    Cografts of testis-derived Sertoli cells

Recipient manipulations

Immunosuppression

Induction of tolerance
    Non-ablative T cell therapy
    Haematopoietic chimerism

---

potential strategies to overcome the T cell response is given in Table 1. Only a few of these strategies have been tested in neural xenotransplantation.

A low-immunogenic strain of pigs could serve as a universal donor for xenotransplantation, but has not been found. Introduction of human genes into the pig germline has been accomplished (Cozzi & White 1995), but so far no transgenic pig has been produced to give tissues tolerated by human T cells. Embryonic stem cells are not available for the pig, and knockouts are thus not an option yet. However, production of a knockout donor by nuclear transfer does not require embryonic stem cells, and may solve this problem in the near future (Wolf et al 1998). Masking of MHC class I antigens on porcine embryonic brain cells by divalent antigen-binding fragments of antibodies enhances survival after transplantation into rat brain, but is less effective than cyclosporin treatment, particularly in terms of graft volume (Pakzaban et al 1995). Encapsulation of the donor cells can effectively isolate grafts from the immune system of the host, but so far at the expense of making axon outgrowth and innervation of host brain impossible (Emerich et al 1992). Cografting of testis-derived Sertoli cells, which secrete immunosuppressive factors, such as Fas ligand, improves the survival of bovine adrenal chromaffin cells in rat brain (Sanberg et al 1996). Induction of immunological tolerance, i.e. antigen-specific non-responsiveness, to xenogeneic cells may be possible in humans in the future, e.g. by short-term blocking of T cell costimulation pathways by antibodies (Elwood et al 1998), or by making the recipient a human/pig haematopoietic chimera prior to transplantation (Auchincloss & Sachs 1998).

We have taken the approach of depleting the donor tissue of APCs. However, because MHC antigens are not expressed in fresh brain tissue, these molecules are not optimal targets for pretreatments aiming at depleting immunogenic cells from the donor material. Treatment of cultured porcine embryonic brain cells, grown under conditions favouring astrocytes and microglia, with human serum, which contains a high titre of natural antibodies against the α-galactosyl epitope, and complement reduces their ability to induce human T cell proliferation (Brevig et al 1997). This is consistent with more recent studies showing that the α-galactosyl epitope is expressed by microglial precursor cells and endothelial cells in embryonic pig brain (E. B. Pedersen & D. Møller, unpublished work, Sumitran et al 1999). Treatment of the mixed glial cultures with purified human antibodies against the α-galactosyl epitope and complement reduces the content of microglia and abolish direct recognition of the brain cells by human CD4 T cells *in vitro* (T. Brevig, M. Meyer, T. Kristensen, J. Zimmer & J. Holgersson, unpublished work). A pre-treatment of porcine donor tissue with antibodies against the α-galactosyl epitope and complement may not only reduce direct graft recognition by human T cells, but may also reduce antibody and natural killer-cell responses, which at least in part are directed against the α-galactosyl epitope (Galili 1993, Inverardi et al 1997).

Concluding remarks

Although neural allografts survive well in hosts receiving standard immuno-suppression, these grafts might be at continuous risk of being rejected, which could be a result of microglial activation following injury or other types of neurodegenerative stimuli. Neural tissue transplanted between species is promptly rejected, but transplantation of low-immunogenic porcine tissue with reduced content of the α-galactosyl epitope and microglial precursor cells, will supposedly reduce the immediate risk of rejection in humans. However, no strategy has been developed to deal with indirect graft recognition by host T cells, which might be particularly important to secure the survival of already established porcine grafts repopulated with host microglia. The absence of hyperacute rejection of neovascularized cellular xenografts, the promising donor tissue pretreatments, and the great effort presently being invested in overcoming the immunological barriers in xenotransplantation give us strong reasons to believe that neural xenografting may be of benefit to patients with neurodegenerative diseases in the near future.

Acknowledgements

Supported by the EU Biomed II program (BMH4-CT-97-2596), the Danish Parkinson Foundation, the P. Carl Petersen Foundation, the Danish Multiple Sclerosis Society, the Danish MRC and University of Southern Denmark–Odense University.

References

Auchincloss H Jr, Sachs DH 1998 Xenogeneic transplantation. Annu Rev Immunol 16:433–470

Bachoud-Lévi A, Bourdet C, Brugières P et al 2000 Safety and tolerability assessment of intrastriatal neural allografts in five patients with Huntington's disease. Exp Neurol 161:194–202

Barker CF, Billingham RE 1977 Immunologically privileged sites. Adv Immunol 25:1–54

Bartlett PF, Rosenfeld J, Bailey KA, Cheesman H, Harvey AR, Kerr RSC 1990 Allograft rejection overcome by immunoselection of neuronal precursor cells. Prog Brain Res 82:153–160

Batten P, Yacoub MH, Rose ML 1996 Effect of human cytokines (IFN-γ, TNF-α, IL-1β, IL-4) on porcine endothelial cells: induction of MHC and adhesion molecules and functional significance of these changes. Immunology 87:127–133

Bechmann I, Mor G, Nilsen J, Eliza M, Nitsch R, Naftolin F 1999 FasL (CD95L, Apo1L) is expressed in the normal rat and human brain: evidence for the existence of an immunological brain barrier. Glia 27:62–74

Björklund A, Stenevi U, Dunnett SB, Gage FH 1982 Cross-species neural grafting in a rat model of Parkinson's disease. Nature 298:652–654

Brevig T, Pedersen EB, Kristensen T, Zimmer J 1997 Proliferative response of human T lymphocytes to porcine fetal brain cells. Cell Transplant 6:571–577

Brevig T, Kristensen T, Zimmer J 1999 Expression of major histocompatibility complex antigens and induction of human T-lymphocyte proliferation by astrocytes and macrophages from porcine fetal brain. Exp Neurol 159:474–483

Broadwell RD, Baker BJ, Ebert PS, Hickey WF 1994 Allografts of CNS tissue possess a blood–brain barrier: III. Neuropathological, methodological, and immunological considerations. Microsc Res Tech 27:471–494

Cozzi E, White DJ 1995 The generation of transgenic pigs as potential organ donors for humans. Nat Med 1:964–966

Dalmau I, Finsen B, Tønder N, Zimmer J, Gonzalez B, Castellano B 1997 Development of microglia in the prenatal rat hippocampus. J Comp Neurol 377:70–84

Deacon T, Schumacher J, Dinsmore J et al 1997 Histological evidence of fetal pig neural cell survival after transplantation into a patient with Parkinson's disease. Nat Med 3:350–353

De Simone R, Giampaolo A, Giometto B et al 1995 The costimulatory molecule B7 is expressed on human microglia in culture and in multiple sclerosis acute lesions. J Neuropathol Exp Neurol 54:175–187

Elwood ET, Larsen CP, Cho HR et al 1998 Prolonged acceptance of concordant and discordant xenografts with combined CD40 and CD28 pathway blockade. Transplantation 65:1422–1428

Emerich DF, Winn SR, Christenson L, Palmatier MA, Gentile FT, Sanberg PR 1992 A novel approach to neural transplantation in Parkinson's disease: use of polymer-encapsulated cell therapy. Neurosci Biobehavioral Rev 16:437–447

Finsen BR, Sørensen T, Castellano B, Pedersen EB, Zimmer J 1991 Leukocyte infiltration and glial reactions in xenografts of mouse brain tissue undergoing rejection in the adult rat brain. A light and electron microscopical immunocytochemical study. J Neuroimmunol 32:159–183

Finsen B, Lehrmann E, Castellano B, Kiefer R, Zimmer J 1996 The role of microglial cells and brain macrophages in transient global cerebral ischemia. In: Ling E-A, Tan CK (eds) Topical issues in microglial research. Humanities Press, Singapore, p 297–318

Finsen B, Pedersen EB, Lehrmann L, Jensen MB, Aznar S, Zimmer J 1997 Microglial and astroglial activation patterns in neural graft rejection and neuronal and axonal degeneration. In: Jeserich G, Althaus HH, Richter-Landsberg C, Heumann R (eds) Molecular signalling and regulation in glial cells: a key to remyelination and functional repair. Springer Verlag, Heidelberg, p 213–229

Freeman TB, Olanow CW, Hauser RA et al 1995a Bilateral fetal nigral transplantation into the postcommissural putamen in Parkinson's disease. Ann Neurol 38:379–388

Freeman TB, Sanberg PR, Nauert GM et al 1995b The influence of donor age on the survival of solid and suspension intraparenchymal human embryonic nigral grafts. Cell Transplant 4:141–154

Frei K, Siepl C, Groscurth P, Bodmer S, Schwerdel C, Fontana A 1987 Antigen presentation and tumor cytotoxicity by interferon-γ-treated microglial cells. Eur J Immunol 17:1271–1278

Friedrich MJ 1999 Fetal pig neural cells for Parkinson disease. JAMA 282:2198–2199

Galili U 1993 Interaction of the natural anti-Gal antibody with α-galactosyl epitopes: a major obstacle for xenotransplantation in humans. Immunol Today 14:480–482

Gill RG, Wolf L 1995 Immunobiology of cellular transplantation. Cell Transplant 4:361–370

Hart DNJ, Fabre JW 1981 Demonstration and characterization of Ia-positive dendritic cells in the interstitial connective tissues of rat heart and other tissues, but not brain. J Exp Med 153:347–361

Inverardi L, Clissi B, Stolzer AL, Bender JR, Sandrin MS, Pardi R 1997 Human natural killer lymphocytes directly recognize evolutionarily conserved oligosaccharide ligands expressed by xenogeneic tissues. Transplantation 63:1318–1330

Kopyov OV, Jacques D, Lieberman A, Duma CM, Rogers RL 1996 Clinical study of fetal mesencephalic intracerebral transplants for the treatment of Parkinson's disease. Cell Transplant 5:327–337

Kordower JH, Styren S, Clarke M, DeKosky ST, Olanow CW, Freeman TB 1997 Fetal grafting for Parkinson's disease: expression of immune markers in two patients with functional fetal nigral implants. Cell Transplant 6:213–219

Lawrence JM, Morris R J, Wilson D J, Raisman G 1990 Mechanisms of allograft rejection in the rat brain. Neuroscience 37:431–462

Lawson LJ, Perry VH, Gordon S 1992 Turnover of resident microglia in the normal adult mouse brain. Neuroscience 48:405–415

Lehrmann E, Kiefer R, Kristensen T et al 1998 Microglia and macrophages are major sources of locally produced transforming growth factor-β1 mRNA after transient middle cerebral artery occlusion in rats. Glia 24:437–448

Lindvall O, Sawle G, Widner H et al 1994 Evidence for long-term survival and function of dopaminergic grafts in progressive Parkinson's disease. Ann Neurol 35:172–180

Lopez-Lozano J J, Bravo G, Brera B et al 1997 Regression of parkinsonian fetal ventral mesencephalon grafts upon withdrawal of cyclopsorin A immunosuppression. Transplant Proc 29:977–980

Lund RD, Rao K, Kunz HW, Gill T J III 1988 Instability of neural xenografts placed in neonatal rat brains. Transplantation 46:216–223

Mason DW, Charlton HM, Jones A J, Lavy CBD, Puklavec M, Simmonds S J 1986 The fate of allogeneic and xenogeneic neuronal tissue transplanted into the third ventricle of rodents. Neuroscience 19:685–694

Matyszak MK, Lawson LJ, Perry VH, Gordon S 1992 Stromal macrophages of the choroid plexus situated at an interface between the brain and peripheral immune system constitutively express major histocompatibility class II antigens. J Neuroimmunol 40:173–181

Medawar PB 1948 Immunity to homologous grafted skin. III. The fate of skin homografts transplanted to the brain, to subcutaneous tissue, and to the anterior chamber of the eye. Br J Exp Pathol 29:58–69

Neumann H, Schmidt H, Cavalié A, Jenne D, Wekerle H 1997 Major histocompatibility complex (MHC) class I gene expression in single neurons of the central nervous system: differential regulation by interferon (IFN)-γ and tumor necrosis factor (TNF)-α. J Exp Med 185:305–316

Nicholas MK, Antel JP, Stefansson K, Arnason BG 1987 Rejection of fetal neocortical neural transplants by H-2 incompatible mice. J Immunol 139:2275–2283

Nicholas MK, Chenelle AG, Brown MM, Stefansson K, Arnason BGW 1990 Prevention of neural allograft rejection in the mouse following *in vivo* depletion of L3T4+ but not Lyt-2+ T lymphocytes. Prog Brain Res 87:161–167

Oehmichen M, Grüninger H, Wiethölter H, Gencic M 1979 Lymphatic efflux of intracerebrally injected cells. Acta Neuropathol (Berl) 45:61–65

Pakzaban P, Deacon TW, Burns LH, Dinsmore J, Isacson O 1995 A novel mode of immunoprotection of neural xenotransplants: masking of donor major histocompatibility complex class I enhances transplant survival in the central nervous system. Neuroscience 65:983–996

Pedersen EB 1997 Transplantation immunology in the rodent central nervous system. PhD thesis, Odense University, Odense, Denmark

Pedersen EB, Zimmer J, Finsen B 1997a Triple immunosuppression protects murine intracerebral, hippocampal xenografts in adult rat hosts: effects on cellular infiltration, major histocompatibility complex antigen induction and blood–brain barrier leakage. Neuroscience 78:685–701

Pedersen EB, McNulty JA, Castro AJ, Fox LM, Zimmer J, Finsen B 1997b Enriched immune-environment in blood–brain barrier deficient areas of the adult rat brain. J Neuroimmunol 76:117–131

Perry VH, Lund RD 1989 Microglia in retinae transplanted to the central nervous system. Neuroscience 31:453–462

Peschanski M, Defer G, N'Guyen JP et al 1994 Bilateral motor improvement and alteration of L-dopa effect in two patients with Parkinson's disease following intrastriatal transplantation of foetal ventral mesencephalon. Brain 117:487–499

Sanberg PR, Borlongan CV, Saporta S, Cameron DF 1996 Testis-derived Sertoli cells survive and provide localized immunoprotection for xenografts in rat brain. Nat Biotechnol 14:1692–1695

Sloan DJ, Baker BJ, Puklavec M, Charlton HM 1990 The effect of site of transplantation and histocompatibility differences on the survival of neural tissue transplanted to the CNS of defined inbred rat strains. Prog Brain Res 82:141–152

Spencer DD, Robbins RJ, Naftolin F et al 1992 Unilateral transplantation of human fetal mesencephalic tissue into the caudate nucleus of patients with Parkinson's disease. N Engl J Med 327:1541–1548

Streilein JW 1993 Unraveling immune privilege. Science 270:1158–1159

Sumitran S, Liu J, Czech KA, Christensson B, Widner H, Holgersson J 1999 Human natural antibodies cytotoxic to pig embryonic brain cells recognize novel non-Galα1,3Gal-based xenoantigens. Exp Neurol 159:347–361

Wekerle H, Linington C, Lassmann H, Meyermann R 1986 Cellular immune reactivity within the CNS. Trends Neurosci 6:271–277

Widner H, Möller G, Johansson BB 1988 Immune response in deep cervical lymph nodes and spleen in the mouse after antigen deposition in different intracerebral sites. Scand J Immunol 28:563–571

Widner H, Tetrud J, Rehncrona S et al 1992 Bilateral fetal mesencephalic grafting in two patients with parkinsonism induced by 1-methyl-4-phenyl-1,2,3,6-tetrahydropyridine (MPTP). N Engl J Med 327:1556–1563

Wolf E, Zakhartchenko V, Brem G 1998 Nuclear transfer in mammals: recent developments and future perspectives. J Biotechnol 65:99–110

Wood MJA, Sloan DJ, Wood KJ, Charlton HM 1996 Indefinite survival of neural xenografts induced with anti-CD4 monoclonal antibodies. Neuroscience 70:775–789

Zimmer J, Finsen B, Sørensen T, Poulsen PH 1988 Xenografts of mouse hippocampal tissue. Exchange of laminar and neuropeptide specific nerve connections with the host rat brain. Brain Res Bull 20:369–379

DISCUSSION

Barker: Can I clarify your purging technique? Essentially, you seem to be removing the α-galactosyl-positive cells from the cell suspension, and this epitope is predominantly expressed on the microglia and the endothelial cells in the suspension. Is that right?

Finsen: That is correct.

Barker: And the astrocytes and the neurons don't express it?

Finsen: No. We have tried also to look for MHC class I and II expression. The astrocytes express just class I, but the microglial cells express both. Thomas Brevig has tried to run the T cell proliferation assay with freshly isolated cultures. At this time point the T cells are not stimulated very well: they need to be cultured for 14 days in order for the MHC expression be up-regulated to stimulate the human T cells.

Björklund: You showed one slide where you listed various cells in the brain that expressed MHC class I and II. There were numerous astrocytes, oligodendrocytes and microglia. What about the endothelial cells?

Finsen: It depends on the species. In rats I don't see MHC class II. It is the same in humans.

Gray: Hugh Perry, would you like to comment on what you have heard from the point of view of someone who studies inflammatory processes?

Perry: It is a complicated issue. There is no doubt that depleting the resident cells is going to be beneficial in a xenograft. But this is not of itself a sufficient condition to render these transplants now resistant to attack. The problem is that when one injects the transplant, antigens are released and these will drain to the draining lymph nodes. Activated T cells will the find their way to the brain and this will then initiate a secondary destruction. The problem will always be that a xenograft will be fragile relative to an allograft. However, it is clear that human allografts can survive if people are given immunosuppression. In essence one might therefore say that it is not really a problem until you get to xenografts. With xenografts it will always be a case of the level of immunosuppression you have to keep in place in order for these xenografts to survive. I think this will be true for the brain just as it is for xenografts to other sites. Withdrawing immunosuppression will be much more difficult with a xenograft.

As regards what happens with cell lines, I think this is a very interesting question. Then there is the separate issue of what happens using a virus. It is possible to deliver this to the brain, and it is not like a soluble antigen. There are a number of experiments in the literature showing that if you put a virus into the brain parenchyma so that none of the virus gets to the ventricles or meninges, this virus can remain undetected by the immune system in the brain parenchyma. In essence, there is almost an absolute privilege under the appropriate conditions, because the brain parenchyma does not have true APCs, the dendritic cells. These are the only cells that will present antigen to a naïve T cell, and are the cells that initiate completely *de novo* immune reactions. Once you have primed T cells, however, they can find their way into the brain. Once you have become sensitized to any transplant antigen, it is now potentially available for immunological assault. In conclusion, I think xenografts will pose huge immunological problems, but it will be interesting to see what happens with cell lines.

Gray: Can we predict what the immune response to cell lines might be?

Snyder: We have now used the same mouse clone in thousands of mouse recipients of all different strains, ages and diseases, without any evidence of immunorejection or the need for immunosuppression. The interesting finding is that the developmental state in which we transplant the cells is one in which the cells don't express MHC class I or II on their surface, a surprising preliminary observation. It is not that these cells don't have the ability to express them — they can be induced to express them, particularly by treatment with IFN-γ — but they don't express it at the differentiation stage at which we do the transplantation. Therefore, these mouse clones act like 'universal donor cells' for mice. It might be that it is not the brain but rather the neural stem cell that is immunologically privileged at certain stages in its development.

Gray: Have you tried those cells in species other than the mouse?

Snyder: We have tried them in rat and fetal goat. If we go across species we may start to see evidence of rejection, particularly in older animals, though this aspect requires more systematic evaluation because it is not an invariant observation.

Annett: Helen Hodges reported putting mouse cell lines into marmosets, and even though they were immunosuppressed, the levels of cyclosporin would not have been sufficient to protect xenografts. It seems that these cells are protected.

Hodges: We think that they must be somewhat protected, even in that huge cross-species jump. We had one monkey where we didn't include the behavioural data, because there was no recovery, and this animal had been given no cyclosporin. There were still some β-galactosidase-positive cells, but they seemed very immature and they didn't migrate up through the CA1 field, although they survived.

Gage: When one takes human haemopoietic cells, these need to be put into an immune-suppressed mouse for reconstitution to occur. There is clearly not any privilege in this context.

Snyder: I can't say what would happen if we put our murine neural stem cell clones outside the CNS. They may be more vulnerable to immune attack in those areas.

Finsen: Also, within the CNS rejection depends on the location. The spinal cord may be a more hostile environment. Additionally, among inbred strains of rats or mice, there are high responders and low responders.

Some years ago Widner & Brundin (1993) did an experiment in which they did sequential grafting. They found that if they first transplanted one allogeneic graft into one side of the brain, followed by a second allograft into the contralateral side, then the first allograft always survived better than the second allograft. These observations are potentially very interesting. A contributing factor that the first graft remained relatively unaffected by the immune response elicited by the second graft might be that the cells/antigens (i.e. microglia) which the host immune cells are educated to target no longer are present within the primary graft.

However, both allografts were rejected if the re-grafted animal was challenged with a peripheral skin allograft, which is known to give rise to a very strong sensitization of the recipient immune system.

Sinden: We looked at a human differentiated neuroblastoma graft in the rat, and by injecting the cells peripherally we got rejection of the human neuroblastoma cells which had initially survived without immunosuppression.

Olson: You mentioned that there might be a difference between the spinal cord and the brain. When we transplant different brain areas versus spinal cord tissue to the anterior chamber of the eye, there seems to be such a difference. The spinal cord tissue is more easily rejected and evokes more of an immune response than brain tissue grafts.

Finsen: This could be because of a larger proportion of white matter in spinal cord. White matter glial cells are highly responsive to injury.

Blakemore: There are big differences in the reaction to a replication-defective adenovirus that is put into the brain or spinal cord (O'Leary & Charlton 1999). The spinal cord is on the twitch all the time. I wanted to pursue the question of what is actually surviving with the neurons, and to what extent the glia populations are exchanged. In other words, do you lose all the donor microglia, which would be a good thing? Do you also lose the donor astrocytes? In these long-term grafts, how many cell types survive and integrate? Is it just the neurons?

Finsen: In the MHC class I staining I showed, after three weeks presumably all cells, except the microglial cells and sporadic T cells, are donor cells. This means that neurons as well as astrocytes and oligodendrocytes are of donor-origin, and that all donor cell types except the neurons express MHC class I.

Perry: The problem with cells and transplants (and the reason why we did it with bacteria and viruses) is that you have rather poor control over precisely what you inject, what gets to the periphery, and how you measure it. The reason we use BCG (Matyszak & Perry 1995) is that we can study these things in rather more detail than you can if you inject cell suspensions which contain soluble antigens and bits of cells. The precise method which you use to do your injection—whether you touch the ventricles, whether some antigen escapes to the meninges, whether enough antigen to evoke an immune response drains to the meninges and so on—will make a difference and they are not issues that people doing transplants normally worry about.

Gray: Could someone summarize the state of play on the human clinical Parkinson's cases?

Freeman: From the allograft point of view, I took my lead from Professors Lindvall and Björklund, based on the concept that in kidney transplants, multiple unrelated allografts did not influence the survival rate of subsequent allografts. The clinical hypothesis was that multiple unrelated donors would not cause an adverse second set rejection, even in a staged transplant paradigm. Our transplants were a week to a month apart, and the positron emission tomography (PET) data from our Parkinson's disease patients with grafts that were four weeks apart showed presumptive continuous survival of the grafts based on the surrogate marker of the PET scan. At autopsy we have now reported 13 unrelated allografts that all survived.

Gray: Did those patients have an initial period of immunosuppression?

Freeman: Ours have had initial immunosuppression for only six months.

Gray: Is it yet known whether that is a critical feature of transplants?

Freeman: Our guess is that it is probably a minor variable, on the basis of the animal data where allografts survive well in rodents and primates with no immunosuppression. The rationale for immunosuppression was weak. The only data we have are preliminary, and come from Curt Freed's work (Freed et al 1997, 1999). He did not use immunosuppression, and his survival rate is about half what we have reported, but he also stored tissue in culture for up to one month. Therefore one would expect a lower viability on the basis of his transplant methodology, not necessarily on an immunological basis.

Lindvall: The data from Curt Freed suggest that immunosuppression may not be necessary for survival of dopamine neurons after grafting. It has been well documented by several groups that immunosuppression can be withdrawn and that grafts can still survive for many years. The question is, if you want to re-graft the patient, is it then important to have immunosuppression during the first grafting session and for a short period thereafter? In our own patients, who were re-grafted between 10 and 56 months after the first transplantation and who showed good survival of both the first and the second graft, we used immunosuppression up to at least two years after the second graft.

Freeman: One other piece of evidence that immunosuppression is not needed is that in our protocol we have used the immunosuppression, but we have stopped it in cases where kidney function is threatened. One of our patients developed a rise in creatine and BUN between the two staged procedures, and in the second operation was given a transplant without immunosuppression. His PET scan fluorodopa uptake is one of the highest in our group. We are awaiting to accumulate information on a medical necessity basis before changing our protocol. However, this does not address the question as to whether immunosuppression is needed during the first transplant if staged procedures are anticipated.

Gray: Bente Finsen, is there anything in our understanding of the kind of issue you were describing to us that would lead one to say that immunosuppression at the time of surgery would have a critical difference to immunosuppression being given later on? Does this procedure that has been used for a long time make rational sense?

Finsen: Yes. I would prefer to use immunosuppression at the time of grafting and for a short while after until everything has settled down. From the animal studies we know that in both allografts and syngeneic grafts there is a period where inflammatory cells accumulate within and around the graft and where donor APCs may be drained away to the lymphoid organs. We also know that this is accompanied by up-regulation of MHC antigens on the graft. During this period it would be desirable to completely immunosuppress the host and prevent accumulation of host T cells.

Gray: I had a naïve understanding — which is quite clearly wrong in the light of the nice paper you gave — that a critical part of the brain's privileged immune status is because of the BBB. Because this barrier is opened to some extent during surgery, it would appear to be critical at that time to have immune suppression. Your data showed that the BBB does not play a major role in protecting the transplants from rejection. If that is so, my naïve understanding of the rationale for this initial period of immune suppression is wrong. However, I'm not sure that I see an alternative.

Finsen: In a study published a few years ago we compared using a mouse-to-rat xenograft model, the survival of mouse xenografts without immune suppression, with cyclosporin A only, and with conventional triple immune suppressive therapy with cyclosporin A, aziotroprine and methylprednisolone (Pedersen et al 1997). We obtained much better graft survival in the triple immune-suppressed group than in the others. When we looked at these grafts after long-term survival, we found healthy grafts with no MHC antigen expression or T cell infiltration. In this case we have not tried to withdraw the immunosuppression, and we may have been lucky and prevented T cell stimulation in the first place. This is why one should give immunosuppression, and not because of the BBB. If the T cells are activated they will sooner or later find their way to the graft.

References

Freed CR, Trojanowski JQ, Galvin JE et al 1997 Embryonic dopamine cells cultured as strands show long term survival without immunosuppression in a patient with advanced Parkinson's disease. Soc Neurosci Abstr 23:1682

Freed CR, Breeze RE, Greene PE et al 1999 Double-blind controlled trial of human embryonic dopamine cell transplants in advanced Parkinson's disease. Am Soc Neural Transplantation & Repair, Conference Abstracts 5/6:20

Matyszak MK, Perry VH 1995 Demyelination in the central nervous system following a delayed-type hypersensitivity in response to bacillus Calmette–Guèrin. Neuroscience 64:967–977

O'Leary MT, Charlton HM 1999 A model for long-term transgene expression in spinal cord regeneration studies. Gene Ther 6:1351–1359

Pedersen EB, Zimmer J, Finsen B 1997 Triple immunosuppression protects murine intracerebral, hippocampal xenografts in adult rat hosts: effects on cellular infiltration, major

histocompatibility complex antigen induction and blood–brain barrier leakage. Neuroscience 78:685–701
Widner H, Brundin P 1993 Sequential intracerebral transplantation of allogeneic and syngeneic fetal dopamine-rich neuronal tissue in adult rats: will the first graft be rejected? Cell Transplant 2:307–317

Porcine neural xenografts:
what are the issues?

Roger A. Barker

Cambridge Centre for Brain Repair, Robinson Way, Cambridge CB2 2PY, UK

Abstract. The allografting of embryonic neural tissue into the CNS of animals with experimental lesions and patients with neurodegenerative conditions has shown that this tissue survives, makes and receives synapses, and ameliorates behavioural deficits without inducing a significant rejection process. There are though, major problems with the use of aborted human tissue in clinical programmes of transplantation which has lead to the search for alternative sources of cells, including embryonic porcine tissue. However there are two major issues relating to the use of this tissue: (a) the risk of zoonotic infection especially with porcine endogenous retroviruses (PERVs); and (b) the loss of the tissue to an immunologically based rejection process, and it is this latter issue that forms the basis of this chapter. The rejection of neural xenografts has clearly been shown to involve T cell-directed processes although there is now increasing evidence that complement and humoral immune mediators may also play a role. This suggests that transgenic pigs expressing regulators of the human complement cascade may offer an advantage over normal porcine tissue in any clinical neural xenograft programmes. However the extent to which these different immune processes are interdependent, and the contribution of each of them to the actual loss of the grafted tissue is currently unresolved.

2000 Neural transplantation in neurodegenerative disease. Wiley, Chichester (Novartis Foundation Symposium 231) p 184–201

The allografting of embryonic neural tissue into the CNS of animals has now reached the level of clinical trials with Parkinson's disease (PD) and more recently Huntington's disease (HD) (Freeman & Widner 1998, Olanow et al 1996). This is based on a background of experimental work which has shown that embryonic neural tissue allografted into the CNS survives, makes and receives synapses, and ameliorates behavioural deficits without inducing a significant rejection process (Barker & Dunnett 1999). However there are major practical and ethical problems with the use of aborted human tissue in clinical programmes of transplantation which prevents its widespread adoption and has lead to the search for alternative sources of cells, including embryonic porcine tissue. However this tissue, whilst having several obvious advantages, also has its

TABLE 1   Advantages and disadvantages of using porcine donor tissue for neural transplantation

Advantages	*Disadvantages*
(i) The size and development of its brain is similar to that seen in humans	(i) The risk of zoonotic infection, especially with PERVs
(ii) It is relatively easy to breed and produces large litters of embryos	(ii) Immunological rejection
(iii) It can be genetically modified to produce transgenic animals	(iii) The transplanted tissue will always be different to that originally lost in the host human CNS
(iv) It has long been considered as a possible source of peripheral whole organ transplants	
(v) Xenotransplanted, over allografted, tissue may have the primary advantage of a greater potential for sending fibres into the host brain — possibly through the avoidance of species specific barriers to axonal growth	

own unique problems, of which the main two are the risk of infection, especially from porcine endogenous retroviruses (PERVs) and the loss of the xenografted tissue to an immune rejection process (see Table 1).

Xenografted porcine neural tissue is rejected even when placed in the relatively immunologically privileged site of the brain, and it is becoming clear that this process is complex and involves a number of immune processes.

This relative immunological privilege of the CNS has been shown to be in need of redefinition as (i) antigen placed into the CNS can drain into the deep cervical lymph nodes; (ii) activated lymphocytes can cross the intact blood–brain barrier (BBB); and (iii) microglia, as well as possibly astrocytes, can act as antigen presenting cells (reviewed in Sloan et al 1991). Therefore, it is not surprising that xenografted neural tissue can be rejected when placed into the CNS, especially given the fact that the BBB is disrupted during the implantation procedure. It is clear that neural xenografts placed into the brain induce a T cell response (both CD4 and CD8) that is apparent 5–10 days post-implantation. At this time the normally low or absent MHC expression seen with embryonic neural tissue, increases within the graft. This change in epitope expression coupled to the T cell infiltrate leads to rejection of the xenografted neural tissue over the ensuing 3–4 weeks in the majority of cases, although there are occasional reports of long-term survival of such tissue in the non-immunosuppressed host (reviewed in Pakzaban & Isacson 1994). However the rejection of such grafts can be abrogated, although not always abolished, by the use of cyclosporin A (CyA) as well as other immunosuppressive regimes, of which the most successful to date have been monoclonal antibody therapy to CD4 lymphocytes and the interleukin (IL)-2 receptor (Honey et al 1990, Wood et al 1996). Whilst these studies have clearly shown a role for T cell-directed processes in the rejection of neural xenografts, there is increasing recent evidence that humoral immune mediators may play a part.

The role of complement in the rejection of cellular, including neural, xenografts is unresolved unlike the hyperacute rejection of peripheral whole-organ xenografts where complement plays a critical role (Auchincloss & Sachs 1998). In this latter situation with pig-to-human whole organ vascularized xenografts, there is immediate binding of immunoglobulin (Ig)M to the major xenoantigen, α-Gal (1,3) Gal, on the endothelial cells, which triggers the complement cascade. This leads to the formation of the membrane attack complex (MAC) with lysis or activation of the endothelial cells with the generation of a procoagulative state within the graft. The graft is thus lost within minutes due to fibrin deposition and microvascular thrombosis and haemorrhage, with little in the way of an inflammatory cellular infiltrate.

In this chapter we will recap on the complement system and the expression of its components within the CNS, followed by an analysis of its role in the rejection of peripheral xenografts of islet cells. Finally we will discuss the rejection of neural xenografts and the evidence that antibodies and complement may play a role in their rejection which raises the possibility that transgenic porcine tissue expressing human complement regulatory proteins may offer an advantage in clinical xenograft programmes. Issues relating to infection and more especially PERVs have recently been discussed elsewhere (Weiss 1999).

Complement and the CNS

The complement cascade consists of 30 fluid-phase and cell membrane proteins, and a grossly simplified schematic of this is shown in Fig. 1. The activation of the cascade can be through a number of routes — the classical pathway is activated through C1 and is antibody-dependent; the alternative pathway is through antibody-independent binding of C3b to the pathogen and a third pathway is activated by the binding of mannan-binding lectin (MBL) to mannose groups present on many bacterial cell walls (Taylor et al 1998). The cascade is also regulated through a number of membrane and secreted regulatory proteins including CR1 (CD35), DAF (CD55), MCP (CD46), CD59 on the membrane and a host of secreted factors such as C1 inhibitor, C4 binding protein, Factor H and Factor I.

The majority of the secreted proteins in the complement system are derived from the hepatocyte, although other cells that are capable of producing some, if not all, of these proteins include monocytes/macrophages, fibroblasts, endothelial cells, leukocytes, cells of the renal glomerulus and synovial lining cells, and more recently cells of the nervous system (see below). This local synthesis of

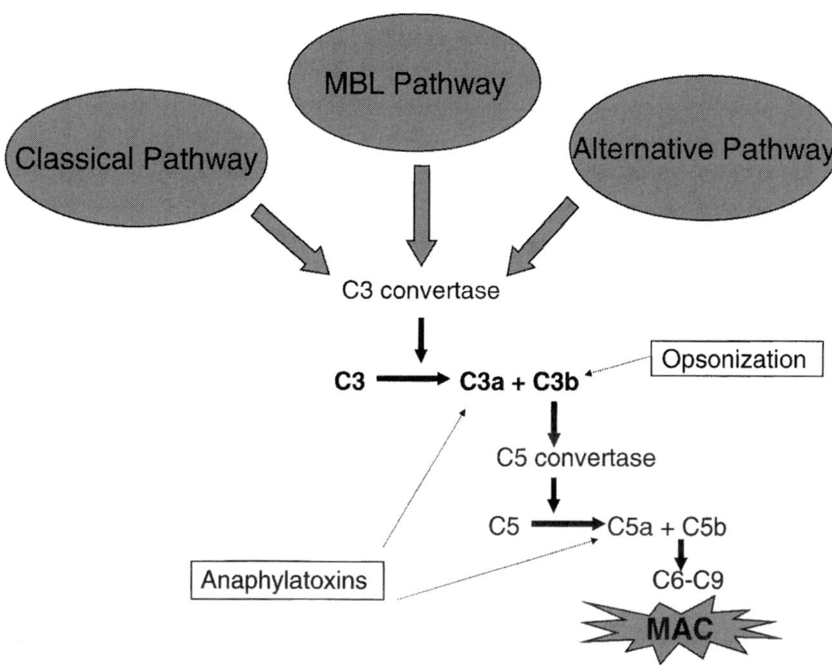

FIG. 1.   Simplified schematic figure of complement cascade. The classical pathway is activated by antibody binding whilst the mannan-binding lectin (MBL) and alternative pathways are directly activated, typically by pathogenic organisms. All pathways converge on the C3 convertase which splits C3 into C3a and C3b, and C3b adheres to specific complement receptors on phagocytic cells which facilitates the removal of the cell that has bound C3b (opsonization). C3a with C5a (anaphylatoxins) on the other hand are responsible for the generation of the full inflammatory response, with activation and recruitment of phagocytes and vasodilatation with increased vascular permeability. Ultimately the cascade leads to the formation of a membrane attack complex (C6–9; MAC) that inserts into the cell membrane causing lysis of the cell.

complement may be important in triggering and perpetuating inflammation locally.

In the periphery complement mediates the following events, many of which rely on the binding of complement components to specific receptors:

(1)   Opsonization of cells with C3b deposition on cell surface for phagocytosis and clearance.

(2)   Anaphylatoxins which attract and activate mast cells, polymorphonuclear lymphocytes and macrophages and by so doing lead to the release of a host of cytokines and vasoactive substances which generates the acute inflammatory response with increasing vascular permeability.

(3)   MAC causing cell lysis.
(4)   Activation and proliferation of B and T cells.
(5)   Clearance of apoptotic cells.
(6)   Clearance of antigen–antibody immune complexes.

In the normal and damaged CNS complement biosynthesis can occur, which means that the BBB does not need breaching for complement activation to occur. *In vitro* the major cell in the CNS that is responsible for complement production is the astrocyte as, at least in the human, they express all components of complement cascade — albeit at very low levels, although inducible by γ-interferon (IFN-γ) as well as tumour necrosis factor (TNF)α and IL-1β (reviewed in Morgan & Gasque 1996). Microglia, oligodendrocytes and neurons may be induced to produce complement although the extent to which this occurs *in vivo* is unresolved as is the significance of neurons expressing anaphylatoxin receptors (Nataf et al 1999). Indeed astrocytes may even function to switch on their own complement system through an autocrine effect by releasing cytokines. In addition human astrocytes can express decay accelerating factor (DAF), membrane cofactor protein (MCP), CR1 and CD59, whilst rat astrocytes express CD59 and an MCP analogue and so are very resistant to complement lysis unless these molecules are neutralized, especially CD59. Even then complement, whilst not actually lysing the cells, may induce dysfunction and damage to neighbouring cells such as oligodendrocytes and neurons.

Overall the production of complement by astrocytes may serve similar functions in the CNS compared to the periphery in that it may lead to opsonization of pathogens, and chemotaxis and activation of cells, including astrocytes and microglia. The relevance of this to neural xenografts is that the placement of immunogenic tissue whilst recruiting a humoral response from circulating factors may equally well evoke a local response from cells of the CNS which may perpetuate the local rejection process.

Cellular xenografts in the periphery: the role of antibodies and complement in islet cell transplants

Xenografted islet cells have been studied as a possible therapy for the treatment of insulin-dependent diabetes mellitus. This has lead to early clinical trials even though issues of their rejection are unresolved (Groth et al 1994). These cells when implanted experimentally are rejected not in a hyperacute fashion, as is seen with whole organ xenotransplants, but acutely over days (Wallgren et al 1995). This rejection is clearly a T cell-dependent process given that nude mice display indefinite islet cell xenograft survival (Korsgren et al 1991) and anti-CD4 treatment not only prolongs islet cell survival but can induce tolerance

TABLE 2 Comparison of porcine islet and neural xenografts with respect to the humoral responses they can evoke

Experimental paradigm	*Porcine islet cells*	*Porcine neural tissue*
B cell-deficient or IgKO mice	Significantly prolonged survival time of islet cell xenografts (Mirenda et al 1997)	Prolonged survival (Larsson et al 1999)
IgM/C3 deposition in grafted cells	Yes (Deng et al 1994)	Yes*
Effects of cobra venom factor	Prolonged islet cell xenograft survival although rejection will still occur (Oberholzer et al 1999)	Delayed cellular infiltration of the graft*
Human immunoglobulin binding to cells	Yes (Korbutt et al 1996)	Yes (Sumitran et al 1999)
Human complement mediated lysis of cells	Yes (Schaapherder et al 1996)	Yes (Sumitran et al 1999, *)
Host antibody response when grafted	Yes (Galili et al 1995)	Unknown
Epitope	*Porcine islet cell*	*Porcine neural tissue*
α-Gal (1,3) Gal	+ (McKenzie et al 1995)	+ (Sumitran et al 1999, *)
MHC I	+ (Auchincloss & Sachs 1998)	+/− (but inducible) (Brevig et al 1999, *)
MHC II	+/− (Auchincloss & Sachs 1998)	+/− (but inducible) (Brevig et al 1999, *)

*Unpublished data from our laboratory (R. Barker, T. Harrower, E. Ratcliffe, A. Richards) and Barker et al (2000).

(Simeonovic et al 1990). Furthermore porcine islet cell xenografts are lost equally quickly in wild-type and Ig or F_c knock-out mice (Benda et al 1996). However whilst the rejection of these cells is clearly a T cell-directed phenomenon, the effector cell may be the macrophage. Wallgren et al (1995) have shown that islet cell grafts induce a macrophage infiltrate that is initially positive for the surface markers ED1/CD4 but which switches in time to ED2/CD8. In the rat CD4 is mainly confined to the T helper (Th) lymphocytes and some macrophages, whilst CD8 is present on cytotoxic T cell (Tc), macrophages and the majority of rat natural killer (NK) cells. However macrophages can only stimulate a specific immune response if they are linked to the target structure by antibodies and/or complement (unless the target expresses certain lectins as occurs with some bacteria) which suggests that islet cell xenografts may induce a humoral response of significance, a suggestion that has been supported by a number of other studies (Table 2).

The uncertainty of the relative role of any effector humoral response in porcine islet cell xenograft rejection is also seen with porcine neural tissue given the fact that they are both grafted as a cellular suspension and both have similar epitope expression (Table 2).

The rejection of neural xenografts

The first neural xenografts in the modern era were performed by Björklund et al (1982), with the grafting of mouse embryonic ventral mesencephalon (VM) tissue into a cavity in the rat striatum. The tissue survived in almost two-thirds of cases (10/18) and produced functional benefit with no immunosuppression, although most of graft had been resorbed with low numbers of cells surviving 6 months following grafting (Björklund et al 1982). Subsequently Inoue et al (1985) and Brundin et al (1985) showed that CyA enhanced the survival of mouse to rat xenografts with loss of the graft in the non-immunosuppressed animals (Brundin et al 1985, 1989, Inoue et al 1985), although xenograft survival without immunosuppression can still be seen on occasions (e.g. Daniloff et al 1985).

The mechanisms underlying the rejection of neural xenografts were first investigated by Mason et al (1986) using rat–mouse paradigms. They demonstrated that by 5 days the grafts exhibited a leukocyte infiltrate that was mainly perivascular and consisted of CD4- and CD8-positive lymphocytes in equal numbers along with major histocompatibility complex (MHC) class II-expressing macrophages and a few polymorphonuclear lymphocytes (Mason et al 1986). Subsequently a number of other studies have shown that xenografts induce an initial non-specific inflammatory response followed by a more specific lymphocytic infiltration which coincides with increased MHC expression within the graft (reviewed in Sloan et al 1991). However whilst many of these studies confirmed that CyA was helpful in promoting graft survival, a significant number of xenografts were still lost to a presumed immune-mediated process (reviewed in Pakzaban & Isacson 1994). This lead to the use of other immunosuppressive regimes including FK 506 (Sakei et al 1991) and 15-deoxyspergualin (DSG) (Zhou et al 1993) as well as specific monoclonal antibodies to components of the immune system. In this respect anti-CD4 treatment for 10 days with rat–mouse xenografts of hypothalamic tissue prolongs survival although at 60 days there is evidence of rejection (Wood et al 1996), in contrast anti-IL-2R treatment for 10 days prevents human–rat VM xenograft rejection (Honey et al 1990). Furthermore, triple therapy consisting of CyA with prednisolone and azathioprine offers a survival advantage with xenografts, over CyA alone (Pedersen et al 1995).

These studies raise issues, as with the islet cell grafts, about whether the xenografted tissue may be generating a humoral response which may account for the failure of CyA to offer 100% protection for such grafts; a point that has been previously raised. Brundin et al (1989) with mouse–rat xenografts showed antibodies to mouse MHC in serum of grafted rats irrespective of whether they received CyA (Brundin et al 1989). There was no quantitative difference in antibody binding between rats that exhibited graft survival and functional effects and those that did not, similar to that which they found with human to rat xenografts (Brundin et al 1989). Finsen et al (1990) demonstrated that mouse–rat xenografts induce an antibody response which did not correlate with the use of CyA nor the state of the graft and furthermore the cellular infiltrate into the graft was of T cell and macrophage origin with only very few B cells (Finsen et al 1990). Finally Duan et al (1995) postulated that the rejection of neural xenografts may occur in two phases, an initial early antibody response causing some graft cavities followed by a second more prolonged T cell-mediated rejection process (Duan et al 1995). Subsequently a number of studies have addressed this specific issue of the role of antibodies and complement.

Cellular xenografts in the CNS: the role of antibodies and complement in porcine neural cell transplants

Porcine neural tissue has been grafted experimentally, as well as into patients with PD and HD (Deacon et al 1997, Edge et al 1998). However whilst these grafts can survive, there is evidence that in some cases they are lost to an immune process even when the animals have received CyA (Edge et al 1998).

The evidence that humoral factors may play a role in neural xenograft rejection are summarized in Table 2 and has lead us, amongst others, to explicitly address the issue of complement and humoral effector systems in neural xenograft rejection.

Porcine neural tissue is known to express a number of immunogenic epitopes including the major xenoantigen α-Gal (1,3) Gal (see Table 2). However other epitopes are found on these cells and all can bind human Ig and evoke antibody-dependent cell-mediated cytotoxicity (ADCC) *in vitro* (Sumitran et al 1999; see also Deacon et al 1998, R. A. Barker, unpublished data). However the relevance of this to the grafting situation is not clear, especially given the commonly used pig–rat paradigm. In terms of mammals, only old world primates and humans do not express α-Gal (1,3) Gal and thus have preformed antibodies, hence in pig–rat xenografts no such antibodies should be present. Indeed rats have only very low levels of naturally occurring antibodies to pig tissue (R. A. Barker, unpublished data). Nevertheless porcine neural cells when injected intraperitoneally into rats generate a systemic antibody response (A. Richards, unpublished data), so that this tissue is known to express other immunogenic epitopes which could recruit an antibody response and thus complement activation through the classical pathway.

In order to address this, we xenografted embryonic porcine ventral mesencephalic tissue into the 6-hydroxydopamine (6-OHDA)-lesioned, non-immunosuppressed rat (an animal model of PD), followed its rejection profile histologically and compared this to that seen with isografts and sham grafts. In addition, the behaviour of the grafts was monitored using amphetamine-induced rotation—a surrogate marker of dopaminergic innervation within the striatum. Over the first 10 days post-implantation the xenograft matured with identifiable tyrosine hydroxylase (TH) neurons within it and pig-specific neurofilament fibres extending out from it along host white matter tracts. Unlike isografts, these xenografts had no effect on drug-induced rotation. However during this period of time both a CD8-cell response and humoral (IgM and C3) response was observed within the graft, which was then rejected over the next 25 days (see Fig. 2). This was not seen in either stab wounds or isografts, implying that the deposition of IgM and C3 was specific for the xenograft (Barker et al 2000).

In order to further address this issue, the effect of complement depletion using cobra venom factor (CVF) was addressed in this model using xenografted porcine VM tissue and a 21 day post-implantation period of follow-up. Unfortunately total complement depletion could only be maintained for 7 days using systemic CVF treatment in our standard strain of rat (Sprague–Dawley), and thus the effects of complement depletion at different times relative to the implantation of the xenograft was undertaken. This study showed that CVF administration in the period immediately before and after grafting delayed, but did not prevent, the cellular immune response induced by the graft (Barker et al 2000). This suggests that xenografted neural tissue can activate the complement cascade and that this plays a role in the rejection process, possibly by the recruitment of a full cellular response.

In parallel with these studies Widner and colleagues have studied the survival of porcine xenografts in immunologically modified mice, more specifically immunoglobulin knockout (IgKO) animals (Larsson et al 1999). In this study they have shown that in the normal wild-type mice, xenografted porcine VM tissue survived poorly with the majority of the grafts being lost within two weeks of implantation. In contrast similarly grafted tissue in the IgKO mouse survived for longer periods of time, with the majority of the grafts being lost 4–6 weeks after implantation. Furthermore, the two different hosts appear to mount different T cell responses, with the wild-type animals showing an early CD4+ T cell response, and the IgKO mice a later CD8+ T cell infiltrate. This latter response was associated with more intense microglia staining, whilst non-specific immunoglobulin binding was seen in and around the grafts of wild-type hosts. Thus this study suggests that immunoglobulins may be important in the early stages of neural xenograft rejection, in conjunction with a CD4+ T cell response,

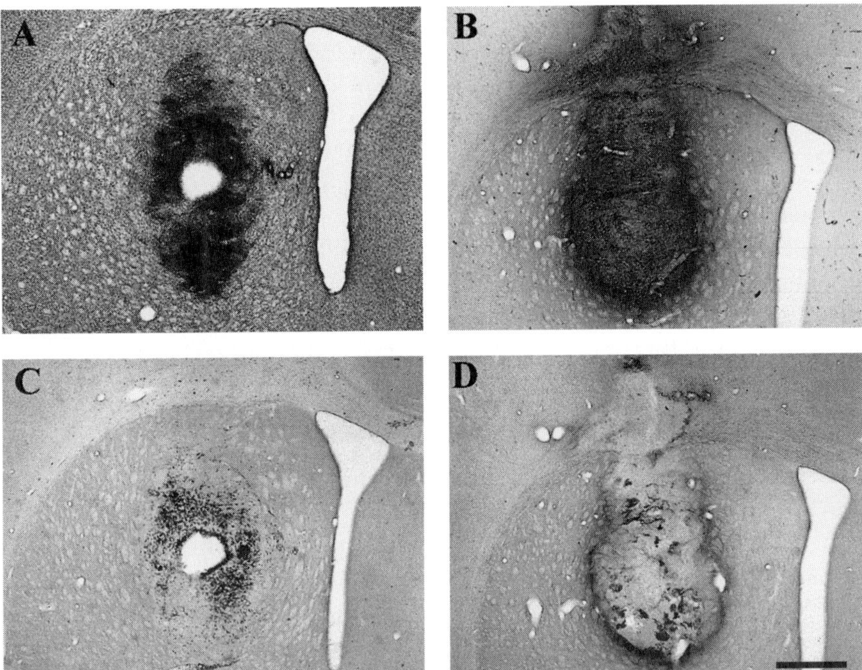

FIG. 2.   An embryonic day (E)26 VM graft in the non-immunosuppressed 6-OHDA lesioned
rat, 10 days after grafting. (A) Cresyl violet staining of the graft which is very cellular with some
necrosis at the centre of it. (B) Pig-specific neurofilament staining showing dense fibres within
the graft, illustrating that the graft at this stage contains abundant viable pig neuronal processes.
(C) CD8 staining shows an infiltrate of cells with cavitation of the graft as it is rejected. (D) C3
staining in and around the graft showing that elements within it have bound complement. Scale
bar = 1 mm.

whilst a later rejection event is the activation of CD8+ T cells in association with, or
as a result of, microglial activation in the graft site.

All of these studies therefore suggest, as with islet cells, that xenografts of
porcine neural tissue are capable of recruiting an antibody/complement response
and that this may play a role in the rejection of this tissue. However whilst the
mechanisms by which this may occur are unresolved, these studies raise
fundamental issues on xenoantigen handling within the CNS as well as having
implications for the use of transgenic porcine tissue in any clinical trials.

Transgenic porcine tissue and neural xenografts

A number of transgenic pigs are now available that have been developed to
overcome hyperacute rejection and thus express either regulators of the human

complement system or mask the α-Gal (1,3) Gal epitope. Whole organ transplants from these animals have been shown to have prolonged survival in the xenograft paradigm (Cozzi & White 1995), but their relevance to neural xenografts is unresolved.

Recently Deacon et al (1998) have demonstrated that grafts of embryonic VM tissue derived from transgenic pigs expressing the human CD59 cell surface complement inhibitor, survive and have a functional effect following transplantation in the CyA-treated rat. However the expression of the transgene in embryonic neural tissue needs to be shown and its effects on complement activation known for the species into which it is grafted. This is currently being undertaken by us for the transgenic pig expressing the human DAF.

Conclusion

The ethical and practical limitations of using human fetal tissue has lead to the search for alternative sources of cells, of which embryonic porcine tissue offers many attractions. However, one of the major problems with this tissue is its immunological rejection and whilst this has traditionally been thought to be a T cell-mediated process, there is now emerging evidence for a role for antibodies and complement. More work needs to be done on the interaction of the cellular and humoral arms of the rejection process, and the advantage that transgenic pig tissue may have in any clinical programme of porcine neural xenografting. Furthermore, whilst studies on neural xenografts have clear clinical implications, they may also provide a more fundamental understanding of CNS immunological processes.

Acknowledgements

RAB is an MRC Clinician Scientist. Work cited in this chapter has been supported by the MRC (UK) and Imutran Ltd (a Novartis Pharma AG Company). I would like to thank Richard Armstrong, Tim Harrower and Andy Richards for their critical comments and Emma Ratcliffe for the histology.

References

Auchincloss H Jr, Sachs DH 1998 Xenogeneic transplantation. Annu Rev Immunol 16:433–470
Barker RA, Dunnett SB 1999 Neural repair, transplantation and rehabilitation. Psychology Press, Hove
Barker RA, Ratcliffe E, McLaughlin M, Richards A, Dunnett SB 2000 A role for complement in the rejection of porcine ventral mesencephalic xenografts in a rat model of Parkinson's disease. J Neurosci 20:3415–3424
Benda B, Karlsson-Parra A, Ridderstad A, Korsgren O 1996 Xenograft rejection of porcine islet-like clusters in immunoglobulin- or Fc-receptor γ-deficient mice. Transplantation 62:1207–1211

Björklund A, Stenevi U, Dunnett SB, Gage FH 1982 Cross-species neural grafting in a rat model of Parkinson's disease. Nature 298:652–654

Brevig T, Kristensen T, Zimmer J 1999 Expression of major histocompatability complex antigens and induction of human T-lymphocyte proliferation by astrocytes and macrophages from porcine fetal brain. Exp Neurol 159:474–483

Brundin P, Nilsson OG, Gage FH, Björklund A 1985 Cyclosporin A increases survival of cross-species intrastriatal grafts of embryonic dopamine-containing neurons. Exp Brain Res 60:204–208

Brundin P, Widner H, Nilsson OG, Strecker RE, Björklund A 1989 Intracerebral xenografts of dopamine neurons: the role of immunosuppression and the blood–brain barrier. Exp Brain Res 75:195–207

Cozzi E, White D 1995 The generation of transgenic pigs as potential organ donors for humans. Nat Med 1:964–966

Daniloff JK, Low WC, Bodony RP, Wells J 1985 Cross-species neural transplants of embryonic septal nuclei to the hippocampal formation of adult rats. Exp Brain Res 59:73–82

Deacon T, Schumacher J, Dinsmore J et al 1997 Histological evidence of fetal pig neural cell survival after transplantation into a patient with Parkinson's disease. Nat Med 3:350–353

Deacon T, Fodor W, Rollins S et al 1998 Xenotransplantation of transgenic fetal pig dopamine neurons to rats and systemic prevention of host complement-mediated cell lysis. Soc Neurosci Abstr 421:9

Deng S, Bühler L, Lou J et al 1994 Study of concordant xenografted islets of Langerhans rejection: humoral or cellular mechanism? Transplant Proc 26:1184–1185

Duan WM, Widner H, Brundin P 1995 Temporal pattern of host responses against intrastriatal grafts of syngeneic, allogeneic or xenogeneic embryonic neuronal tissue in rats. Exp Brain Res 104:227–242

Edge SB, Gosse ME, Dinsmore J 1998 Xenogeneic cell therapy: current progress and future developments in porcine cell transplantation. Cell Transplant 7:525–539

Finsen BR, Pedersen EB, Sørensen T, Hokland M, Zimmer J 1990 Immune reactions against intracerebral murine xenografts of fetal hippocampal tissue and cultured cortical astrocytes in the adult rat. Prog Brain Res 82:111–128

Freeman TB, Widner H (eds) 1998 Cell transplantation for neurological disorders: toward reconstruction of the human central nervous system. Humana Press, Totowa, NJ

Galili U, Tibell U, Samuelson B, Rydberg L, Groth CG 1995 Increased anti-Gal activity in diabetic patients transplanted with fetal porcine islet cell clusters. Transplantation 59:1549–1556

Groth CG, Korsgren O, Tibell A et al 1994 Transplantation of porcine fetal pancreas to diabetic patients. Lancet 344:1402–1404

Honey CR, Clarke DJ, Dallman MJ, Charlton HM 1990 Human neural graft function in rats treated with anti-interleukin II receptor antibody. Neuroreport 1:247–249

Inoue H, Kohsaka S, Yoshida K, Ohtani M, Toya S, Tsukada Y 1985 Cyclosporin A enhances the survivability of mouse cerebral cortex grafted into the third ventricle of rat brain. Neurosci Lett 54:85–90

Korbutt GS, Aspeslet L, Ao Z et al 1996 Porcine islet cell antigens are recognized by xenoreactive natural human antibodies of both IgG and IgM subtypes. Transplant Proc 28:837–838

Korsgren O, Jansson L, Eizirik D, Andersson A 1991 Functional and morphological differentiation of fetal porcine islet-like cell clusters after transplantation into nude mice. Diabetologia 34:379–386

Larsson LC, Czech KA, Widner H, Korsgren O 1999 Discordant neural tissue xenografts survive longer in immunoglobulin deficient mice. Transplantation 68:1153–1160

Mason DW, Charlton HM, Jones AJ, Lavy BD, Puklavec M, Simmonds SJ 1986 The fate of allogeneic and xenogeneic neuronal tissue transplanted into the third ventricle of rodents. Neuroscience 19:685–694

McKenzie IFC, Koulmanda M, Mandel TE, Xing P-X, Sandrin MS 1995 Pig to human xenotransplantation: the expression of Gal α(1,3) Gal epitopes on pig islet cells. Xenotransplantation 2:1–7

Mirenda V, Sigalla J, Fiche M et al 1997 Pig pancreatic islet xenografts in a B-cell-deficient mouse model. Transplant Proc 29:762–763

Morgan BP, Gasque P 1996 Expression of complement in the brain: role in health and disease. Immunol Today 17:461–466

Nataf S, Stahel PF, Davoust N, Barnum SR 1999 Complement anaphylatoxin receptors in neurons: new tricks for old receptors? Trends Neurosci 22:397–402

Oberholzer J, Yu D, Triponez F et al 1999 Decomplementation with cobra venom factor prolongs survival of xenografted islets in a rat to mouse model. Immunology 97:173–180

Olanow CW, Kordower JH, Freeman TB 1996 Fetal nigral transplantation as a therapy for Parkinson's disease. Trends Neurosci 19:102–109

Pakzaban P, Isacson O 1994 Neural xenotransplantation: reconstruction of neuronal circuitry across species barriers. Neuroscience 62:989–1001

Pedersen EB, Poulsen FR, Zimmer J, Finsen B 1995 Prevention of mouse–rat brain xenograft rejection by a combination of cyclosporin A, prednisolone and azathioprine. Exp Brain Res 106:181–186

Sakei K, Date I, Yoshimoto Y et al 1991 The effect of a new immunosuppressive agent, FK-506, on xenogeneic neural transplantation in rodents. Brain Res 565:167–170

Schaapherder AFM, Wolvekamp MCJ, te Bulte MTJ, Bouwman E, Gooszen HG, Daha MR 1996 Porcine islet cells of Langerhans are destroyed by human complement and not by antibody-dependent cell-mediated mechanisms. Transplantation 62:29–33

Simeonovic CJ, Wilson JD, Ceredig R 1990 Antibody-induced rejection of pig proislet xenografts in CD4[+] T-cell depleted diabetic mice. Transplantation 50:657–662

Sloan DJ, Wood MJ, Charlton HM 1991 The immune response to intracerebral neural grafts. Trends Neurosci 14:341–346

Sumitran S, Liu J, Czech KA, Christenson B, Widner H, Holgersson J 1999 Human natural antibodies cytotoxic to pig embryonic brain cells recognize novel non-Gal-α1,3-Gal-based xenoantigens. Exp Neurol 159:347–361

Taylor P, Botto M, Walport M 1998 The complement system. Curr Biol 8:R259–R261

Wallgren AC, Karlsson-Parra A, Korsgren O 1995 The main infiltrating cell in xenograft rejection is a CD4[+] macrophage and not a T lymphocyte. Transplantation 60:594–601

Weiss RA 1999 Xenografts and retroviruses. Science 285:1221–1222

Wood MJA, Sloan DJ, Wood KJ, Charlton HM 1996 Indefinite survival of neural xenografts induced with anti-CD4 monoclonal antibodies. Neuroscience 70:775–789

Zhou J, Date I, Sakai K et al 1993 Suppression of immunorejection against rat fetal dopaminergic neurons in a mouse brain by 15-deoxyspergualin. Brain Res 621:155–160

DISCUSSION

Gray: Could you extrapolate what you have said to the current trials using porcine tissue in the treatment of HD and PD?

Barker: My understanding is that the phase I trial in the USA involved 12 patients with moderate-to-severe PD receiving porcine VM tissue into three sites. They were either immunosuppressed with CyA or the tissue-treated with a masking antibody to MHC I. Of these 12, two have improved up to two years post-implantation. There is also one post-mortem study showing poor dopaminergic cell survival in a grafted patient. Ten HD patients also received grafts, but I am not sure what immunosuppression they had. A phase II trial for PD is taking place, which I think Tom Freeman knows more about.

Freeman: The surgical arm of that trial has been completed; it is a double-blind placebo-controlled trial with a total of 17 patients with PD. The clinical data should be available in eight months. The immunotherapy involves both CyA and prednisone, with doses typically used in kidney transplant programmes. The placebo surgical group does not receive immunosuppression.

Perry: I was interested in the absence of the antibody response to the porcine tissue in the first 10 days. What happens to the antibody levels later? As your grafts are being rejected there are presumably all sorts of antigens released.

Barker: We don't know. We have serum samples from slightly later time points, but we have not analysed them for antibody levels.

Isacson: In the rat, the antibody response also takes a bit longer. One would expect an antibody response. Since it is present with allografts, one would very likely get it with xenotransplants.

Aebischer: Have you performed *in vitro* cytotaxic assays using human serum or human cerebrospinal fluid (CSF), to see whether you could kill pig neural tissue *in vitro* to assess the effect of complement antibodies?

Barker: Porcine embryonic neural tissue can bind human Ig and activate complement with cell lysis. We have shown this, as has Sumitran and colleagues at the Karolinska Institute in Sweden. We haven't tried CSF.

Aebischer: In examining the safety of our cell lines, we can have a positive cytotoxic assay with serum but never with CSF, which shows that pre-existing antibodies are not present in the CSF.

Finsen: We tried to add serum and rat complement to porcine brain cell cultures. The viability is quite high—about 87%. The cells which disappear are the endothelial cells and microglial cells, but the astrocytes survive.

Aebischer: That is in 2D. Whenever you go in 3D with cell aggregates, the best you can do is have the first cell layer killed. It is very difficult to kill a 3D structure just with antibodies and complement. The probability of this system being important in the xenograft kill is rather small.

Barker: But one could argue that if it targets the outer cells and kills them, then the next layer of cells is vulnerable to attack. In humans we certainly know that we have high levels of circulating naturally occurring antibodies to porcine xenoantigens which will be exposed to the implanted tissue in the grafting situation with BBB disruption.

Aebischer: But we don't have them in the CSF. The BBB may be open for a while but I'm not sure the timing in issue is in favour of a cell kill by this mechanism.

Barker: In the case of an inflammatory immune response to the graft, the BBB may not seal up again, but remain leaky for an indefinite period of time, unlike the situation with the iso- or allografts.

Perry: It will be leaking for days. I would think, however, that complement is a relatively minor player compared with the next phase of the immune response involving the T cells.

Isacson: We have some data on that. We do a red blood cell lysis assay with human or primate serum. The problem with these complement lysis assays is that they are usually carried out for only one or two hours. However, when we added human or primate sera to primary fetal pig neurons, we also had some loss. My thinking was that if we have a BBB breakage for 7–14 days, even the 10–20% cell lysis we saw for 1–2 weeks would accumulate over time. Thus, in principle, Roger Barker's work and our work suggest that complement does play an immunological role in CNS xenograft rejection. It does not, however, explain away the T cell role, which is dominant in all these situations. If you don't block the T cells these xenografts will be destroyed. The complexity of this situation is extraordinary. In his early work on mouse-to-rat xenografts, Anders Björklund showed that occasional xenografts could survive even without any immunosuppression (Björklund et al 1982). In our work we have a fairly constant frequency of 10–15% of pig-to-rat xenograft survival without any immunosuppression. This suggests that in some conditions, a graft getting in behind the BBB and not expressing much MHC class I molecules will survive because of lack of T cell recognition, even if you get the humoral response. It is a complex issue.

Perry: There is another aspect that we have studied (Ohmoto et al 1999). This not only depends on the strain of the rat but also the state of the animal house. The cleaner the animal house, the easier it is to get things behind the BBB and they will survive. We have studied this with both adenovirus and BCG. BCG is a 1 mm bug, so you need a larger gauge needle to stick it into the brain. When it is put into the brain parenchyma, there is a typical acute inflammatory response, but it seals up over the next few days and these bugs remain there for a year undetected by the immune system. This doesn't happen every time: occasionally we get escape, probably because we have injected too many bugs. The reason a small percentage of your transplants survive in the absence of immunosuppression may well be because in a clean rat with very little damage, the inflammatory response is low and the BBB hides the graft away.

Isacson: Yes, such data, which are consistent across laboratories, inform us about the complexity of the immunological responses (Isacson & Breakefield 1997).

Freeman: To throw one more complexity in, there are now two experiments where xenografts without immunosuppression survived when transplanted on microcarriers that were about 300 µm in diameter (Saporta et al 1997, Subramanian et al 2000). These glass beads served as a substrate and tight junctions were formed before the transplants were done. In one case this was a human mesencephalic transplant into a rat; in the other case it was human retinal pigmented epithelium cells into rats and monkeys. These survived without immunosuppression. Substrate and tight junctions therefore play and important part in the mechanism of xenograft survival.

Barker: One of the major stumbling blocks of this field is the inconsistency of what is seen experimentally with xenografts. If we get six out of 10 grafts surviving that is great, but if we are ever going to take this to clinical trials we need to have a better understanding of what is going on so that we can achieve 100% survival. The complexity of the rejection process means that different mechanisms may underlie different phases of graft rejection, and one of the great problems facing any xenograft programme is getting consistent survival of the grafted tissue in the long term.

Isacson: There is a great consistency between research groups. We had the same rate of over 80% xenograft survival as Bente Finsen's group, as did Steve Dunnett's with the standard CyA immunosuppression protocol. However, there is a difference between transplanting xenografts to a rat and transplanting xenografts to a monkey or human hosts, although I don't think it is an all or none situation, as has been suggested. There is complement activation also in the rat, but it is of a smaller magnitude. In the final analysis, you need to have data on specific species as donor–host combinations to determine empirically the immunological reactions and responses.

Perry: Rats are different. The amount of adjuvant you have to inject into even a susceptible strain to give it experimental autoimmune encephalitis (EAE) is huge. If I did it to you, you would be extremely unhappy! In a similar manner, the amount of lipopolysaccharide (LPS) you can put into a rat is enormous. These animals are the great survivors — they live in sewers.

Isacson: When we did the first xenotransplantation trial of porcine cells in humans with PD, we put in as mild CyA levels as possible, and there were no data on complement activation for these types of transplants in 1994 when this was IND and FDA filed. Our data today suggest that complement is something we have to pay attention to, even though it is not as vigorous as the xenograft kidney or islet situation.

Lindvall: There is another issue with embryonic porcine cells that we haven't really discussed — that is, the growth capacity of these cells as compared to that of their equivalents in the human embryo. If we take primary embryonic porcine dopamine neurons, and implant these into the striatum of a patient, what are the growth characteristics of these porcine cells? What volume can they reinnervate? How many pig donors do you have to use in order to have a sufficient number of surviving dopamine neurons in each patient? How many tracts do you need in order to reinnervate the human putamen? There are some figures available on the number of dopamine neurons in the pig mesencephalon from Karen Østergaard, and these are in the order of 40 000–50 000.

Isacson: Those figures have now been revised upwards to at least 200 000.

Barker: And more recently, Arne Möller from Denmark reports that in the mini pig there are at least 700 000 TH-positive neurons in the midbrain.

Lindvall: Much of the concern was based on Karen Østergaard's figures, which were relatively low. Assuming that the survival rate of embryonic porcine dopamine neurons after grafting is similar to that in other transplants of human or rodent tissue, one would need a lot of donors.

The figures we are talking about here are that you may need tissue from up to as many as 20 pig donors for one side of the brain in a PD patient. However, I don't see this as the major problem, and if there are more dopamine neurons in each pig donor, it would make the logistics more feasible. Another issue relates to the fact that if you are going to reinnervate the human putamen, we know quite well that the human embryonic dopamine neurons can grow about 7 mm. But we don't know how far pig dopamine neurons can grow. There is a maximum number of implantation sites one can have in the human putamen. An important question is, therefore, how much of the volume of this structure will one be able to reinnervate using porcine dopamine neurons?

Isacson: If the situation was indeed as you have painted it, it wouldn't work. In the human striatum, where we do implantation in PD and HD (Deacon et al 1997), the 115 d gestational period may not be sufficient to grow really long axons. But the pig neurons, according to my calculations, will be able to grow sufficiently, even if it is necessary to graft into a few more sites than with human donor neurons. We know that forebrain pig axons can grow in the adult rat all the way down to the spinal cord.

Lindvall: I am talking about the growth capacity of pig dopamine neurons within the grey matter of the human striatum. Do we know if the terminals can extend more than 2–3 mm from the graft? We hope this is the case, but do we know it?

Dunnett: Arne Møller (unpublished) has these data with his pig-to-pig allografts.

Gray: But you cannot necessarily assume that these are the critical data.

Isacson: I think Olle Lindvall has asked a good question about species-specific axonal capacity. These data do exist; these are the pig-to-PD patient data (Deacon et al 1997). I saw donor porcine fibres with specific neurofilament markers extending for about a halo of 7–8 mm. TH dopaminergic fibres cannot be labelled specifically to distinguish between the human and the pig.

Freeman: In our porcine transplant program, we had no proof, and presuming that the donor plays an important role in determining growth from the graft, we know that the neuritic outgrowth in rodent grafts is between 0.5 and 2 mm, outgrowth from human grafts is between 2 and 7 mm, so we estimated that the outgrowth from porcine grafts is somewhere in between. The best evidence we had was from the pig into rat xenografts, in which neural outgrowth in grey matter was at least 2 mm. Our best guess was that the pig neurons, if they survive as a xenograft, would extend neuritic processes for 2–3 mm, so if we put the deposits 5 mm apart we are likely to saturate the striatum. It is possible, in theory, to saturate the entire striatum with 8 tracts. In our clinical protocol we used only 5 tracts in the postcommisural putamen, spaced 5 mm apart, and one tract in the caudate.

References

Björklund A, Stenevi U, Dunnett SB, Gage FH 1982 Cross-species neural grafting in a rat model of Parkinson's disease. Nature 298:652–654

Deacon T, Schumacher J, Dinsmore J et al 1997 Histological evidence of fetal pig neural cell survival after transplantation into a patient with Parkinson's disease. Nat Med 3:350–353

Isacson O, Breakefield XO 1997 Benefits and risks of hosting animal cells in the human brain. Nat Med 3:964–969

Ohmoto Y, Wood M JA, Charlton HM, Kajiwara K, Perry VH, Wood K J 1999 Variation in the immune response to adenoviral vectors in the brain: influence of mouse strain, environmental conditions and priming. Gene Ther 6:471–481

Saporta S, Borlongan C, Moore J et al 1997 Microcarrier enhanced survival of human and rat fetal ventral mesencephalon cells implanted in the rat striatum. Cell Transplant 6:579–584

Subramanian T, Marchionini D, Potter EM, Cornfeldt ML 2000 Striatal transplantation of human retinal pigmented epithelium attached to microcarriers in hemiparkinsonian rats. Exp Neurol, submitted

Gene transfer techniques for the delivery of GDNF in Parkinson's disease

Jean-Luc Ridet, Nicole Déglon and Patrick Aebischer[1]

Division of Surgical Research and Gene Therapy Center, Lausanne University Medical School, CHUV, Pavillon 4, CH-1011 Lausanne, Switzerland

Abstract. Parkinson's disease (PD) is a neurodegenerative disorder characterized by motor disturbances caused by an alteration of the dopaminergic nigrostriatal system. Current symptomatic treatments for PD include dopaminergic drug administration, deep brain stimulation, ablative surgery and fetal cell transplantation. Though these approaches have significant beneficial effects, they are hampered by limiting side-effects, but more importantly they do not change the disease progression. Alternative restorative and neuroprotective strategies have therefore to be considered. Neuroprotective effects of neurotrophic factors, anti-apoptotic and antioxidant molecules are currently being investigated for this purpose. Among neurotrophic molecules, the potential of the glial cell line-derived neurotrophic factor (GDNF) to protect the nigral dopaminergic neurons and/or rescue striatal dopamine levels has been extensively documented. For GDNF to become a clinical reality, appropriate delivery techniques will have to be developed. This chapter focuses on the potential of encapsulated cells and viral vectors to locally release neurotrophic factors in experimental models of PD.

2000 Neural transplantation in neurodegenerative disease. Wiley, Chichester (Novartis Foundation Symposium 231) p 202–219

Parkinson's disease (PD), a progressive neurodegenerative disease with a prevalence of 100–200 per 100 000 persons, affects several million individuals around the world. The major clinical symptoms, including tremor, muscle rigidity, bradykinesia, gait and postural deficits, are related to dopamine deficiency within the striatum following degeneration of dopaminergic neurons of the substantia nigra. Current symptomatic treatments include L-dopa administration, deep brain stimulation, ablative surgery and fetal cell transplantation. Though these approaches have significant beneficial effects, they

---

[1]This chapter was presented at the symposium by Professor Aebischer, to whom correspondence should be addressed.

also lead to limiting side-effects after few years (see references in Dunnett & Björklund 1999, Hallett et al 1999, Krack et al 1999). For instance, the systemic administration of L-dopa leads over time to daily 'on–off' fluctuations and dyskinesias. The efficacy of deep brain stimulation (thalamic, pallidal or subthalamic nuclei) is today well established. Although indicated for late parkinsonism, deep brain stimulation is quite invasive and not devoid of side effects (Hallett et al 1999, Krack et al 1999). Furthermore, most of these therapies do not change the disease progression. The development of strategies capable of preventing or even reversing the degeneration process early in the course of the disease is therefore needed. These include the local administration of neurotrophic factors and anti-apoptotic or antioxidant molecules (see Alexi et al 2000). Numerous *in vitro* and *in vivo* studies suggest that members of the glial cell line-derived neurotrophic factor (GDNF) family, especially GDNF itself, are the most potent survival factors for mesencephalic dopaminergic neurons (see Collier & Sortwell 1999, Alexi et al 2000).

Sustained administration of therapeutic molecules to the brain is however challenged by stability and distribution issues. The development of an efficient drug delivery system represents, therefore, a major challenge for the treatment of neurodegenerative disorders such as PD. Since the intraventricular delivery of large boluses of GDNF lead to severe side-effects, the use of encapsulated cells and viral vectors is being investigated for its sustained and local delivery.

This chapter describes these two powerful systems, cell encapsulation and lentiviral vectors, for the delivery of GDNF family members and reviews *in vivo* studies that have illustrated their efficacy for the neuroprotection of dopaminergic nigral neurons.

Cell encapsulation

The transplantation of fetal mesencephalic neurons constitutes a promising approach for the ectopic replacement of the nigral dopaminergic neurons predominantly affected in PD. However, this approach is limited by tissue procurement and ethical issues (Dunnett & Björklund 1999). In order to overcome these limitations, various alternatives to fetal transplantation techniques are being developed. Cell encapsulation constitutes one option. It consists of surrounding cells by a permselective polymer membrane shielding them from the host immune system. It allows the use of cell lines or primary cells either from allo- or xenogeneic donor origin without immunosuppression (Hottinger & Aebischer 1999a,b, Lysaght & Aebischer 1999, Bensadoun et al 2000a). The molecular weight cut-off of this the encapsulating membrane is determined set to prevent (i) the inward diffusion of immunoglobulins and lytic factors of the complement, and (ii) interactions of the host immunocompetent

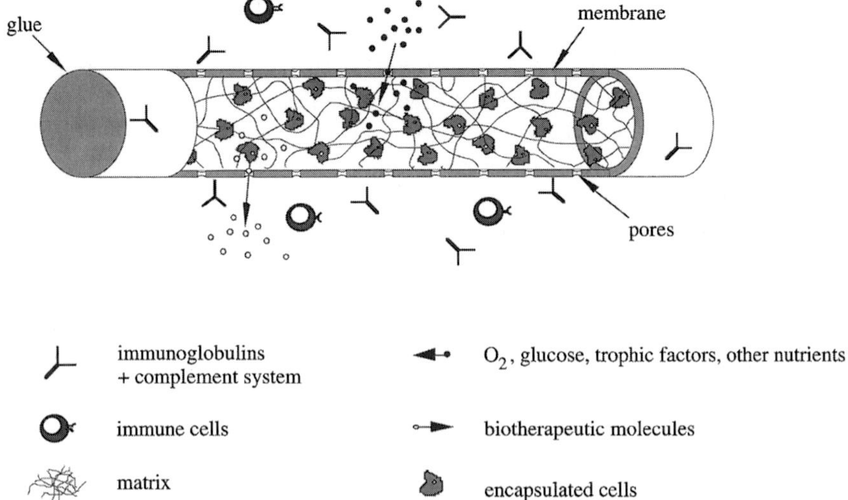

FIG. 1.   Schematic representation of a macrocapsule. The genetically engineered cells are surrounded within a permselective polymer membrane preventing the inward diffusion of immunoglobulins and lytic factors of the complement, but allowing the inward diffusion of nutrients and the outward diffusion of therapeutic molecules.

cells with the grafted cells, but (iii) still allow the inward diffusion of oxygen, glucose and other nutrients as well as the outward diffusion of biotherapeutic molecules released by the encapsulated cells (Fig. 1).

Microencapsulation allows the encapsulation of small cell clusters within a thin, spherical, semipermeable membrane. Such microcapsules containing dopamine-producing cells, when intrastriatally implanted have been shown to reduce behavioural deficits in experimental models of PD (Bensadoun et al 2000a). However, the mechanical and chemical fragility of these microcapsules as well as their unretrievability after implantation constitute major biosafety limitations for clinical use. *Macroencapsulation* is an alternative cell immunoisolation system involving preformed hollow, cylindrical, permselective polymer membranes (Fig. 1). During the past decade, considerable efforts have been devoted to adapt macrocapsule technology for use in the CNS. The major advantages of these macrocapsules are their biocompatibility, chemical stability, durability and appropriate mechanical properties. Provided adequate geometry, macrocapsules can be retrieved, an important feature for clinical application.

Experimental studies demonstrated that encapsulated PC12 cells, a catecholaminergic cell line, exhibit long-term survival and improve behavioural deficits when implanted within the brain of parkinsonian rats (Tresco et al 1992, Emerich et al 1996) and non-human primates (Aebischer et al 1994, Kordower et al

1995a). Importantly, no significant immunological problems or host tissue reactions have been reported. However, intraventricular implantation of encapsulated PC12 cells appears less efficient than intraparenchymal placement to improve parkinsonian symptomatology (Emerich et al 1996). Further studies might will be necessary to improve the amount of dopamine released by the capsule. However, such an increase in dopamine levels may lead to severe side effects if diffusing dopamine reaches other brain areas.

The most promising application of encapsulation for PD is the development of neuroprotective and/or restorative strategies based on the local delivery of neurotrophic factors such as GDNF. Genetically engineered cell lines can be encapsulated and implanted into the brain. Baby hamster kidney (BHK) cells have been transfected with expression vectors carrying the cDNA coding for human GDNF (Tseng et al 1997). The neuroprotective properties of these encapsulated GDNF-releasing BHK cells have been evaluated in a rat model of PD (Tseng et al 1997). After perinigral implantation of BHK-GDNF cells and subsequent axotomy of the medial forebrain bundle, rats exhibited significant improvement in amphetamine-induced rotational behaviour, as compared to controls. Furthermore, the release of GDNF permitted a higher survival rate of the nigral dopaminergic neurons (65% versus 27% in controls) (Tseng et al 1997). Using the same experimental paradigm, neuroprotective effects were obtained after implantation of encapsulated neurturin-releasing BHK cells, a member of the GDNF family (Tseng et al 1998).

The restorative potential of encapsulated BHK-GDNF cells has also been evaluated in late-stage parkinsonian baboons (Palfi & Hantraye, unpublished data). In this study, monkeys were chronically lesioned with MPTP (1-methyl-4-phenyl-1,2,3,6-tetrahydropyridine) for 12–18 months and then implanted bilaterally in the ventricles with a single capsule containing BHK-GDNF cells, releasing approximately 200 ng per capsule. GDNF treatment almost completely reversed MPTP-induced hypokinesia. Histological analyses revealed that GDNF induced sprouting of the remaining TH-positive neurites in the substantia nigra and in the striatum. Importantly, no side-effects were observed (Palfi & Hantraye, unpublished data). These results strongly suggest that long-term intracerebroventricular delivery of small amounts of GDNF *via* encapsulated cells constitutes a promising therapeutical strategy for clinical applications.

Perhaps the most promising perspective for cell encapsulation is the increase of cell survival in the co-implantation paradigm. Limited cell survival of fetal mesencephalic neurons has been reported in animal models of PD as well as in parkinsonian patients. Only 5–20% of the implanted fetal mesencephalic neurons survive the transplantation procedure (Kordower et al 1995b, Lindvall 1998). Neurotrophic factors, free radical scavengers, antioxidants and anti-apoptotic molecules are candidates to improve grafted cell survival (Alexi et al 2000). In this context, the effect of encapsulated genetically engineered cells releasing low amounts of neurotrophic factors have been evaluated in co-grafting experiments (Sautter et al 1998). GDNF was selected to test this approach as it had previously been shown to increase the survival of transplanted ventral mesencephalic cells when administered through repeated bolus injections close to grafts (Rosenblad et al 1996). Furthermore, the study involved the striatal placement, one week before transplantation of fetal ventral mesencephalic tissue, of a single capsule containing BHK-GDNF (Sautter et al 1998). GDNF triggered a 2.6-fold increase in the number of dopaminergic neurons within the transplants and a 1.5-fold increase in the dopaminergic fibre network surrounding the graft. Amphetamine-induced rotating behaviour was also significantly improved at 3 and 6 weeks after co-grafting with GDNF-releasing capsules as compared to graft alone or GDNF alone (Sautter et al 1998). These results demonstrate that continuous delivery of GDNF by encapsulated cells constitutes an efficient support for long-term survival and function of intracerebral dopaminergic transplants in rats. Furthermore, such an approach may reduce the amount of fetal tissue required for transplantation into PD patients. Therefore, a clinical trial based on striatal co-transplantation of GDNF-releasing capsule and fetal mesencephalic tissue is being considered.

Viral vectors

Gene therapy has emerged as a promising approach to the treatment of neurodegenerative diseases and traumatic injuries. Both direct (*in vivo*) and indirect (*ex vivo*) gene transfer have been developed. In the context of *ex vivo* gene therapy of the CNS, cell encapsulation or direct cell transplantation of genetically engineered cells have been investigated (Gage 1998, Lysaght & Aebischer 1999). *In vivo* gene therapy approaches include direct naked DNA injection and the use of viral and non-viral vectors. To date, all non-viral vectors encounter limitations in terms of transduction level and long-term expression of the transgene. Several viral vectors have been designed for gene transfer, i.e. adenovirus (Barkats et al 1998, Benihoud et al 1999, Wickham 2000), adeno-associated virus (AAV) (Rabinowitz & Samulski 1998, Snyder 1999, Monahan & Samulski 2000), baculovirus (Kost & Condreay 1999), herpes simplex virus (Fink et al 2000), lentivirus (Naldini 1998, Federico 1999, Trono 2000) and RNA virus (Lundstrom et al 1999, Schlesinger & Dubensky 1999, Hewson 2000). The potential of these viral vectors has been tested in various experimental models of neurodegenerative disorders and traumatic injuries (Hottinger & Aebischer 1999b, Costantini et al 2000). So far, according to the transduction efficiency and safety of the currently available versions, the most promising candidates for CNS gene therapy are the adenoviral, AAV and lentiviral vectors.

The first generation of adenoviral vectors have been widely used in various experimental models of neurodegenerative disorders, especially in PD models. Both restorative and neuroprotective strategies using adenoviral vectors have been shown to protect nigral dopaminergic neurons and/or rescue striatal dopamine levels (Horellou & Mallet 1997, Barkats et al 1998). These vectors are however hampered by a rather strong immune host reaction accompanied by a loss of transgene expression. Recently, it has been reported that *gutless* versions of adenoviral vectors are less immunogenic and thus sustain higher transduction levels than the first generation vectors when injected into rat striatum (Thomas et al 2000).

Beneficial effects of AAV vectors carrying aromatic amino acid decarboxylase and/or tyrosine hydroxylase, or GDNF (AAV–GDNF) genes have been reported in experimental models of PD (Mandel et al 1997, 1999a,b, During et al 1998, Fan et al 1998, Leff et al 1999). However, *in vivo*, a 40% decrease of the GDNF levels is observed over time (Mandel et al 1997). It has been shown that a perinigral injection of AAV–GDNF in rats protects dopaminergic neurons against 6-hydroxy-dopamine (OHDA)-induced toxicity (Mandel et al 1997, 1999b). Interestingly, these neuroprotective effects are observed in two different paradigms: AAV–GDNF injected before (Mandel et al 1997) or just after a 6-OHDA lesion (after onset of degeneration) (Mandel et al 1999b). AAV diffusion of the vector is limited within brain parenchyma, which is either an advantage or a disadvantage depending on the experimental paradigm. The small (4.5 kb) cloning capacity may also constitute a limitation of the AAV system. Stability and long-term expression from AAV vectors seem also to depend on brain area (Costantini et al 2000).

Replication-defective lentiviral vectors have been developed from retroviruses, of human, feline, simian or equine origin (Naldini 1998, Federico 1999). Lentiviral vectors derived from HIV-1 transduce both dividing and non-dividing cells, allowing efficient delivery of therapeutic genes to haematopoietic cells and neurons (Naldini 1998, Federico 1999). For the last few years, major advances have been accomplished to optimize the biosafety and efficacy of lentiviral vectors. Replicative-defective and multiply attenuated versions have been designed (Zufferey et al 1997, 1998, Dull et al 1998, Miyoshi et al 1998; see for review Naldini 1998) without affecting the efficiency of transgene expression. Available versions of lentiviral vectors allow an efficient and sustained expression of a transgene in rodent (Naldini et al 1996a, Miyoshi et al 1997, Blömer et al 1998, Takahashi et al 1999, Bensadoun et al 2000b, Déglon et al 2000, Rosenblad et al 2000) and primate (Kordower et al 1999) CNS (Fig. 2). In addition, lentiviral vectors permit infection of large brain areas since they can diffuse over 2–3 mm from the injection site, allowing the transduction of a high number of cells within the striatum or the substantia nigra in of rodents (Bensadoun et al 2000b, Déglon et al 2000, Rosenblad et al 2000).

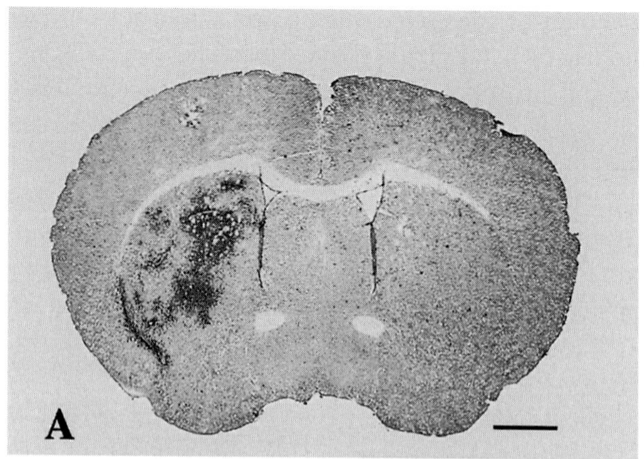

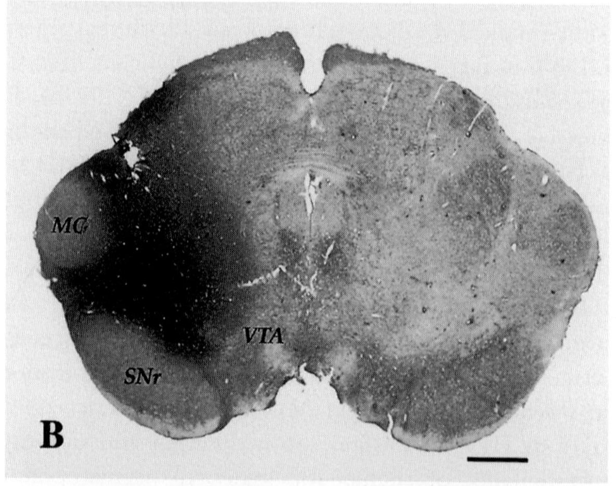

MC
VTA
SNr

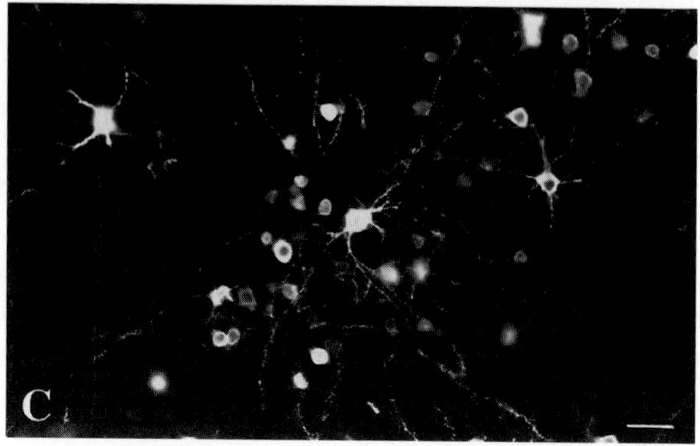

It has been documented that lentiviral vectors preferentially transduce neurons, e.g. 90–100% in the rat (Naldini et al 1996a,b, Blömer et al 1998, Déglon et al 2000, Rosenblad et al 2000) and mice striatum (J. C. Bensadoun, unpublished data) (Fig. 2 A,B), and 80–88% in the striatum of non-human primates (Kordower et al 1999) (Fig. 2C). More recently, we have shown that a single injection of 2 μl (200 000 ng p24/ml) of a lentiviral vector carrying the reporter gene *lacZ* (LV–*lacZ*) into the rat substantia nigra permitted the transduction of 40% of the dopaminergic neurons, as compared to 5% with an earliery version of lentiviral vectors (Déglon et al 2000). In mice, the injection of 1 μl of LV–*lacZ* (100 000 ng p24/ml) above the substantia nigra allowed the transduction of 20% (maximum 50% surrounding the needle tract) of the nigral dopaminergic cells (Bensadoun et al 2000b). In non-human primate, the injection of LV–*lacZ* (200 000– 250 000 ng p24/ml) permits the transduction of 1–1.5 million cells when injected into the striatum (40 μl total/5 sites), and the transduction of 190 000 cells when injected into the substantia nigra (5 μl/1 site) (Kordower et al 1999) (Fig. 2). Furthermore, no major immune response or tissue reaction has been detected after brain inoculation of lentiviral vectors.

The ability of lentiviral vectors to efficiently transduce neuronal cells in the striatum or substantia nigra highlights their potential for the treatment of neurodegenerative disorders, especially PD. For such purpose, a self-inactivating and multiply attenuated lentiviral vector containing the post-transcriptional regulatory element of the woodchuck hepatitis virus and the cDNA for human GDNF has been designed (Déglon et al 2000). In a rat model of Parkinson's disease, LV–GDNF protects nigral dopaminergic neurons from axotomy-induced cell death (55.8% remaining dopaminergic neurons as compared to 23.9% in LV–*lacZ* control group) (Déglon et al 2000). The neuroprotective effects of GDNF family members, i.e. GDNF, artemin, neublastin, delivered *via* lentiviral vectors have been confirmed in the 6-OHDA model of PD in rats (Rosenblad et al 2000). In the latter study, a lentiviral vector injection into both striatum and substantia nigra leads to a 80–90% nigral dopaminergic neuron protection, as compared to 20% in controls (Rosenblad et al 2000). More recently, the neuroprotective potential of LV–GDNF has been evaluated in mice (Bensadoun

---

FIG. 2.   Transduction of neuronal cells via lentiviral vectors (LV–*lacZ*, A,C; LV–GDNF, B) in the mouse (A, B) or primate (C) brain. Transduced cells are identified by Xgal enzymatic staining (A) or β-galactosidase immunostaining (C). (A) The diffusion of lentiviral vectors over 2–3 mm within the striatum. (B) Note the large distribution of the therapeutic molecule (here GDNF) after injection of LV–GDNF into the mouse substantia nigra pars compacta. (C) Numerous neurons exhibiting extensive neuritic network express the transgene three months after the injection of LV–*lacZ* into the caudate of a Rhesus monkey. Scale bar = 1 mm (A), 600 μm (B) or 35 μm (C)

et al 2000b). LV–GDNF vectors were injected unilaterally above the substantia nigra, two weeks before the ipsilateral striatal injection of 6-OHDA. In LV–GDNF injected animals, 69.5% of the dopaminergic neurons were protected as compared to 33.1% in the control mutated GDNF (muGDNF) group. The dopaminergic fibre network was also clearly preserved within the nigra in the presence of GDNF. Furthermore, these anatomical benefits in the LV–GDNF were associated with a significant 50% reduction of the apomorphine-induced rotating behaviour, as compared to the muGDNF group (Bensadoun et al 2000b).

Efforts are currently devoted to further increasing both the number of transduced neurons and transgene expression by improving the lentiviral vector design and the injection procedures. For instance, Zennou and colleagues (2000) recently demonstrated the key role of a central 99 nucleotide-long sequence in the nuclear import of HIV-1 DNA. Furthermore, lentiviral vectors containing the central DNA flap increase both transduction levels and the number of neural cells expressing green fluorescent protein (GFP) reporter gene, as compared to vectors lacking this sequence (Serguera et al 1999a). Taken together, these experimental results emphasize the potential of lentiviral vectors for the sustained and continuous delivery of GDNF for the protection of nigral dopaminergic neurons in PD. Further studies in non-human primates demonstrating neuroprotective effects of lentivirally delivered GDNF are currently being conducted.

Conclusions

Restorative and/or protective strategies have demonstrated their anatomical and functional benefits in experimental PD models. To date, two delivery systems allow for a local and sustained release of therapeutic molecules within the brain, i.e. polymer encapsulation of genetically engineered cell lines and viral vectors. The first one is sufficiently developed to allow its use in the clinic. The transplantation of polymer-encapsulated genetically engineered cells has indeed already been attempted in humans. Our group has reported the cerebrospinal fluid implantation of encapsulated BHK cells genetically engineered to release ciliary neurotrophic factor (CNTF) in patients suffering from amyotrophic lateral sclerosis (Aebischer et al 1996a,b). This study demonstrated the survival of the encapsulated cells as well as the sustained release of CNTF within the cerebrospinal fluid of these patients. Based on the excellent safety record of this initalinitial trial and the preclinical data accumulated in rodents (Sautter et al 1998), We we are currently designing a trial combining the delivery of GDNF secreted by encapsulated C_2C_{12} cells with the transplantation of fetal mesencephalon in late PD patients.

In contrast, several biosafety issues need to be assessed before any clinical trial involving viral vectors will occur. First, a packaging cell line has to be established to scale-up the technology and to produce clinical batches of lentiviral vectors. Furthermore, sensitive methods have to be designed to (i) detect recombinant competent viral particles, and (ii) to evaluate the biodistribution of the vector and its germline transmission in patients treated with lentiviral vectors.

The possibility of recombination between lentiviral vector and the wild-type HIV or endogenous retroviruses constitute another major biosafety issue. Recently, it has been shown that no adverse effect, such as vector mobilization or recombination, infectivity or spread of HIV-1, was observed with self-inactivated versions of lentiviral vectors (Bukovsky et al 1999). This has to be tested *in vivo* after intracerebral injection of lentiviral vectors. Furthermore, the possibility of seroconversion of patients treated with lentiviral vectors has to be considered.

Another level of biosafety consists of controlling of transgene expression to either (i) avoid undesirable transgene overexpression ('off' versions), or (ii) induce transgene expression within a limited time-window ('on' versions), depending on the physiopathological circumstances. Although several regulatable systems have been developed (Miller & Whelan 1997, Harvey & Caskey 1998, Rossi & Blau 1998), the most appropriate and potent for gene therapy is, so far, the tetracycline (tet)-dependent system. The proof of principle for its uses in encapsulation paradigms (Serguera et al 1999b) and viral contexts (Corti et al 1999a,b, Ridet et al 1999), have already been demonstrated. Adaptation of the tet system to lentiviral vectors is underway.

We conclude that the recent developments of delivery techniques should allow, in the foreseeable future, the delivery of biotherapeutic molecules in the brain parenchyma of patients suffering from neurodegenerative diseases. However, extensive work still has to be conducted in order to identify the molecules capable of affecting the outcome of these debilitating diseases.

Acknowledgements

The authors wish to acknowledge laboratory members for helpful discussions, especially Drs Anne D. Zurn and Jean-Charles Bensadoun. The authors also thank Drs Jack Tseng, Luis Pereira de Almeida and Diana Zala for their contributions to these studies, and Nicolas Bouche, Dana Hornfeld, Anne Maillard, Viviane Padrun, Fabienne Pidoux, Maria Rey, Lilianne Schnell and Laurence Winkel for their technical expertise. This work was supported in part by Swiss National Science Foundation and the Swiss Priority Programs on Gene Therapy and Neurological Diseases.

References

Aebischer P, Goddard M, Signore AP, Timpson RL 1994 Functional recovery in hemiparkinsonian primates transplanted with polymer-encapsulated PC12 cells. Exp Neurol 126:151–158

Aebischer P, Pochon NAM, Heyd B et al 1996a Gene therapy for amyotrophic lateral sclerosis (ALS) using a polymer encapsulated xenogenic cell line engineered to secrete hCNTF. Hum Gene Ther 7:851–860

Aebischer P, Schluep M, Déglon N et al 1996b Intrathecal delivery of CNTF using encapsulated genetically modified xenogeneic cells in amyotrophic lateral sclerosis patients. Nat Med 2:696–699 (erratum: 1996 Nat Med 2:1041)

Alexi T, Borlongan CV, Faull RL et al 2000 Neuroprotective strategies for basal ganglia degeneration: Parkinson's and Huntington's diseases. Prog Neurobiol 60:409–470

Barkats M, Bilang-Bleuel A, Buc-Caron MH et al 1998 Adenovirus in the brain: recent advances of gene therapy for neurodegenerative diseases. Prog Neurobiol 55:333–341

Benihoud K, Yeh P, Perricaudet M 1999 Adenovirus vectors for gene delivery. Curr Opin Biotechnol 10:440–447

Bensadoun JC, Widmer HR, Zurn AD, Aebischer P 2000a Polymer-encapsulated cells as a tool for drug delivery and neural transplantation in Parkinson's disease. In: Krauss JK, Jankovic J, Grossman RG (eds) Principles of surgery for Parkinson's disease and movement disorders. Lippincott-Raven Press, Philiadelphia, in press

Bensadoun JC, Déglon N, Tseng JL, Ridet JL, Zurn AD, Aebischer P 2000b Lentiviral vectors as a gene delivery system in the mouse midbrain: cellular and behavioural improvements in a 6-OHDA model of Parkinson's disease using GDNF. Exp Neurol 164:15–24

Blömer U, Kafri T, Randolph-Moore L, Verma IM, Gage FH 1998 Bcl-xL protects adult septal cholinergic neurons from axotomized cell death. Proc Natl Acad Sci USA 95:2603–2608

Bukovsky AA, Song JP, Naldini L 1999 Interaction of human immunodeficiency virus-derived vectors with wild-type virus in transduced cells. J Virol 73:7087–7092

Collier TJ, Sortwell CE 1999 Therapeutic potential of nerve growth factors in Parkinson's disease. Drugs Aging 14:261–287

Corti O, Sabaté O, Horellou P et al 1999a A single adenovirus vector mediates doxycycline-controlled expression of tyrosine hydroxylase in brain grafts of human neural progenitors. Nat Biotechnol 17:349–354

Corti O, Sánchez-Capelo A, Colin P, Hanoun N, Hamon M, Mallet J 1999b Long-term doxycycline-controlled expression of human tyrosine hydroxylase after direct adenovirus-mediated gene transfer to a rat model of Parkinson's disease. Proc Natl Acad Sci USA 96:12120–12125

Costantini LC, Bakowska JC, Breakefield XO, Isacson O 2000 Gene therapy in the CNS. Gene Ther 7:93–109

Déglon N, Tseng JL, Bensadoun JC et al 2000 Self-inactivating lentiviral vectors with enhanced transgene expression as potential gene transfer system in Parkinson's disease. Hum Gene Ther 11:179–190

Dull T, Zufferey R, Kelly M et al 1998 A third-generation lentivirus vector with a conditional packaging system. J Virol 72:8463–8471

Dunnett SB, Björklund A 1999 Prospects for new restorative and neuroprotective treatments in Parkinson's disease. Nature (suppl) 399:A32–A39

During MJ, Samulski RJ, Elsworth JD et al 1998 In vivo expression of therapeutic human genes for dopamine production in the caudates of MPTP-treated monkeys using an AAV vector. Gene Ther 5:820–827

Emerich DF, Winn SR, Lindner MD 1996 Continued presence of intrastriatal but not intraventricular polymer-encapsulated PC12 cells is required for alleviation of behavioral deficits in Parkinsonian rodents. Cell Transplant 5:589–596

Fan DS, Ogawa M, Fujimoto KI et al 1998 Behavioral recovery in 6-hydroxydopamine-lesioned rats by cotransduction of striatum with tyrosine hydroxylase and aromatic L-amino acid decarboxylase genes using two separate adeno-associated virus vectors. Hum Gene Ther 9:2527–2535

Federico M 1999 Lentiviruses as gene delivery vectors. Curr Opin Biotechnol. 10:448–453

Fink D J, DeLuca NA, Yamada M, Wolfe DP, Glorioso JC 2000 Design and application of HSV vectors for neuroprotection. Gene Ther 7:115–119

Gage FH 1998 Cell therapy. Nature (suppl) 392:18–24

Hallett M, Litvan I, and the task force on surgery for Parkinson's disease 1999 Evaluation of surgery for Parkinson's disease. Neurology 53:1910–1921

Harvey DM, Caskey CT 1998 Inducible control of gene expression: prospects of gene therapy. Curr Opin Chem Biol 2:512–518

Hewson R 2000 RNA viruses: emerging vectors for vaccination and gene therapy. Mol Med Today 6:28–35

Horellou P, Mallet J 1997 Gene therapy for Parkinson's disease. Mol Neurobiol 15:241–256

Hottinger AF, Aebischer P 1999a Treatment of diseases of the central nervous system using encapsulated cells. Adv Tech Stand Neurosurg 25:3–20

Hottinger AF, Aebischer P 1999b Strategies for administering neurotrophic factors to the central nervous system. In: Hefti F (ed) Neurotrophic factors. Springer-Verlag, Berlin (Handbook of experimental pharmacology, vol 134) p 255–280

Kordower JH, Liu YT, Winn S, Emerich DF 1995a Encapsulated PC12 cell transplants into hemiparkinsonian monkeys: a behavioral, neuroanatomical, and neurochemical analysis. Cell Transplant 4:155–171

Kordower JH, Freeman TB, Snow B J et al 1995b Neuropathological evidence of graft survival and striatal reinnervation after the transplantation of fetal mesencephalic tissue in a patient with Parkinson's disease. N Engl J Med 332:1118–1124

Kordower JH, Bloch J, Ma SY et al 1999 Lentiviral gene transfer to the nonhuman primate brain. Exp Neurol 160:1–16

Kost TA, Condreay JP 1999 Recombinant baculoviruses as expression vectors for insect and mammalian cells. Curr Opin Biotechnol 10:428–433

Krack P, Hamel W, Mehdorn HM, Deuschl G 1999 Surgical treatment of Parkinson's disease. Curr Opin Neurol 12:417–425

Leff SE, Spratt SK, Snyder RO, Mandel R J 1999 Long-term restoration of striatal L-aromatic amino acid decarboxylase activity using recombinant adeno-associated viral vector gene transfer in a rodent model of Parkinson's disease. Neuroscience 92:185–196

Lindvall O 1998 Update on fetal transplantation: the Swedish experience. Mov Disord (suppl) 13:83–87

Long Z, Lu P, Grooms T et al 1999 Molecular evaluation of biopsy and autopsy specimens from patients receiving in vivo retroviral gene therapy. Hum Gene Ther 10:733–740

Lundstrom K, Schweitzer C, Richards JG, Ehrengruber MU, Jenck F, Mülhardt C 1999 Semliki Forest virus vectors for *in vitro* and *in vivo* applications. Gene Ther Mol Biol 4:23–31

Lysaght M J, Aebischer P 1999 Encapsulated cells as therapy. Sci Am 280:76–82

Mandel R J, Spratt SK, Snyder RO, Leff SE 1997 Midbrain injection of recombinant adeno-associated virus encoding rat glial cell line-derived neurotrophic factor protects nigral neurons in a progressive 6-hydroxydopamine-induced degeneration model of Parkinson's disease in rats. Proc Natl Acad Sci USA 94:14083–14088

Mandel R J, Rendahl KG, Snyder RO, Leff SE 1999a Progress in direct striatal delivery of L-dopa via gene therapy for treatment of Parkinson's disease using recombinant adeno-associated viral vectors. Exp Neurol 159:47–64

Mandel R J, Snyder RO, Leff SE 1999b Recombinant adeno-associated viral vector-mediated glial cell line-derived neurotrophic factor gene transfer protects nigral dopamine neurons after onset of progressive degeneration in a rat model of Parkinson's disease. Exp Neurol 160:205–214

Miller N, Whelan J 1997 Progress in transcriptionally targeted and regulatable vectors for genetic therapy. Hum Gene Ther 8:803–815

Miyoshi H, Takahashi M, Gage FH, Verma IM 1997 Stable and efficient gene transfer into the retina using an HIV-based lentiviral vector. Proc Natl Acad Sci USA 94:10319–10323

Miyoshi H, Blömer U, Takahashi M, Gage FH, Verma IM 1998 Development of a self-inactivating lentivirus vector. J Virol. 72:8150–8157

Monahan PE, Samulski RJ 2000 AAV vectors: is clinical success on the horizon? Gene Ther 7:24–30

Naldini L 1998 Lentiviruses as gene transfer agents for delivery to non-dividing cells. Curr Opin Biotechnol 9:457–463

Naldini L, Blömer U, Gage FH, Trono D, Verma IM 1996a Efficient transfer, integration, and sustained long-term expression of the transgene in adult rat brains injected with a lentiviral vector. Proc Natl Acad Sci USA 93:11382–11388

Naldini L, Blömer U, Gallay P et al 1996b *In vivo* gene delivery and stable transduction of nondividing cells by a lentiviral vector. Science 272:263–267

Rabinowitz JE, Samulski J 1998 Adeno-associated virus expression systems for gene transfer. Curr Opin Biotechnol 9:470–475

Ridet JL, Corti O, Pencalet P et al 1999 Towards autologous *ex vivo* gene therapy for the CNS with human adult astrocytes. Hum Gene Ther 10:271–280

Rosenblad C, Martinez-Serrano A, Björklund A 1996 Glial cell line-derived neurotrophic factor increases survival, growth and function of intrastriatal fetal nigral dopaminergic grafts. Neuroscience 75:979–985

Rosenblad C, Grønborg M, Hansen C et al 2000 *In vivo* protection of nigral dopamine neurons by lentiviral gene transfer of the novel GDNF-family member neublastin/artemin. Mol Cell Neurosci. 15:199–214

Rossi FM, Blau HM 1998 Recent advances in inducible gene expression systems. Curr Opin Biotechnol 9:451–456

Sautter J, Tseng JL, Braguglia D et al 1998 Implants of polymer-encapsulated genetically modified cells releasing glial cell line-derived neurotrophic factor improve survival, growth, and function of fetal dopaminergic grafts. Exp Neurol 149:230–236

Schlesinger S, Dubensky Jr TW 1999 Alphavirus vectors for gene expression and vaccines. Curr Opin Biotechnol 10:434–439

Serguera C, Zennou V, Sarkis C et al 1999a Study of the effect of central triplex sequence for transduction in the nervous tissue by using lentiviral vectors. 4th Meeting of the French Society for Neuroscience: J54

Serguera C, Bohl D, Rolland E, Prevost P, Heard JM 1999b Control of erythropoietin secretion by doxycycline or mifepristone in mice bearing polymer-encapsulated engineered cells. Hum Gene Ther 10:375–383

Snyder RO 1999 Adeno-associated virus-mediated gene delivery. J Gene Med 1:166–175

Takahashi M, Miyoshi H, Verma IM, Gage FH 1999 Rescue from photoreceptor degeneration in the rd mouse by human immunodeficiency virus vector-mediated gene transfer. J Virol 73:7812–7816

Thomas CE, Schiedner G, Kochanek S, Castro MG, Lowenstein PR 2000 Peripheral infection with adenovirus causes unexpected long-term brain inflammation in animals injected intracranially with first-generation, but not with high-capacity, adenovirus vectors: toward realistic long-term neurological gene therapy for chronic diseases. Proc Natl Acad Sci USA 97:13 7482–7487

Tresco PA, Winn SR, Tan S, Jaeger CB, Greene LA, Aebischer P 1992 Polymer-encapsulated PC12 cells: long-term survival and associated reduction in lesion-induced rotational behavior. Cell Transplant 1:255–264

Trono D 2000 Lentiviral vectors: turning a deadly foe into a therapeutic agent. Gene Ther 7:20–23

Tseng JL, Baetge EE, Zurn AD, Aebischer P 1997 GDNF reduces drug-induced rotational behavior after medial forebrain bundle transection by a mechanism not involving striatal dopamine. J Neurosci 17:325–333
Tseng JL, Bruhn SL, Zurn AD, Aebischer P 1998 Neurturin protects dopaminergic neurons following medial forebrain bundle axotomy. Neuroreport 9:1817–1822
Wickham TJ 2000 Targeting adenovirus. Gene Ther 7:110–114
Zennou V, Petit C, Guetard D, Nerhbass U, Montagnier L, Charneau P 2000 HIV-1 genome nuclear import is mediated by a central DNA flap. Cell 101:173–185
Zufferey R, Nagy D, Mandel RJ, Naldini L, Trono D 1997 Multiply attenuated lentiviral vector achieves efficient gene delivery *in vivo*. Nat Biotechnol 15:871–875
Zufferey R, Dull T, Mandel RJ et al 1998 Self-inactivating lentivirus vector for safe and efficient *in vivo* gene delivery. J Virol 72:9873–9880

DISCUSSION

Dunnett: As you think about clinical trials, are you going to be constrained to intraventricular placement, or will intraparenchymal placements be possible? In the animal models, are there clear differences between the outcomes depending on where the capsule is placed?

Aebischer: So far, all clinical trials have dealt with implantation of capsules in the cerebrospinal fluid, either in the ventricles or the intrathecal lumbar space. Intraparenchymal implantation was studied only in animals, however extensively. We would feel comfortable placing a capsule in the parenchyma of humans, but we would not feel comfortable moving it in and out as we do with capsules placed in the intrathecal space. In amyotrophic lateral sclerosis (ALS), changing the device every six months is not a big deal. You couldn't do this in the brain parenchyma. This, however, will be a problem for all the gene transfer approaches. If the molecules are needed for 10 years, do you need 10 years' animal work before you can go to the clinic? This is where the co-transplantation of fetal mesencephalon and GDNF-releasing implants in the context of PD becomes interesting, as we believe that the trophic factor presence is needed for a relatively short period of time, a couple of months at most.

Dunnett: Of course, behind my question is just that issue: most of the animal data involve intraparenchymal administration. For example, when co-grafting GDNF-producing cells to enhance the survival of nigral grafts, do we know that this will be as effective if GDNF-producing cells are put in the ventricle rather than into the parenchyma?

Aebischer: The co-transplantation work was performed only in the rat where the differences between ventricular versus parenchyma cannot be studied due to size limits. In primates, we have shown that GDNF released from the ventricles improves the behaviour of primates chronically lesioned with MPTP. Side by side comparison between intraventricular versus parenchymal release of GDNF was, however, not performed.

Dunnett: That is exactly the point. A repeated issue in these discussions is whether we can apply the animal models to the human situation. Your model seems not to match with what you are planning to do in patients.

Aebischer: The experiments planned in humans were indeed performed in the rat where the GDNF capsules were placed in the parenchyma.

Gray: But in the human case you are not going to put capsules into the parenchyma.

Aebischer: In humans we intend to place the capsules in the parenchyma.

Gage: I think what Steve Dunnett is getting at is that you should put the GDNF in the ventricle of the rat along with the fetal striatal graft.

Aebischer: It is difficult to do this in rats, the capsules are too big.

Dunnett: You could do this in the monkeys.

Aebischer: I have no problems putting capsules in the parenchyma in humans.

Dunnett: But can you believe from the animal studies that you have a sufficient basis to implant capsules intraventrically in patients?

Aebischer: We are hesitating between two trials. One is to add the encapsulated cells with the fetal graft, which we would do in the parenchyma because we do not believe that we need a long-term release of GDNF. However, as we have observed an effect with intraventricular delivery of GDNF alone in MPTP parkinsonian monkeys we could envision a trial based on the intraventricular delivery of GDNF where replacement of implants, once a year for example, is conceivable.

Bohn: Jeff Kordower has recently published the results of a post-mortem case from a study in which they infused GDNF protein into the lateral ventricle of a patient with PD (Kordower et al 1999). This study showed that diffusion of GDNF protein into the parenchyma was very limited. Whether you inject GDNF protein into the brain or implant a capsule of cells containing GDNF, there will be limited diffusion of the protein.

Aebischer: You have to be very careful there. The case you are referring to was based on bolus injections. Continuous release is different and the kinetics are not comparable.

Freeman: What was the sphere of influence intraparenchymally in the primate, and how does this relate to the distance between the ventricular wall and the nigra in human?

Aebischer: These experiments were performed with intraparenchymal injection of lentiviral vectors. At the immunohistochemical level, we seem to affect a very large portion of the striatum, using four injections. The sphere of influence was up to a centimetre.

Freeman: So you would at least expect to influence the medial half of the nigra.

Aebischer: That would be our assumption.

Olson: On the issue of where to deliver trophic factors, we have some limited experience of delivering nerve growth factor (NGF) to patients using a pump and a catheter. In three patients with PD, we pumped NGF into the caudate putamen to support intraparenchymal adrenal medullary autografts, and there were no noticeable side effects of NGF. In Alzheimer's disease we delivered NGF into the lateral ventricle to obtain a more global spread of NGF. Although there were some positive effects, there were two major negative side effects: loss of appetite and pain elicited by movements (perhaps because NGF will also spread down the central canal and influence dorsal root ganglia and/or the spinal cord). However, relatively large amounts of NGF infused intraparenchymally had no side effects.

Gray: Has there been any observation of reduced food intake in the animals given NGF?

Olson: Yes.

Gray: That is an expected side-effect, then.

Aebischer: With all trophic factors the first side effect usually seen is weight loss. This occurs with brain-derived neurotrophic factor (BDNF), GDNF, CNTF and NGF, whenever they are delivered into the ventricle.

Bohn: Until recently, it has been almost impossible to get widespread expression and stability of a transgene protein by a viral vector. The lentiviral data you showed in the monkey are phenomenal. This raises the issue of what is going to happen when you express large amounts of a potent growth factor in many brain areas? Jeff Kordower injected into caudate, putamen and substantia nigra and the whole nigrostriatal system was filled with GDNF. What should we start worrying about? How would you distinguish the effects of the growth factor on other types of neurons, or even on the dopamine neurons in the other brain areas?

Aebischer: That is a good point. Until now, we had the opposite problem. We have currently the pleasant difficulty of trying to see whether we can limit the system. This is possible by altering the number of injections, the viral vector titre, and most importantly by using an inducible promoter system. Today, however, lentiviral vectors are not sufficiently developed so as to use them in clinical experiments. The current versions will lead to long-term expression, and without a possibility for turning the expression off. Versions including inducible promoters are being developed. The interesting thing is that our primates didn't seem to show any side effects. I understand that humans and primates are different, but if you do the same thing with CNTF, we observe limiting side effects in primates. The fact that we do not see any side effect with GDNF in the primates suggests GDNF has a better safety profile, as long as it is given only in the appropriate areas.

Gray: What other systems are likely to be affected by GDNF apart from the dopaminergic?

Aebischer: GDNF is a trophic factor for some cholinergic neurons such as motoneurons. It is also a trophic factor for dorsal root ganglia neurons.

Freeman: In terms of GDNF being distributed widely, you showed a slide with transport from the striatal injection site to the pallidum. Is there retrograde transport from the striatum to the nigra?

Aebischer: We have looked at this, and it doesn't seem to be very important.

Price: Overexpression is a much better problem to be faced with than underexpression. Trying to think ahead towards potential problems downstream, natural substances such as hormones and neurotransmitters don't make good drugs. In general, you have to generate an artificial compound that has some of the properties of the natural substances but which lacks others. I don't see any reason why protein growth factors should be different in this respect. In other words, the brain has a whole set of processes to protect itself against over-stimulation by these factors, and these defensive processes will kick in. If you generate a drug you usually have to overcome these processes. I suspect the biggest problem downstream with this approach will be that the brain will not simply stand by and allow you to bombard it with a growth factor, continuing to respond in the way that it otherwise would to this factor.

Raisman: If you use a long-term neurotrophic virus *in vivo*, what way have you got of assessing its cytotoxicity? Is there an established test?

Aebischer: You count the cells that are infected and look at their morphology over time.

Raisman: That is quite a crude measure. You could be losing 10–20% of cells, given the variation between injections.

Gage: Experimentally you can attempt to address that by fusing the factor to a marker gene like GFP. When we use lentivirus or AAV, we fuse it to a marker gene and look to see how many cells are expressing this marker gene at early times versus later times. Depending on whether or not you are using an intrinsically active molecule like Bcl-x as a modulator of cell survival, versus a secreted molecule like NGF, you would be looking for the local effect on the cell expressing the transgene versus the effect that might occur on cells that don't even express the gene. There are two issues that need facing: what is the effect of long-term expression of a trophic factor within a cell, and what is the effect of the protein being secreted and stimulating the local environment, independent of whether or not these neighbouring cells make the gene or not? The initial question at least can be answered by tagging the gene and monitoring its expression in the cell over long periods to see whether or not there is a subsequent reaction in the cell that is carrying this gene.

Annett: You showed some behavioural data of maximum distance travelled. Could you comment any more on the Parkinsonian symptoms of these monkeys? I'm interested because we know from the transplantation work with allografts that recovery is incomplete. Is it the case that with your GDNF strategy you can get more complete recovery?

Aebischer: I don't think any detailed clinical rating was done in those experiments.

Reference

Kordower JH et al 1999 Clinicopathological findings following intraventricular glial-derived neurotrophic factor treatment in a patient with Parkinson's disease. Ann Neurol 46:419–424

Neurogenesis in the adult hippocampus

Gerd Kempermann*† and Fred H. Gage*[1]

*The Salk Institute for Biological Studies, Laboratory of Genetics, 10010 North Torrey Pines Road, La Jolla, CA 92037, USA, and †Neurologische Universitätsklinik, Universitätsstr. 84, D-93053 Regensburg, Germany

Abstract. The surprising finding that the adult hippocampus produces new neurons throughout life has challenged many old views about the brain, because the brain appears to be plastic enough to integrate new neurons. Research on adult hippocampal neurogenesis also allows one to study neuronal stem or progenitor cells in the mature and working brain. It therefore will provide key information necessary for any attempt to use neuronal stem cells *in situ* to treat neurological disease. Although this new strategy holds great promise, a large number of questions, some of which are discussed herein, remain to be addressed.

2000 Neural transplantation in neurodegenerative disease. Wiley, Chichester (Novartis Foundation Symposium 231) p 220–241

The biggest question about neurogenesis in the adult brain used to be whether it occurred at all. When this question was convincingly answered in the affirmative (Altman & Das 1965, Cameron et al 1993, Kaplan & Hinds 1977, Kuhn et al 1996, Kempermann et al 1997a, Eriksson et al 1998), the focus moved to whether adult neurogenesis had any tangible biological relevance.

In the hippocampus of adult mammals, a population of proliferating precursor cells resides within the subgranular zone, the border between the granule cell layer of the dentate gyrus and the hilus. Progeny from these cells migrate into the granule cell layer and differentiate into neurons that become, by all measures so far investigated, indistinguishable from the surrounding granule cells. Although neurogenesis has been described in numerous mammalian species, including humans (Eriksson et al 1998), its function and therefore biological significance has remained elusive. Enough is known about the activity-dependent regulation of adult hippocampal neurogenesis, however, to reject the assumption that adult neurogenesis is a mere atavism, playing no integrated functional role.

---

[1]This chapter was presented at the symposium by Professor Gage, to whom correspondence should be addressed.

Conceptually, the fact that adult neurogenesis does occur introduces considerable obstacles to some old views of how the hippocampus and, more generally, the brain function.

Research on adult hippocampal neurogenesis therefore serves two goals. The first is the understanding of an intrinsic and currently poorly understood quality of the brain to produce new neurons during adulthood and use them in the hippocampal neuronal network. Secondly, adult hippocampal neurogenesis serves as an intriguing model system that, if used cleverly, allows one to examine fundamental aspects of the stem cell biology of the adult brain.

Both aspects are inseparable, and results from studies with a 'systems' focus might substantially influence progress in 'basic cellular' research, and vice versa. Both the intellectual, almost philosophical *relevance* driving hippocampus-oriented research and the medical implications that primarily come from the broader, stem-cell oriented approach have sparked ever-increasing interest in adult hippocampal neurogenesis. In this review several unanswered questions are identified which have only surfaced because of the recent interest in adult hippocampal neurogenesis.

Is adult neurogenesis a more general phenomenon than we think?

The finding that neurons in the adult brain are post-mitotic has lead to a generally pessimistic view of the adult brain's ability to produce new neurons. Part of the explanation for this pessimism was that the concept of stem cells in the adult organism was not accepted in the field of neuroscience. However, it has been convincingly demonstrated that neuronal stem cells can be extracted from the adult brain (Richards et al 1992, Vescovi et al 1993, Kilpatrick & Bartlett 1995, Reynolds et al 1992, Lois & Alvarez-Buylla 1993, Ray et al 1993, Palmer et al 1997, Johansson et al 1999). Two brain regions, the lateral ventricular walls as part of a neurogenic apparatus in the olfactory system (Corotto et al 1993, Luskin 1993, Goldman 1995) and the hippocampal dentate gyrus, are known to be privileged sites, in that stem cells not only reside in these areas, but also give rise to new neurons. Stem cells have been found not only in these regions, but also in areas that under normal conditions are not neurogenic: the striatum and septum (Palmer et al 1995), the spinal cord (Shihabuddin et al 1997), and most recently the cerebral cortex and corpus callosum (Palmer et al 1997).

While neurogenesis does not seem to occur physiologically outside the known neurogenic regions, it is likely that other, if not all, brain regions retain some regenerative potential because stem cells exist in these areas. This finding raises several important issues. For example, how homogeneous is the population of neuronal stem cells in the adult brain? How similar with respect to their potential and their biological properties are stem cells derived from different brain regions, and how many different types of stem cells can be found in one region at a given time? Clonal hippocampal progenitor cells were found to be multipotent but, in related *ex vivo* experiments, no lineage-restricted populations were found (Palmer et al 1997). Therefore, it remains unclear whether the differentiated phenotypes develop directly from one multipotent cell or from lineage-restricted intermediates.

With regard to 'spatial multipotentiality,' transplantation experiments have yielded interesting results. Hippocampus-derived precursor cells have been shown to integrate not only into the hippocampus (Gage et al 1995) but also into the olfactory system after transplantation into the migratory stream between lateral ventricles and olfactory bulb, and to develop phenotypes not present in the hippocampus (Suhonen et al 1996). After implantation into the developing retina the cells showed morphologically key characteristics of several types of retinal neurons (Takahashi et al 1998).

Taken together these experimental data suggest that neuronal stem cells derived from the adult mammalian brain retain a high degree of multipotentiality. This finding raises the question, how far from totipotency are the cells that can be isolated from the brain? The demonstration that neuronal progenitor cells can repopulate experimentally depleted murine bone marrow and reconstitute the haematopoietic system (Bjornson et al 1999) indicates that neuronal stem cells might be even more multipotent than previously assumed.

Partially along these lines, some researchers have begun attempts to merge concepts from haematopoiesis and 'neuropoiesis' (Scheffler et al 1999). Without doubt, many important lessons will be learned from haematology. However, the analogy should not be stressed beyond its limits (Weiss & Van Der Kooy 1998): haematological stem cells *in vitro* do not form spheres as do some neuronal precursor cells. Furthermore, neuronal stem cells can be propagated *in vitro* with relative ease, and the anatomical structure in which 'poiesis' occurs *in vivo* is so fundamentally different (parenchymatous organ vs. loose trabecular structure of bone marrow or the liquidity of blood) that labelling the regions of neuronal stem cell activity 'brain marrow' (Scheffler et al 1999) remains problematic.

Research will be much easier once stem cell-specific antigens are characterized, thus allowing their unambiguous identification *in vivo*. Currently the picture is complex. Some researchers argue that, in the subventricular zone, two different precursor cell populations are present: one rarely reproducing stem cell population, and the offspring of that population, the progenitor cells, which are more restricted in their multipotentiality and their ability for self-renewal (Morshead et al 1994). Subventricular stem cells have been identified as both ependymal cells (Johansson et al 1999) and, more convincingly, as a population of astrocytes in and below the ependymal ventricular lining (Doetsch et al 1999). To establish the nature of the hippocampal neuronal stem cell *in vivo* and to describe their relation to stem cells from other brain and body regions will be among the challenges that lie ahead.

What is the function of adult neurogenesis?

Early theories of brain function fared quite well without needing to integrate the possibility that the adult brain might also be able to generate more neurons. With some analogy to computers, it was assumed that to a large degree the brain was hard-wired and that all plasticity that occurred was due to changes on the level of neuronal connections, the neurites and synapses. Surprisingly, of all the brain regions, it was in the hippocampus, which is highly involved in learning and memory formation, where it was established that neurogenesis occurred in the adult brain (Altman & Das 1965). Although the existence of adult hippocampal neurogenesis has been known for more than 35 years, very little hard data about its functional relevance existed. However, inferential evidence about the functional role of adult hippocampal neurogenesis is increasing. Challenging adult animals with exposure to an enriched environment (Kempermann et al 1997a, 1998a,b, Kempermann & Gage 1999) and the application of focused learning stimuli (Gould et al 1999) result in increased survival of newly generated neurons in the dentate gyrus, suggesting a functional selection process. Voluntary physical exercise (Van Praag et al 1999a) and, in a different inbred strain of mice (Kempermann et al 1998a), living in an enriched environment caused a marked increase in cell proliferation within the subgranular zone. These findings might imply that very general forms of activation, probably through the reticular formation (because inhibition of serotonergic input from the raphe nuclei decreases hippocampal cell proliferation; Brezun & Daszuta 1999), have effects on the hippocampal stem cell population. More specific stimuli such as learning, be it experimentally focussed (Gould et al 1999) or hidden in the complexity of an enriched environment (Kempermann et al 1997a), will then act upon this increased neurogenic potential and select new neurons for integration in the network.

Future experiments will have to test this hypothesis and demonstrate how this functional integration could actually work. There is no doubt that the new hippocampal granule cells send axons along the mossy fibre tracts to area CA3, as do all other granule cells (Markakis & Gage 1999, Stanfield & Trice 1988). The great challenge lies in providing a convincing demonstration that it is the new neurons that enable the stimulated animals to learn better (i.e. to perform better on a learning task). From the observation that animals living in an enriched environment not only had more new neurons than controls but also performed better on a spatial learning task (Kempermann et al 1997a, 1998a,b, Nilsson et al 1999) the hypothesis could be derived that the link between the two parameters is not only correlational but causal. Strong support for this hypothesis comes from the finding that running not only increases adult hippocampal neurogenesis, but also improves acquisition on the water maze task and long-term potentiation (LTP) in the dentate gyrus (Van Praag et al 1999b), providing the first evidence of electrophysiologically measurable changes in a region of adult neurogenesis.

With respect to the use of adult hippocampal neurogenesis as a model system for neuronal stem cell biology in the adult brain, direct evidence of functional gain attributable to these neurons would increase the chances that neuroregeneration, by recruiting the activity of quiescent neuronal stem cells in other regions, could result in functional benefit. Again, however, intimate knowledge about the factors that control adult neurogenesis within the hippocampal neurogenic region will be crucial for understanding the requirements for functionally effective neurogenesis to take place.

What is the role of adult neurogenesis in concepts of plasticity?

Plasticity is the ability of the adult brain to change its anatomy in response to external or internal stimuli, and neurons are the principal units in most theories of brain function. Adding more neurons to the existing network must therefore appear as the highest degree of plasticity imaginable. For this reason it has been hard to reconcile adult neurogenesis with the presumed necessity of stability and conservation in a neuronal network (Rakic 1985). Most aspects of plasticity have accordingly been described on the level of synapses (Hebb 1949, Kleim et al 1996, Anderson et al 1994), defined synaptic sub-structures (Greenough et al 1978, Comery et al 1996) and on neurite formation (Comery et al 1996, Juraska et al 1985, Greenough & Volkmar 1973). 'Maps' are functional representations in the brain, and they rely on patterns of excitation in connected neurons. Experimental interaction with this map formation leads to spatial shifts of these representations and to some degree these shifts can be followed on a morphological level (Stryker 1999, Merzenich et al 1984).

The key question here is, how does adult neurogenesis fit into these concepts? While it is not likely that, under ordinary conditions, stem cell activity outside the known neurogenic regions contributes to plasticity through neurogenesis, the potential should not be underestimated. Current knowledge about neuronal stem cells in the adult brain must at least be seen as a challenge to the old understanding of what 'plasticity' can possibly mean. Adult hippocampal neurogenesis will serve here as a proof of principle, showing that neuronal cellular plasticity with functional consequences is generally possible. One will then have to demonstrate how plasticity on a cellular level is related to the better understood plasticity on subcellular levels, and how both lead to a functional plasticity that can be measured as a behavioural outcome. The findings that running enhances neurogenesis in the dentate gyrus, improves water maze performance and increases LTP in perforant path-to-dentate gyrus synapses have, for the first time, related cellular plasticity and behavioural outcome to a standard measure of plasticity on an electrophysiological level (Van Praag et al 1999b).

How does adult neurogenesis react under pathological conditions?

If the regenerative potential of adult neurogenesis is ever to be used in clinically effective strategies for neuronal repair, knowledge about how the intrinsic mechanisms that govern the biology of neuronal stem cells *in situ* react to pathological conditions will be crucial. These studies will also answer the question of whether there is any attempt at stem cell-based self repair in the adult brain. It might well be that abortive responses exist which for some reasons do not lead to true regeneration and functional benefit. If so, the reasons for failure will have to be identified. Extending the interest in the role of adult neurogenesis in physiological plasticity as an integrative part of the way the brain works, another equally important question is, how does this plasticity react under pathological conditions? For example, induction of hippocampal seizures as a model of temporal lobe epilepsy results in a massive stimulation of proliferative activity in the dentate gyrus (Parent et al 1997, 1999, Bengzon et al 1997). Ischaemia (Liu et al 1998) and trauma (Gould & Tanapat 1997) have similar results, but it is not yet clear what the net consequences are of these pathological stimuli on the actual production of new neurons.

Obviously, in this context, studying adult hippocampal neurogenesis is of particular interest with regard to hippocampal pathology. There is an anecdotal report of cells that stain for a proliferation marker in the dentate gyrus of Alzheimer's patients (Nagy et al 1997a,b). Whether this finding indicates a neurogenic response to signals related to the degenerating neurons remains to be established, as does why such a regenerative attempt, if it exists, fails.

It might even be that some cellular regeneration is actually taking place but has not yet been identified. Experiments that stimulate a regenerative mechanism by inducing a defined pathology but specifically eliminate neuronal stem cells in this response are one way to test how great the contribution is of stem cells to regeneration (Parent et al 1999).

How is adult neurogenesis regulated?

Evidence that adult hippocampal neurogenesis is regulated in an activity-dependent manner (Kempermann et al 1997a, Gould et al 1999, Van Praag et al 1999a) leads to the question, which factors mediate this regulation? From the external stimulus to gene regulation, a cascade of controlling events has to unfold. All results so far indicate that adult neurogenesis is not regulated in an on/off way but by a multi-step process with dynamic control over the end result. Many of the known stimulators of adult hippocampal neurogenesis induce proliferation of progenitor cells in the subgranular zone, whereas, for example, learning and environmental complexity increase survival of newborn cells (Kempermann et al 1997a, Gould et al 1999). From strain comparison studies we know that these different steps are differentially influenced by background genes (Kempermann et al 1997b), which also control the varying involvement of these steps in a neurogenic response (Kempermann et al 1998a). Other regulatory steps beyond proliferation, survival and differentiation include migration, neuritogenesis, synaptogenesis and the establishment of functioning network connections, none of which have yet been subject to detailed study in this context of activity-dependent regulation.

The fact that regulation of adult neurogenesis is a very complex process should come as no surprise, because we know that neurogenesis during development is very complex — although how far adult neurogenesis recapitulates embryonic development remains to be investigated. Although our knowledge about external manipulations and about molecules that can influence regulation of adult hippocampal neurogenesis is constantly increasing, almost nothing is known about how the regulatory cascade works, which molecules are involved at which stage and by what means one identified stimulus acts on different regulatory events. But single effectors have been identified *in vivo*. For example, glutamatergic input to the dentate gyrus seems to limit neurogenesis (Cameron et al 1995, Gould 1994), whereas serotonergic afferents increase neurogenesis (Brezun & Daszuta 1999). On a hormonal level, it has been shown that glucocorticoids inhibit neurogenesis (Gould et al 1992, Gould 1994), a fact that has been brought into context of a down-regulation of adult hippocampal neurogenesis by stress (Gould et al 1997). Among the growth factors, fibroblast growth factor (FGF) 2 and epidermal growth factor (EGF) show effects on cell proliferation and differentiation after intraventricular infusion, both in the subventricular zone and in the dentate gyrus (Craig et al 1996, Kuhn et al 1997). Brain-derived neurotrophic factor (BDNF) increases the number of new neurons in the adult olfactory bulb (Zigova et al 1998).

The finding that environmental stimulation has a survival-promoting effect on newborn cells in the subgranular zone of mice (Kempermann et al 1997a) and rats (Nilsson et al 1999) and that, in the subgranular zone of stimulated animals, fewer apoptotic nuclei could be found (Young et al 1999), suggests that adult neurogenesis is to some degree regulated through apoptotic/anti-apoptotic mechanisms.

Although many studies are seeking to establish the effects of one molecule or another on adult hippocampal neurogenesis — the neuroleptic haloperidol, for example, seems to increase (or disinhibit) cell proliferation in the subgranular zone (Dawirs et al 1998)—it should be remembered that a larger task lies ahead: to describe regulation in its multitude of involved events, from a system level down to cellular mechanisms and the genes involved.

Which genes govern adult neurogenesis?

Many factors have been identified as showing interaction with adult neurogenesis, and the number of reports that will name new effective agents will continue to grow. It is likely that many surprising compounds will have some effect on adult neurogenesis. The problem will be that, in most of such experiments, one will not know how close to the level of direct regulation the new compound actually got. Some of these experiments will be very useful, but the key to the regulation of adult neurogenesis (and thereby the transfer of knowledge to non-neurogenic brain regions) will lie in identifying and manipulating the key genes that define a microenvironment that is permissive for neurogenesis.

Ultimately, no single gene will be identified that rules adult neurogenesis and whose successful manipulation is the key to the therapeutic potential of neuronal stem cells *in vivo*. It is far more likely that only the coordinated sequence of activity of several genes will lead to new neurons, which makes any attempt to artificially imitate natural conditions a daunting task. Strategies that make use of the intrinsic programs of neuronal development and rely on the inborn coordination of gene activation are more likely to succeed. To achieve this, many lessons from embryonic development have to be learned.

Strain comparisons in mice have shown that the different levels in the regulation of adult hippocampal neurogenesis are differently influenced by inheritable traits (Kempermann et al 1997b). In 129/SvJ mice, up-regulation of adult hippocampal neurogenesis after exposure to an enriched environment included an increase in proliferative activity in the subgranular zone, whereas in C57BL/6 mice the increase was due to a survival-promoting effect (Kempermann et al 1997b, 1998b). These results imply that several key genes are regulated in adult hippocampal neurogenesis. Classical genetics might help to narrow in on the relevant gene loci.

In years to come, a flood of studies will use the alternative approach, i.e. examining adult neurogenesis in knockout and transgenic animals. Although this approach will increase our knowledge of possible regulators, much of this knowledge will be incidental and will await integration into larger concepts. Most importantly, studies of adult neurogenesis in a mutant that has disturbed embryonic neurogenesis may produce results that are severely confounded. Conditional and regulatable knockouts will open an entire new field of research.

At the same time we will profit from *in vitro* studies that describe signal transduction in developing neurons. Events such as entering the cell cycle, leaving the cell cycle, fate choice, induction of apoptosis, migration and neurite extension can be studied *in vitro* and lead to the identification of relevant candidate genes.

Some genes have received considerable interest in the recent past because of their possible relevance in neurogenic regulation. For example, Notch is involved in the cell fate decision against becoming a neuroblast (Cabrera 1990, Weinmaster 1998), and Notch1 can be activated in cultured hippocampal neurons and inhibits neurite growth (Berezovska et al 1999). Nothing is known about the relevance of Notch for adult hippocampal neurogenesis and its expression in neuronal stem cells from the adult brain. NeuroD, in contrast, has already been studied *in vivo*; its deficiency results in a lack of hippocampal and cerebellar granule cells (Miyata et al 1999). On the level of cell migration in the olfactory system, the putative role of Slit has been studied (Wu et al 1999). Generally, however, the demonstration that a certain gene or molecule can exert a certain regulative function does not necessarily mean that it indeed plays this role under physiological conditions.

What is the relation between adult neurogenesis and the genesis of other cell types?

As neurogenesis *in vitro* relies on the presence of very defined culture media (Kilpatrick & Bartlett 1995, Reynolds et al 1992, Ray et al 1993), adult neurogenesis *in vivo* depends on a defined and highly specialized microenvironment. While the microanatomy of the subventricular zone has already been described in great detail (Doetsch et al 1999), such knowledge is still lacking for the subgranular zone. Which cell types are present in this region and what roles they play in adult neurogenesis are not entirely known. As mentioned above, it is also not known how homogeneous the population of dividing progenitor cells in the subgranular zone is. Subpopulations with different potentials and different proliferation kinetics might be present, as has been suggested for the subventricular zone (Morshead et al 1994). While in the subventricular zone the hypothesis has been raised of an identity between stem cells and ependymal cells (Johansson et al 1999) or—more convincingly—a population of astrocytes (Doetsch et al 1999), so far no such ideas exist for the subgranular zone. *In vitro* studies on cell–cell interactions required for neurogenesis also indicate that astrocytes support or even stimulate neurogenesis from neuronal precursor cells from the subventricular zone (Lim & Alvarez-Buylla 1999).

In the past, excitement about adult neurogenesis led to a somewhat 'neuronocentric' perspective. But both neurogenesis and gliogenesis occur in the subgranular zone (Cameron et al 1993, Kuhn et al 1996) and many factors that influence neurogenesis also interact with gliogenesis: experience of an enriched environment, for example, not only leads to more neurons but also to more astrocytes in the dentate gyrus of mice (Kempermann et al 1997a). Intraventricular infusion of EGF and FGF2 had effects on both gliogenesis and neurogenesis (Kuhn et al 1997). In the context of adult hippocampal neurogenesis, gliogenesis largely means the generation of astrocytes. Hardly anything is known about the role of new oligodendrocytes in this area. Proliferating cells that exist in other brain regions, such as the neocortex, seem to generate primarily oligodendrocytes (Levison et al 1999).

The concept of multipotent neural stem cells links neurogenesis with gliogenesis. The finding, however, that brain-derived stem cells have a haematopoietic potential (Bjornson et al 1999) raises the question, how many more links exist with other cell types? The relation to microglia, to endothelium and to extracerebral cell types remains to be examined. The key questions become: how primordial actually are the detected cells that are still rather uniformly labelled as 'stem cells'? How multipotent are they and which lineage restrictions are introduced at which level of differentiation?

The finding that neuronal stem cells in the subventricular zone might mask as astrocytes or are astrocytes (Doetsch et al 1999) implies that neuronal stem cells *in vivo* might not appear as undifferentiated as previously thought. This could help to explain why markers specific for neuronal stem cells have not yet been found, but also raises another key issue: can mature brain cells physiologically de-differentiate in order to undergo mitosis?

How can one successfully intervene in the regulation of adult neurogenesis?

In principal, there are two approaches to induction of neurogenesis: a pharmacological, direct intervention (here including gene transfer and transplantation of cells, native or engineered to release active substances), and strategies that are based on the indirect activation of intrinsic regulation. The former approach is more targeted; the latter makes use of the existing complexity of regulatory pathways and does not interfere as much with natural balances of forces. Useful strategies will probably have to employ both approaches and combine selected gene activation with techniques of bringing the brain into a state of activity that allows or even demands neurogenesis. To date no quantitative data exist on how much neurogenesis can be achieved under each condition. One of the key requirements will be to develop a standardized assay system that allows the quantitative comparison of different types of intervention. Quantitative data will have to be linked with behavioural or other functional parameters to allow a final evaluation. 'Success' does not necessarily lie in the greatest number of new neurons, but only in a resulting gain of function.

How could targeted neurogenesis be used for therapy?

Ideas to use neuronal stem cells for therapy have generally followed two basic scenarios (Shihabuddin et al 1999, Fisher 1997). One is the implantation of cultured stem cells in an *ex vivo* approach, in which stem cells are placed into the diseased tissue and one relies on intrinsic or extrinsic factors to guarantee development into functioning neurons. An experimentally successful strategy of this type has been used to prevent metabolic disease in mice (Lacorazza et al 1996, Snyder et al 1995). The other is an *in vivo* approach, where the intrinsic progenitor cells are trained to replace damaged or lost cells.

With regard to clinical relevance, most efforts have gone into new ways to allow the repopulating of the nigrostriatal system with dopaminergic neurons to treat Parkinson's disease. So far, however, it has not been possible to drive cultured neuronal stem cells down a dopaminergic lineage.

All *ex vivo* approaches generally suffer from the difficulty that the microenvironmental conditions at the implantation site might not be neurogenic at all. One would have to combine these strategies, therefore, with manipulations to make the site permissive for neurogenesis. One could argue that it might not be necessary to implant cells at all, if a way were found to recruit local, quiescent stem cells. So far, little information exists about whether the neurogenic or at least proliferative response in neurogenic regions that follows insults such as stroke (Liu et al 1998), trauma (Gould & Tanapat 1997) or epilepsy (Parent et al 1997, 1999) has a measurable benefit. Similarly, one does not know yet whether the local production of new neurons would be of real use in situations of hippocampal pathology, although intuitively this seems likely.

It seems even more likely that stimulation of adult neurogenesis, both in naturally neurogenic regions and in regions where neurogenesis would have to be induced, could have a preventive effect and, at the very least, delay the onset of many, mostly chronic neurological disorders. The underlying assumption is that the more flexible, more plastic brain would be able to better cope with neuronal cell loss.

What are the consequences if adult neurogenesis is disturbed or fails?

If there is neurogenesis in the adult brain, there also must be disease related to it. There are two levels of pathology that might exist.

First, as the hippocampus contains a higher density of neuronal stem cells, it might be prone to stem cell-related disease, most notably tumours. There is increasing support for the hypothesis that glial tumours could arise from neural stem cells, and experimental data support this idea. Not only have progenitor cells been isolated from glial tumours (Noble et al 1995, Noble & Maier-Proschel

1997), but also successfully transduced to form glial tumours (Barnett et al 1998). This theory could also explain why so few neuronal tumours exist, if one assumes that the default lineage decision for a neural stem or progenitor cell is towards a glial phenotype. Gliomas are particularly numerous in regions that coincide with regions of high stem cell activity, especially the temporal lobe, which contains the hippocampus, and areas close to the lateral ventricles.

Second, disturbed adult hippocampal neurogenesis might be involved in hippocampal disease. Only a model system of temporal lobe seizures has been studied in some detail (Parent et al 1997, Bengzon et al 1997), but no conclusive result has been obtained. Still, seizures do induce neurogenesis (Parent et al 1997, 1999), and in post-mortem studies on patients with hippocampal epilepsy, ectopic granule cell clusters have been found (Houser 1990). Although the hypothesis that it is the new neurons that form aberrant connections perpetuating the epileptogenic process has been dismissed (Parent et al 1999), a pathogenic role of misled neurogenesis cannot be ruled out at the present time.

For other disorders it is more likely that a loss of neurogenesis is involved in the pathogenesis of the disease, if only through futile regenerative attempts. Alzheimer's disease affects the entire brain, but the hippocampus is a primary site and likely linked to the memory deficits in the disease. All involvement of adult neurogenesis here is speculative. but it certainly should be discussed. The same is true for transient global amnesia, a somewhat enigmatic bilateral affliction of the hippocampi.

There are obviously many more questions to be asked. A very interesting challenge, for example, would be to speculate about the evolutionary consequences of adult neurogenesis. The observation that lower animals such as lizards (Pérez-Cañellas & Garcia-Verdugo 1996) or lobsters (Harzsch et al 1999) have very high levels of neurogenesis during adulthood has led to the simplistic conclusion that evolution of the 'higher' brain of mammals, and particularly that of primates and humans, with its more sophisticated and complex cognitive function, would call for stability over cellular plasticity. While this notion certainly has some truth to it, the research outlined above indicates that neurogenesis does occur in complex and fundamentally important brain systems of 'higher' animals, including humans. As a consequence, the argument is at least weakened and speculation about the place of adult neurogenesis in evolution seems somewhat premature.

The issues raised in this paper can for the most part be addressed with knowledge that exists today and an appreciation of what is experimentally feasible now. These questions underscore the fact that research on adult neurogenesis covers a wide range of neurobiological topics. The biology of neuronal stem cells is only now beginning to emerge as a defined field. The diversity of questions and the implications of the possible answers indicate that a challenging, very promising and most rewarding time for research lies ahead.

Acknowledgements

The authors would like to thank A. Hesse, B. Winner and U. Bogdahn for their support during the preparation of this manuscript and M. L. Gage for editing the text.

References

Altman J, Das GD 1965 Autoradiographic and histologic evidence of postnatal neurogenesis in rats. J Comp Neurol 124:319–335

Anderson BJ, Li X, Alcantara AA, Isaacs KR, Glack JE, Greenough WT 1994 Glial hypertrophy is associated with synaptogenesis following motor skill learning, but not with angiogenesis following exercise. Glia 11:73–80

Barnett SC, Robertson L, Graham D, Allan D, Rampling R 1998 Oligodendrocyte-type-2 astrocyte (O-2A) progenitor cells transformed with c-myc and H-ras form high-grade glioma after stereotactic injection into the rat brain. Carcinogenesis 19:1529–1537

Bengzon J, Kokaia Z, Elmér E, Nanobashvili A, Kokaia M, Lindvall O 1997 Apoptosis and proliferation of dentate gyrus neurons after single and intermittent limbic seizures. Proc Natl Acad Sci USA 94:10432–10437

Berezovska O, McLean P, Knowles R et al 1999 Notch1 inhibits neurite outgrowth in postmitotic primary neurons. Neuroscience 93:433–439

Bjornson CRR, Rietze RL, Reynolds BA, Magli MC, Vescovi AL 1999 Turning brain into blood: a hematopoietic fate adopted by adult neural stem cells *in vivo*. Science 283:534–537

Brezun JM, Daszuta A 1999 Depletion in serotonin decreases neurogenesis in the dentate gyrus and the subventricular zone of adult rats. Neuroscience 89:999–1002

Cabrera CV 1990 Lateral inhibition and cell fate during neurogenesis in *Drosophila*: the interactions between scute, Notch and Delta. Development 110:733–742

Cameron HA, Woolley CS, McEwen BS, Gould E 1993 Differentiation of newly born neurons and glia in the dentate gyrus of the adult rat. Neuroscience 56:337–344

Cameron HA, McEwen BS, Gould E 1995 Regulation of adult neurogenesis by excitatory input and NMDA receptor activation in the dentate gyrus. J Neurosci 15:4687–4692

Comery TA, Stamoudis CX, Irwin SA, Greenough WT 1996 Increased density of multiple-head dendritic spines on medium-sized spiny neurons of the striatum in rats reared in a complex environment. Neurobiol Learn Mem 66:93–96

Corotto FS, Henegar JA, Maruniak JA 1993 Neurogenesis persists in the subependymal layer of the adult mouse brain. Neurosci Lett 149:111–114

Craig CG, Tropepe V, Morshead CM, Reynolds BA, Weiss S, van der Kooy D 1996 *In vivo* growth factor expansion of endogenous subependymal neural precursor cell populations in the adult mouse brain. J Neurosci 16:2649–2658

Dawirs RR, Hildebrandt K, Teuchert-Noodt G 1998 Adult treatment with haloperidol increases dentate granule cell proliferation in the gerbil hippocampus. J Neural Transm 105:317–327

Doetsch F, Caillé I, Lim DA, García-Verdugo JM, Alvarez-Buylla A 1999 Subventricular zone astrocytes are neural stem cells in the adult mammalian brain. Cell 97:703–716

Eriksson PS, Perfilieva E, Bjork-Eriksson T et al 1998 Neurogenesis in the adult human hippocampus. Nat Med 4:1313–1317

Fisher LJ 1997 Neural precursor cells: applications for the study and repair of the central nervous system. Neurobiol Dis 4:1–22

Gage FH, Coates PW, Palmer TD et al 1995 Survival and differentiation of adult neuronal progenitor cells transplanted to the adult brain. Proc Natl Acad Sci USA 92:11879–11883

Goldman SA 1995 Neuronal precursor cells and neurogenesis in the adult forebrain. Neuroscientist 1:338–350

Gould E 1994 The effects of adrenal steroids and excitatory input on neuronal birth and survival. Ann NY Acad Sci 743:73–93

Gould E, Tanapat P 1997 Lesion-induced proliferation of neuronal progenitor cells in the dentate gyrus of the adult rat. Neuroscience 80:427–436

Gould E, Cameron HA, Daniels DC, Woolley CS, McEwen BS 1992 Adrenal hormones suppress cell division in the adult rat dentate gyrus. J Neurosci 12:3642–3650

Gould E, McEwen BS, Tanapat P, Galea LAM, Fuchs E 1997 Neurogenesis in the dentate gyrus of the adult tree shrew is regulated by psychosocial stress and NMDA receptor activation. J Neurosci 17:2492–2498

Gould E, Beylin A, Tanapat P, Reeves A, Shors TJ 1999 Learning enhances adult neurogenesis in the hippocampal formation. Nat Neurosci 2:260–265

Greenough WT, Volkmar FR 1973 Pattern of dendritic branching in occipital cortex of rats reared in complex environments. Exp Neurol 40:491–504

Greenough WT, West RW, DeVoogd TJ 1978 Subsynaptic plate perforations: changes with age and experience in the rat. Science 202:1096–1098

Harzsch S, Miller J, Benton J, Beltz B 1999 From embryo to adult: persistent neurogenesis and apoptotic cell death shape the lobster deutocerebrum. J Neurosci 19:3472–3485

Hebb DO 1949 The organization of behavior. Wiley, Chichester

Houser CR 1990 Granule cell dispersion in the dentate gyrus of humans with temporal lobe epilepsy. Brain Res 535:195–204

Johansson CB, Momma S, Clarke DL, Risling M, Lendahl U, Frisén J 1999 Identification of a neural stem cell in the adult mammalian central nervous system. Cell 96:25–34

Juraska JM, Fitch JM, Henderson C, Rivers N 1985 Sex differences in the dendritic branching of dentate granule cells following differential experience. Brain Res 333:73–80

Kaplan MS, Hinds JW 1977 Neurogenesis in the adult rat: electron microscopic analysis of light radioautographs. Science 197:1092–1094

Kempermann G, Gage FH 1999 Experience-dependent regulation of adult hippocampal neurogenesis: effects of long-term stimulation and stimulus withdrawal. Hippocampus 9:321–332

Kempermann G, Kuhn HG, Gage FH 1997a More hippocampal neurons in adult mice living in an enriched environment. Nature 386:493–495

Kempermann G, Kuhn HG, Gage FH 1997b Genetic influence on neurogenesis in the dentate gyrus of adult mice. Proc Natl Acad Sci USA 94:10409–10414

Kempermann G, Brandon EP, Gage FH 1998a Environmental stimulation of 129/SvJ mice results in increased cell proliferation and neurogenesis in the adult dentate gyrus. Curr Biol 8:939–942

Kempermann G, Kuhn GH, Gage FH 1998b Experience-induced neurogenesis in the senescent dentate gyrus. J Neurosci 18:3206–3212

Kilpatrick TJ, Bartlett PF 1995 Cloned multipotential precursors from the mouse cerebrum require FGF-2, whereas glial restricted precursors are stimulated with either FGF-2 or EGF. J Neurosci 15:3653–3661

Kleim JA. Lussnig E, Schwarz ER, Comery TA, Greenough WT 1996 Synaptogenesis and Fos expression in the motor cortex of the adult rat after motor skill learning. J Neurosci 16:4529–4535

Kuhn HG, Dickinson-Anson H, Gage FH 1996 Neurogenesis in the dentate gyrus of the adult rat: age-related decrease of neuronal progenitor proliferation. J Neurosci 16:2027–2033

Kuhn HG, Winkler J, Kempermann G, Thal LJ, Gage FH 1997 Epidermal growth factor and fibroblast growth factor-2 have different effects on neural progenitors in the adult rat brain. J Neurosci 17:5820–5829

Lacorazza HD, Flax JD, Snyder EY, Jendoubi M 1996 Expression of the human beta-hexosaminidase alpha-subunit gene (the gene defect of Tay-Sachs disease) in mouse brains upon engraftment of transduced progenitor cells. Nat Med 2:424–429

Levison SW, Young GM, Goldman JE 1999 Cycling cells in the adult rat neocortex preferentially generate oligodendroglia. J Neurosci Res 57:435–446

Lim DA, Alvarez-Buylla A 1999 Interaction between astrocytes and adult subventricular zone precursors stimulates neurogenesis. Proc Natl Acad Sci USA 96:7526–7531

Liu J, Solway K, Messing RO, Sharp FR 1998 Increased neurogenesis in the dentate gyrus after transient global ischemia in gerbils. J Neurosci 18:7768–7778

Lois C, Alvarez-Buylla A 1993 Proliferating subventricular zone cells in the adult mammalian forebrain can differentiate into neurons and glia. Proc Natl Acad Sci USA 90:2074–2077

Luskin MB 1993 Restricted proliferation and migration of postnatally generated neurons derived from the forebrain subventricular zone. Neuron 11:173–189

Markakis E, Gage FH 1999 Adult-generated neurons in the dentate gyrus send axonal projections to the field CA3 and are surrounded by synaptic vesicles. J Comp Neurol 406:449–460

Merzenich MM, Nelson RJ, Stryker MP, Cynader MS, Schoppmann A, Zook JM 1984 Somatosensory cortical map changes following digit amputation in adult monkeys. J Comp Neurol 224:591–605

Miyata T, Maeda T, Lee JE 1999 NeuroD is required for differentiation of the granule cells in the cerebellum and hippocampus. Genes Dev 13:1647–1652

Morshead CM, Reynolds BA, Craig CG et al 1994 Neural stem cells in the adult mammalian forebrain: a relatively quiescent subpopulation of subependymal cells. Neuron 13:1071–1082

Nagy Z, Esiri MM, Cato AM, Smith AD 1997a Cell cycle markers in the hippocampus in Alzheimer's disease. Acta Neuropathol (Berl) 94:6–15

Nagy Z, Esiri MM, Smith AD 1997b Expression of cell division markers in the hippocampus in Alzheimer's disease and other neurodegenerative conditions. Acta Neuropathol (Berl) 93:294–300

Nilsson M, Perfilieva E, Johansson U, Orwar O, Eriksson P 1999 Enriched environment increases neurogenesis in the adult rat dentate gyrus and improves spatial memory. J Neurobiol 39:569–578

Noble M, Maier-Pröschel M 1997 Growth factors, glia and gliomas. J Neurooncol 35:193–209

Noble M, Gutowski N, Bevan K et al 1995 From rodent glial precursor cell to human glial neoplasia in the oligodendrocyte-type-2 astrocyte lineage. Glia 15:222–230

Palmer TD, Ray J, Gage FH 1995 FGF-2-responsive neuronal progenitors reside in proliferative and quiescent regions of the adult rodent brain. Mol Cell Neurosci 6:474–486

Palmer TD, Takahashi J, Gage FH 1997 The adult rat hippocampus contains premordial neural stem cells. Mol Cell Neurosci 8:389–404

Parent JM, Yu TW, Leibowitz RT, Geschwind DH, Sloviter RS, Lowenstein DH 1997 Dentate granule cell neurogenesis is increased by seizures and contributes to aberrant network reorganization in the adult rat hippocampus. J Neurosci 17:3727–3738

Parent JM, Tada E, Fike JR, Lowenstein DH 1999 Inhibition of dentate granule cell neurogenesis with brain irradiation does not prevent seizure-induced mossy fiber synaptic reorganization in the rat. J Neurosci 19:4508–4519

Pérez-Cañellas MM, Garcia-Verdugo JM 1996 Adult neurogenesis in the telencephalon of a lizard: a [3H] thymidine autoradiographic and bromodeoxyuridine immunocytochemical study. Brain Res Dev 93:49–61

Rakic P 1985 Limits of neurogenesis in primates. Science 227:1054–1056

Ray J, Peterson DA, Schinstine M, Gage FH 1993 Proliferation, differentiation, and long-term culture of primary hippocampal neurons. Proc Natl Acad Sci USA 90:3602–3606

Reynolds BA, Tetzlaff W, Weiss S 1992 A multipotent EGF-responsive striatal embryonic progenitor cell produces neurons and astrocytes. J Neurosci 12:4565–4574

Richards LJ, Kilpatrick TJ, Bartlett PF 1992 *De novo* generation of neuronal cells from the adult mouse brain. Proc Natl Acad Sci USA 89:8591–8595

Scheffler B, Horn M, Blumcke I et al 1999 Marrow-mindedness:a perspective on neuropoiesis. Trends Neurosci 22:348–357

Shihabuddin LS, Ray J, Gage FH 1997 FGF-2 is sufficient to isolate progenitors found in the adult mammalian spinal cord. Exp Neurol 148:577–586

Shihabuddin LS, Palmer TD, Gage FH 1999 The search for neural progenitor cells: prospects for the therapy of neurodegenerative disease. Mol Med Today 5:474–480

Snyder EY, Taylor RM, Wolfe, FH 1995 Neural progenitor cell engraftment corrects lysosomal storage throughout the MPS VII mouse brain. Nature 374:367–370

Stanfield BB, Trice JE 1988 Evidence that granule cells generated in the dentate gyrus of adult rats extend axonal projections. Exp Brain Res 72:399–406

Stryker MP 1999 Sensory maps on the move. Science 284:925–926

Suhonen JO, Peterson DA, Ray J, Gage FH 1996 Differentiation of adult hippocampus-derived progenitors into olfactory neurons *in vivo*. Nature 383:624–627

Takahashi M, Palmer TD, Takahashi J, Gage FH 1998 Widespread integration and survival of adult-derived neural progenitor cells in the developing optic retina. Mol Cell Neurosci 12:340–348

Van Praag H, Kempermann G, Gage FH 1999a Running increases cell proliferation and neurogenesis in the adult mouse dentate gyrus. Nat Neurosci 2:266–270

Van Praag H, Christie BR, Sejnowski TJ, Gage FH 1999b Running enhances neurogenesis, learning and long-term potentiation in mice. Proc Natl Acad Sci USA 96: 13 427–13 431

Vescovi AL, Reynolds BA, Fraser DD, Weiss S 1993 bFGF regulates the proliferative fate of unipotent (neuronal) and bipotent (neuronal/astroglial) EGF-generated CNS progenitor cells. Neuron 11:951–966

Weinmaster G 1998 Notch signalling: direct or what? Curr Opin Genet Dev 8:436–442

Weiss S, Van Der Kooy D 1998 CNS stem cells: where's the biology (a.k.a. beef)? J Neurobiol 36:307–314

Wu W, Wong K, Chen J et al 1999 Directional guidance of neuronal migration in the olfactory system by the protein Slit. Nature 400:331–336

Young D, Lawlor PA, Leone P, Dragunow M, During MJ 1999 Environmental enrichment inhibits spontaneous apoptosis, prevents seizures and is neuroprotective. Nat Med 5:448–453

Zigova T, Pencea V, Wiegand SJ, Luskin MB 1998 Intraventricular administration of BDNF increases the number of newly generated neurons in the adult olfactory bulb. Mol Cell Neurosci 11:234–245

DISCUSSION

Perry: Do you know why the dorsal blade of the dorsal root ganglion (DRG) degenerates when you inject things into it? We have seen this frequently and have no explanation.

Gage: Apparently there is a blood vessel there, and when you inject you often hit this. It is a nice control, because you have an astrocytic glial response in the dorsal leaf, and nothing in the ventral leaf, and cells only turn into neurons in ventral leaf or the intact site.

Perry: Does the total number of cells in the dentate stay constant?

Gage: Over the first year there is a constant but modest increase over time. If you do TUNEL staining and look in the dentate gyrus, you will see more TUNEL-positive cells than in the surrounding area, but no one yet has been able to do a match-up and say whether this is a balancing act of death and replacement or not. But what we do see is that with activity or enrichment, it is possible to elevate the number above that baseline. Thus external experiences can affect the total volume and cell number, and now people are reporting a variety of pharmacological manipulations that can increase proliferation and these events. Whatever baseline we had been looking at before in an isolated cage is one number, and any difference that people see in different labs between dentate gyrus cells may be a housing effect. We don't know what the upper limit of granule cells is. There is dramatic genetic variation, with big differences between strains of mice.

Smith: Am I right in thinking that when you transplant the hippocampal progenitors into the cortex, they don't differentiate?

Gage: They do not differentiate into neurons. Around the edge of the injection site you can see some astrocytes. As they migrate out you might see occasional cells differentiating into astrocytes or oligodendrocytes, but at very low frequency. The majority of the cells don't differentiate.

Smith: Do they continue to divide?

Gage: Not much, if at all. If you come back and pulse the animals, or look for PCNA after two weeks, you won't see any continued cell division.

Smith: Can you pull them back out?

Gage: We are trying to do that. We have cell lines that are tagged which will make it easier for us to FACS out. We have tried doing this in the past, but our yield hasn't been high enough, so we have had to expand the cells. The ideal situation would be to harvest enough fresh cells to be able to graft them back to the brain without expansion.

Smith: On the basis of what you have done before, do you think that these cells are remaining as progenitor cells and that they have just been quiescent in the non-neurogenic site? Your expectation would then be that you could pull them out and expand them again with FGF.

Gage: The hypothesis is that there is a subpopulation of cells that we will be able to pull out. One of the questions that will be important in terms of the expansion experiment is whether or not these cells are quiescent or committed *in vitro* and unable to experience neurogenesis. If we were to reactivate them with FGF, we may be able to expand the population more easily, leading to the concept that de-differentiation might be happening, concomitant with expansion.

Lindvall: I have a question related to the change of LTP in dentate gyrus. How was this done?

Gage: Field potentials.

Lindvall: Was it the induction or the maintenance of LTP?

Gage: Both. There was no increase in baseline, but the induced and maintained responses were increased.

Lindvall: My second question concerns what triggers the increase in neurogenesis. We observe increased neurogenesis under physiological conditions such as running, but also as a consequence of pharmacological states, e.g. seizure activity and cerebral ischaemia. What is the common mechanism that triggers this increase?

Gage: As I review more and more papers, I find an increasing number of things that can increase neurogenesis. The simple answer is that we don't know the mechanism, although my feeling is that there is not going to be one single mechanism. There are a number of possibilities. First, with activity there could be some vascular event: it could be hypervascularization because of the running, for example. Bloodflow-related events might be occurring that affect vascularization, which then secondarily can affect the survival of the cells and/or their proliferation. A second possibility is that we also know now that serotonergic drugs have a dramatic effect on neurogenesis. As you were alluding to, the one thing these animals are doing when they are running is generating theta. It does seem that the enhancement of serotonin can increase neurogenesis, and blockers of serotonin can modulate it.

Gray: I don't follow the logic of that argument. As I recall, the ascending serotonergic pathways actually repress theta (Kitchigina et al 1999). While the animal is running and showing lots of theta, it is probably not having a lot of serotonin release.

Gage: With running, the animals have a lot of neurogenesis, and serotonin agonists will increase neurogenesis, and blockers appear to decrease it.

Gray: The link with theta doesn't make sense, though.

Björklund: It may be relevant in this context that serotonin release in the hippocampus as measured by microdialysis has been shown to increase during ongoing locomotor activity.

Isacson: There is an experiment that I would like to do. If you take these cells that don't differentiate unless you put them into the neurogenic region of the adult, if you put them into a neonate or an embryo where there is neurogenesis, do they then take on or respond to the other main regions and cues in that cellular environment?

Gage: Yes.

Isacson: My second question relates to what is normal and what is deprived. A normal rat would be exposed to a huge number of problems in its normal environment. Do you think that the enrichment paradigm is just a normalization, and the normal rat condition in a cage is more of a deprivation?

Gage: That could be the case.

Blakemore: Is there an age-related shut-off effect? How old were the animals you worked with?

Gage: We have looked in mice and rats out to 22 months. There is a significant decrease in proliferation in the dentate gyrus with age. The subventricular zone proliferation doesn't appear to decrease as much as the dentate gyrus. If we take 19–20-month-old rats that have spent their lives in little cages and put them into an enriched environment, you can triple the number of BrdU cells surviving, though it is still a level way below that of younger animals.

Blakemore: Were the transplant experiments done with a line generated from these cells rather than the primaries?

Gage: We have done both fresh proliferating cells and clonal lines from what we call bulk populations, which are just expanded cells that have a certain number of passages.

Blakemore: Presumably these haven't been transfected, just pushed with growth factors to get enough cells.

Gage: We haven't put any oncogenes in them, but we do put marker genes in them such as green fluorescent protein (GFP) sometimes. When we have got over a certain number of doublings, we have karyotyped our cells. We find that they become anuploid. There are occasions when we had highly passaged cells which formed tumours when we grafted them, so we are cautious.

Price: I wanted to comment on the FGF2 effect and how it apparently broadens the potential of the cells. It is interesting, because one sees a similar phenomenon in embryonic cortical precursor cells. I alluded earlier on to that fact that although the embryonic cortical precursor cells, or a population of them, are multipotential, they are relatively reticent to generate oligodendrocytes. If these cells are treated with FGF2, they give rise to oligodendrocytes much more readily (W. D. Richardson, personal communication). Can you get the same FGF2 effect on other populations of precursor cells?

Gage: We see it in the cortex and optic nerve, spinal cord, septum and middle of striatum away from the ventricular zone. It is not cortex-specific.

Price: The obvious difference between what you have reported with your cells and what Helen Hodges and colleagues reported with the MHP cells, is that a broader range of neurons are generated by the MHP cells than you apparently see.

Gage: We have very little experience with damage. Most of what we have looked at is in intact tissue. That is why I was asking whether you had grafted your cells into the granule cell zone, to see if they respond to the local cues that exist within this zone. We do get neurogenesis in that case. Interestingly, in the developing eye we see plenty of neuronal differentiation. Our working hypothesis is that the cells are quite multipotential. It is just that the local cues aren't there to drive them to specific neural lineages.

Gray: There has been a basic difference in strategy between Gage's work and the research described by Hodges and Price using the MHP cell lines. In order to make a proper comparison between these two lines of research, one needs to see what happens to both types of cell in both intact and damaged brain. In both of those sets of experiments, the proportions of stem cells that can be differentiated *in vitro* into neurons, oligodendrocytes or astrocytes can be varied by the particular growth factors used. Are those shifts in cell fate responding to the same shifts in the media in both sets of experiments? Is the cell type that has been conditionally immortalized in the MHP36 line the same type of cell that you, Fred, are using in its endogenous state?

Gage: My guess is that serum induces astrocytes. Most progenitor cells exposed to serum turn into astrocytes.

Price: John Sinden did the experiments with retinoic acid and got similar results to those you report. The simple conclusion is that there is no reason to believe we are not dealing with very similar cells. I can't think of any major discrepancies.

Smith: How does this direction of differentiation compare with Ron McKay's description of growth factor effects on precursors, and the induction of astrocytes with ciliary neurotrophic factor (CNTF), for example?

Price: In our case it is very similar. We have tried Ron's factors in our cells and get somewhat similar results.

Gage: This is over-ridden dramatically by serum. The proportions differ from line to line. If I take 10 individually cloned lines that we have generated from the parent population, the percentages of each cell type would differ, but they would all generate all three phenotypes. In our hands, I would say that if you took the same line and grew them up and plated them, you would probably get slightly different percentages differentiating into each lineage.

Price: Coming back to the FGF effect, everybody who is trying to immortalize cells throws FGF in one form or another into the culture. This observation we just discussed, where FGF brings everything back to some level, might mean that everyone is working with somewhat similar cells.

Gage: There are investigators who use EGF.

Price: EGF is a bit more of a variable, because I don't think neuroepithelial cells from every source are particularly sensitive to EGF. Our data say that cortical precursors don't react too much to EGF, whereas striatal precursors certainly do (Birling & Price 1998).

Smith: In the FGF-induced neurogenesis, is cell division necessary for neuronal differentiation? If you take the quiescent cells from the cortex, for instance, that won't give you neurons unless you give them FGF; in that situation do those cells have to divide before they will differentiate into neurons?

Gage: Yes. Cells that are Tug1+ are also BrdU labelled. This speaks against the idea of a quiescent population.

Finsen: Is the neurogenesis in normal adult hippocampus dependent on an intact perforant path?

Gage: We have really mixed results on this. There is some modulatory effect of an entorhinal lesion, and others have reported effects of glutamate inhibitors. We have looked very hard and have not seen a profound effect. The lesion effect is tough to interpret, because we are doing so much to the brain by introducing a lesion.

Björklund: I was fascinated by your comments on the normal role of neurogenesis. Is there a continued renewal of granule cells over time? When you activate neurogenesis, and continue to do it, would you see an addition of new functional granule cells, or do the cells turnover? You said that there was a 15% increase in volume of the hippocampus in the running experiment. This is quite a substantial rise over a short time, and if it was to continue over an extended period of time, this would make the hippocampus huge in size! What regulates the total granule cell number?

Gage: The 15% increase was not in the running experiment, it was in the enrichment experiment. Gerd Kempermann has taken animals at young ages and kept them in the enriched environment for six months. There is a 15–20% increase that plateaus in those animals, no matter how long they stay in the enriched environment. There does seem to be a limitation. One interesting experiment is that when he withdrew the animals from the enriched environment and looked at the effects, the total number of cells actually decreased. But the rate of proliferation and the number of proliferating cells was sustained, as though there was a pool of progenitor cells that was elevated, but they were then dying off because there was no increased ability to maintain their survival. It does seem to be reasonably tightly regulated, both in terms of how far it can go up and also how long it can be sustained. We don't know what the specific cues are, but there clearly is an upper limit.

Björklund: What about turnover of granule cells?

Gage: I don't think we have a satisfactory answer. In a small cage the baseline numbers increase in the first year and seem to plateau. The real question is whether there is a balance between cell survival and cell loss.

Björklund: What happens to the newcomers? Since proliferation and survival are independently regulated, it seems possible that new cells are generated, but few will survive as granule cells. The turnover could be in the newly generated pool, so that in the normal life of an animal, few or none of these granule cells will remain as functional granule cells.

Gage: Max Cowan did some studies in the 1980s where he asked whether or not the newly born adult cells were the first ones to die off. This is not the case. What it looks likes now is that the outer rim of the dentate is sloughing off. Over time one sees the granule cells newly generated marching their way up. The older the cell is, the higher up in the granule cell layer it is.

Snyder: I wanted to agree with and expand upon Fred Gage's notion that maintaining cells in or 'kicking' quiescent cells back into the cell cycle preserves their pluripotency and/or forestalls their propensity to differentiate. This observation may even be broader than just an FGF-specific effect, but may touch on the larger issue of those regulatory functions employed for maintaining cells in the cell cycle and how they interact with processes that influence neural stem cell differentiation. Other factors that share signal transduction pathways with FGF in influencing progression through the cell cycle may have the same broad effect as FGF.

Price: That couldn't explain Sally Temple's findings, because those cells are dividing but don't express the potential to generate oligodendrocytes. If you then hit them with FGF, they do (Qian et al 1997).

Snyder: It is true that FGF was sufficient to 'unveil' the multipotency of those cells, but other factors and manipulations that act more distal in the FGF (and other growth factor) signal transduction pathways can have a similar effect.

Price: It can't just be that the cells need to be cycling.

Snyder: True. It is not that any precursor cycling will 'become' multipotent. However, it is true that a multipotent stem cell that *stops* cycling will quickly become restricted in its potency. I think those cells need to be cycling; they then remain susceptible to being influenced by external cues as opposed to cascading towards a restricted differentiation pathway that quickly excludes other pathways.

Olson: It is interesting that you can make neurons from the optic nerve. What happens if you go outside the CNS? Can you make neurons from peripheral nerves, or bone marrow?

Gage: Those experiments of taking mesenchymal or bone marrow cells are being done in many labs. There are some reports of neuronal-like *in vitro* characteristics, and people are transplanting from peripheral sources to the CNS. Over the next few years we'll have a clearer view of whether these cells turn into authentic neurons or not.

References

Birling MC, Price J 1998 A study of the potential of the embryonic rat telencephalon to generate oligodendrocytes. Dev Biol 193:100–113

Kitchigina VF, Kudina TA, Kutyreva EV, Vinogradova OS 1999 Neuronal activity of the septal pacemaker of theta rhythm under the influence of stimulation and blockade of the median raphe nucleus in the awake rabbit. Neuroscience 94:453–463

Qian Z, Davis AA, Goderie SK, Temple S 1997 FGF2 concentration regulates the generation of neurons and glia from multipotent cortical stem cells. Neuron 18:81–93

Neural stem cells are uniquely suited for cell replacement and gene therapy in the CNS

Vaclav Ourednik*, Jitka Ourednik*, Kook I. Park*†, Y.D. Teng*, Karen A. Aboody*, Kurtis I. Auguste*, Rosanne M. Taylor‡, Barbara A. Tate* and Evan Y. Snyder*[1]

*Departments of Neurology (Division of Neuroscience), Pediatrics (Division of Newborn Medicine), & Neurosurgery, Children's Hospital, Harvard Medical School, Boston, MA 02115, USA, †Department of Pediatrics, Yonsei University College of Medicine, Yongdong Severance Hospital, Seoul, Korea and ‡University of Sydney, Department of Animal Science, Sydney, Australia

Abstract. In recent years, it has become evident that the developing and even the adult mammalian CNS contain a population of undifferentiated, multipotent cell precursors, neural stem cells, the plastic properties of which might be of advantage for the design of more effective therapies for many neurological diseases. This article reviews the recent progress in establishing rodent and human clonal neural stem cell lines, their biological properties, and how these cells can be utilized to correct a variety of defects, with prospects for the near future to harness their behaviour for neural stem cell-based treatment of diseases in humans.

2000 Neural transplantation in neurodegenerative disease. Wiley, Chichester (Novartis Foundation Symposium 231) p 242–269

Neurological disorders, whether hereditary or acquired, are typically characterized by a variety of cellular and molecular defects. The situation is aggravated by the fact that, during its maturation, the CNS appears progressively to lose its restorative capacity by establishing a potent inhibitory environment to neural regrowth and the formation of new connections, and by the formation of a blood–brain barrier (BBB) that protects the brain from blood-borne pathogens but also prevents the entrance of many therapeutic substances from the vascular compartment. Current attempts to promote CNS repair address these obstacles using the following strategies: (i) replacing affected cell populations (or structural components like

---

[1]This chapter was presented at the symposium by Professor Snyder, to whom correspondence should be addressed.

myelin) and their connections by neural grafts; (ii) providing trophic support by the introduction of neurotrophins and/or cytokines to diminish or prevent progressive neurodegeneration, stimulate neurite outgrowth, guide growing axons to their targets and promote establishment of functional synapses; and (iii) replacing missing neuroactive molecules, such as enzymes and neurotransmitters.

For several decades, fetal neural transplants have been used to promote CNS repair and formed the basis of an important branch of restorative neurobiology (reviewed in Dunnett & Björklund 1994, Fisher & Gage 1993, 1994). They have not only provided us with a wealth of information about normal CNS development but have generated invaluable information regarding the extent to which the perinatal, juvenile and adult CNS is able to react to growth signals and to mobilize dormant, intrinsic plastic capacities. In the majority of cases, fetal grafts have been used in three ways (Kordower & Tuszynski 1999, Marciano et al 1989): (i) to replace cellular elements, especially neurons, in the degenerating host parenchyma and to reinnervate targets which have lost their proper input; (ii) to act as tissue 'bridges' for host axonal regeneration due to their highly growth-permissive environment; and (iii) to prevent degeneration of host cells. More recently, an additional, and as yet hardly explored, phenomenon concerning graft/host interaction has been described, namely, the graft's potential to evoke robust restorative mechanisms within the juvenile recipient's brain which later result in an unusually well-remodelled cytoarchitecture originating almost exclusively from the host (Ourednik et al 1993, 1998, Ourednik & Ourednik 1994). Nevertheless, despite the fact that fetal grafts are already being used with likely success in human parkinsonian patients (Kordower et al 1995), a routine use of fetal tissue raises significant concerns, both biological and ethical, such as the availability of requisite amounts of suitable material and insuring survival of desired cells in a tissue that is typically heterogeneous. Moreover, with respect to the more and more popular idea of transferring therapeutic genes (or their end metabolic products) to the brain, primary fetal tissue is, due to its heterogeneity, not well suited for the genetic engineering (see below) that might be necessary to provide greater or more stable amounts of a trophic factor or to replace a particular enzyme in a defined cell type.

The transfer of a transgene or a gene product is frequently an important step in the attempt to correct a deficiency in the CNS. For this reason, many methods of gene transfer are under investigation (Breakfield et al 1999). They fall into two categories: mechanical delivery of DNA into cells *in vitro* and introduction of genetic material by virus-based vectors. Mechanical ways of introducing DNA into cells rely on diverse means of particulation and concentration of the DNA around the cell membrane in form of precipitates, liposomes, gold particles or molecular conjugates internalized by the cells in an active (endo- or pinocytosis) or passive (membrane fusion, electroporation or bombardment) process.

Although frequently employed, this methodology is not very efficient and cells may not get transfected in a stable manner.

Virus-based delivery of foreign genes into mammalian cells has several advantages: the small genome of retroviruses (still the most frequently used type of virus) allows relatively easy manipulation and insertion of larger transgene sequences, viruses can be grown to high titres in culture, infection efficiency is extremely high (close to 100% of cultured cells), and the DNA, in most cases, gets stably integrated into the genome in form of a provirus. However, care must be taken that the transgene is inserted into a replication-defective virus where all the transforming oncogene sequences have been removed. All the products necessary for replication and integration of such defective viruses are provided *in trans* by replication-competent but non-transforming helper viruses which later have to be completely removed from the purified vector — often a rather difficult task.

The introduction of DNA by viral vectors can be achieved either by *in situ* application, i.e., direct injection of genetically-altered viruses into the CNS, or by *ex vivo* gene therapy, where vector-mediated gene transfer into cells occurs *in vitro* and these transgenic cells are then transplanted into the brain regions of interest. Besides the technical difficulties inherent to the vectors used and common to both strategies (e.g. expression of viral genes, initiation of an antiviral immune response, reversion of the viral vector to a replication-competent state, and inactivation of transcription and/or expression of foreign genes), both suffer from specific insufficiencies as well. Thus, although progress is being made in targeting post-mitotic neural tissue with viral vectors like lentivirus, adenovirus (AV), adenoassociated virus (AAV), or herpes simplex virus (HSV) expressing therapeutic transgenes under cell type-specific promoters, they still may not address the widespread, extensive lesions characteristic of many neuro-degenerative conditions, particularly those of genetic, perinatal, metabolic, inflammatory, infectious or traumatic origin. Furthermore, such strategies depend on relaying new genetic information through established endogenous neural populations and circuits, which, in fact, may have degenerated or failed to develop.

In the alternative approach, the *ex vivo* gene therapy strategy, the challenge comes in selecting a cellular population that can be easily altered genetically to produce a desired protein and then safely and efficiently introduced into discrete or widespread regions of the brain where they can reside innocuously and continue to deliver their genetic 'payload'. Donor cells may be chosen to act as miniature 'pumps' providing a source of exogenous substances that can diffuse to appropriate targets, to become integral members of the host cytoarchitecture and circuitry, or, ideally, to do both. Neurons would seem to be the appropriate cellular candidate for both delivering products to and integrating within the CNS. However, there are restrictions on the types and ages of neurons that survive grafting in a functionally meaningful way for prolonged periods. Also, because mature neurons irreversibly stop proliferating, they are unsuitable targets for retrovirus-based gene delivery. While improvements in the design of integrating vectors (lentivirus, AAV) and episomal vectors (HSV, AV) may ultimately facilitate genetic manipulation of post-mitotic neurons *ex vivo*, at present, the usefulness of primary neurons as vehicles for gene transfer is minimal. Researchers therefore soon turned towards well-established cultures of non-neuronal cells which do proliferate and can easily be manipulated by retroviruses to express transgenes. Fibroblasts quickly became the ideal candidates and have been modified to produce a variety of neurotransmitter-synthesizing enzymes (e.g. tyrosine hydroxylase and choline acetyltransferase) and trophic proteins (e.g. nerve growth factor). Drawbacks of this technique are, however, that fibroblasts are unable to incorporate functionally into the host brain's cytoarchitecture, damaged circuits cannot be reformed and regulated release of substances may be missing. Thus, investigators started to look for another cell type which would be a source of a homogeneous cell population; which, while proliferating, could easily be maintained and genetically manipulated *in vitro*; and, at the same time, would, after grafting, be able to integrate seamlessly into the cytoarchitecture and circuitry of the host CNS.

For several years, there has been a growing interest in the therapeutic potential of neural stem cells (NSCs) and progenitors for therapy in CNS dysfunctions. This interest derives from the realization that these cells are more than simply a replacement for fetal tissue in transplantation paradigms and yet another vehicle for gene delivery. Rather, the basic biology of these cells endows them with a quality that other vehicles for gene therapy and repair may simply not possess (e.g. Martínez-Serrano & Snyder 1999, Snyder & Senut 1997): the potential to integrate into the neural circuitry after transplantation. With the first recognition that NSCs, propagated in culture, could be reimplanted into mammalian brain where they could reintegrate appropriately and stably express foreign genes, gene therapists and restorative neurobiologists began to speculate how such a phenomenon might be harnessed for therapeutic advantage. These, and the studies which they spawned (Yandava et al 1999, Lundberg et al 1997, Rosario et al 1997, Lacorazza et al 1996, Renfranz et al 1991) provided hope that the use of NSCs, by virtue of their inherent biology, might circumvent some of the limitations of presently available graft material and gene transfer vehicles, and make feasible a variety of novel therapeutic strategies (Table 1).

NSCs are postulated to be immature, uncommitted cells that exist in the developing and even adult nervous system (Gage et al 1995, Reynolds & Weiss 1992) and are responsible for giving rise to the vast array of more specialized cells of the mature CNS. They are operationally defined by their ability to self-renew, their potential to differentiate into various (if not all) neuronal and glial cell

TABLE 1   Properties of neural stem cells that make them appealing vehicles for CNS gene therapy and repair

Genetic manipulability

Progenitor/stem cells easily transduced *ex vivo* by most viral and non-viral gene transfer methods.

Facile engraftability following simple implantation procedures

From engraftment in germinal zones (as well as into parenchyma), can broach BBB unimpeded; no requirement for conditioning regimes (e.g. irradiation as in bone marrow transplantation or opening of BBB).

Sustained foreign (therapeutic) gene expression

Throughout CNS, from fetus to adult, following technically simple and safe reimplantation procedures; CNS levels rise immediately.

Potential for normal reintegration into host cytoarchitecture and circuitry

Differentiate along all CNS cell-type lineages; important for diseases in which neurons and glia are both affected; not only allows direct, stable and perhaps regulated delivery of therapeutic molecules, but also enables replacement of range of dysfunctional neural cells and possible reconstruction of connections and networks.

Ability to migrate

Particularly within germinal zones, enabling replacement of genes and cells to be directed not only to discrete sites but to widely disseminated lesions as well for diseases of a more global nature; for more focal implants, ability of cells to intermingle with host cells rather than clump at injection track insures homogeneous distribution of therapeutic molecules throughout target tissue.

Plasticity

Ability to accommodate to region of engraftment and assume array of phenotypes; obviates necessity for obtaining donor cells from many specific CNS regions, or imperative for precise targeting of donor cells during reimplantation, or need for tissue-specific promoters for foreign gene expression.

Compensatory of transgene non-expression

Low levels of normal neural products expressed intrinsically by progenitor/stem cells (lysosomal enzymes; neurotrophic, matrix, adhesion and homeodomain molecules; myelin) helps safeguard against transgene inactivation; neural cells may sustain expression of foreign neural genes longer than non-neural vehicles; ability to integrate multiple copies of a transgene into its genome (e.g. following repeated sequential retroviral infection) helps thwart loss of expression; may also provide as-yet-unrecognized beneficial neural-specific substances.

One stem cell may carry multiple transgenes

Following multiple transfection events, one cell can transfer multiple gene products simultaneously.

Minimization of side effects

Distribution of gene products restricted to CNS; while proteins may be disseminated by stem cells throughout brain for diseases of global nature, by altering mode of administration, cells can be selectively integrated in proximity to neurons that require given factor without affecting cells for which the molecule might be problematic; conditioning regimes not required prior to transplantation as in bone marrow therapy.

(Continued)

TABLE 1 *(Continued)*

Ability to serve as producer cells for the in vivo dissemination of viral vectors

May help amplify distribution of virus-mediated genes to large CNS regions and numbers of cells.

Immunotolerance

In rodent transplant studies, multiple recipients and mouse strains can integrate the same murine stem cell clone without rejection or the necessity for immunosuppression, suggesting a need for generating very few effective clones (one clone used by many).

Tropism for and trophism within regions of CNS degeneration

When confronted with neurodegenerative environments, stem cells alter their migration & differentiation patterns towards replacement of dying cells; probably a vestigial developmental strategy with therapeutic value.

---

lineages, and to populate developing or degenerating CNS regions in multiple regional and temporal contexts. We can even hypothesize that, whenever the CNS is injured, it may actually try to 'repair itself' with its own endogenous NSC population but that, for most injuries that come to clinical attention, that supply is restricted in the number of available NSCs or insufficiently mobilized and even counteracted by growth-inhibitory environment, specially in adult brain. This unexplored possibility of a 'self-repair' could already be postulated in the context of the regenerative effect of fetal tissue grafts on host tissue (Ourednik et al 1993, 1998, Ourednik & Ourednik 1994) and is corroborated by the fact that such fetal tissues still contain a large pool of endogenous NSCs which are probably responsible for the observed graft-induced remodelling by the post-mitotic host brain. Furthermore, pilot studies in which endogenous progenitors in the suventricular germinal zone (SCZ) are labelled and tracked just as a devastating hypoxic–ischaemic brain injury is experimentally imposed on the cortex, suggests that these progenitors alter their normal stereotypical migratory route to the olfactory bulb and move instead towards the damaged regions to become new neurons in regions where neurogenesis has been conventionally deemed as having been completed. Therefore, to augment such a response with 'pure' exogenous NSCs (transgenic or not), implanted opportunistically at strategic times following injury, may enable an even more significant recovery.

NSC clones have been maintained in a proliferative state by several equally safe and effective strategies: through manipulation of 'internal commands' by genetic means (e.g. transduction of propagating genes that interact with cell cycle regulatory proteins) or by exposure to 'external commands' (e.g. such epigenetic means as chronic mitogen stimulation or co-culture on various cellular membrane substrates). Such manipulations do not subvert the ability of stem cells to respond to normal microenvironmental cues: to withdraw from the cell cycle, interact with host cells and to differentiate. This point has been successfully illustrated by a prototypical model murine NSC clone (designated clone C17.2), which was initially isolated from 4-day-old mouse cerebellum but has the ability to accommodate to most neural regions at most periods throughout the mouse's life (Snyder et al 1992). When transplanted into various germinal zones throughout the brain, these cells participate in normal development of multiple regions at multiple stages along the murine neuraxis (expressing their marker, β-galactosidase, from the bacterial *lacZ* transgene). They intermingle non-disruptively with endogenous neural progenitor/stem cells, responding to the same spatial and temporal cues in a similar manner and differentiating into all neuronal and glial cell types. Crucial for therapeutic considerations, the structures to which they contribute develop normally. Thus, their use as graft material can be considered almost analogous to haematopoietic stem cell-mediated reconstitution. In the following sections, using clone C17.2 as model for NSCs in general, we present examples of their behaviour in several grafting experiments simulating various neuropathological situations.

Non-engineered NSCs correct a variety of CNS defects

In testing the potential of NSCs to replace dying cells and lost neural circuits in degenerating brain, insights have been derived from studying mouse mutant and specific injury paradigms which have served nicely as well-controlled and well-defined models for more complex CNS dysfunctions. In such experiments, NSCs appear well suited for replacing some degenerated or dysfunctional neural cells.

In the *meander tail* (*mea*) mutant, which is characterized by failure of sufficient granule neurons to develop in certain regions of the cerebellum, NSCs, implanted at birth, were capable of 'repopulating' large agranular portions with neurons (Rosario et al 1997). A pivotal observation, with implications for fundamental stem cell biology, was that cells with the potential for multiple fates 'shifted' their mode of differentiation to compensate for a deficiency in a particular cell type. As compared with their differentiation in normal cerebella, a preponderance of these donor NSCs in regions deficient in granule neurons pursued a granule neuronal phenotype in preference to other potential phenotypes, suggesting the presence of environmental signals 'pushing' undifferentiated, multipotent cells towards repletion of the inadequately developed cell type. This phenomenon was observed in more than one study (as will be illustrated in some of the following examples) and presents a possible developmental mechanism with obvious therapeutic value.

Preliminary work in another mutant, the *reeler* (*rl*) mouse, has suggested that NSCs may not only replace developmentally impaired cells, but may also help correct certain aspects of abnormal cytoarchitecture (Auguste et al 1996). The laminar assignment of neurons in *rl* mouse brain is profoundly abnormal due, most likely, to a mutation in a gene encoding the secreted extracellular matrix (ECM) molecule, Reelin. NSCs, implanted at birth into the defective developing *rl* cerebellum, appeared in pilot studies not only to replace missing granule neurons in correct laminar position, but also to restore a more wild-type laminated appearance in engrafted regions by influencing the migration and survival of mutant neurons, most likely by providing molecules (including Reelin) that guide proper histogenesis. These findings therefore suggest a possible stem cell-based strategy for the treatment of CNS diseases characterized by abnormal cellular migration, lamination and cytoarchitectural arrangement.

Many neurologic diseases, particularly those of neurogenetic aetiology, are characterized by global degeneration or dysfunction. Mutants characterized by CNS-wide white matter disease provide an ideal model for testing hypotheses that NSCs might also be useful in neuropathologies requiring widespread neural cell replacement. The oligodendroglia of the dysmyelinated *shiverer* (*shi*) mouse are dysfunctional because they lack myelin basic protein (MBP) essential for effective myelination. Therapy, therefore, requires widespread replacement with MBP-expressing oligodendrocytes. NSCs transplanted at birth (employing an intracerebroventricular implantation technique devised for diffuse engraftment of enzyme-expressing NSCs to treat global metabolic lesions, Yandava et al 1999) resulted in engraftment throughout the *shi* brain with repletion of significant amounts of MBP (Figs 1 and 2). Accordingly, of the many donor cells which differentiated into oligodendroglia, a subgroup myelinated 40% of host neuronal processes. In some recipient animals, the symptomatic tremor decreased. Therefore, 'global' cell replacement seems feasible for some pathologies if cells with stem-like features are employed. This approach is being extended to other poorly myelinated mutants, e.g. mouse models of Krabbe's globoid cell leukodystrophy. The ability of NSCs to remyelinate is of particular importance because dys-/de-myelination plays an important role in many genetic (e.g. leukodystrophies, inborn metabolic errors) and acquired (traumatic, infectious, asphyxial, ischemic, inflammatory) neurodegenerative processes. More broadly, complementation studies in mutants, such as those described above, help support a NSC-based approach, whether with exogenous NSCs or with appropriately mobilized endogenous NSCs, for compensating for neurodevelopmental problems of many aetiologies.

One of the most fascinating characteristics of NSCs is that they indeed can react to neurodegeneration by 'shifting' their pattern of differentiation towards 'replenishing' of the missing cell types. One of the studies demonstrating this phenomenon was performed in a model of experimentally induced apoptosis of selectively targeted pyramidal neurons in the adult mammalian neocortex (Snyder et al 1997). Apoptosis (at least at particular critical phases) is becoming implicated in a growing number of both neurodegenerative and normal developmental processes. When transplanted into this neuron-specific degenerative environment, 15% of NSCs 'altered' the differentiation path they otherwise would have taken under normal developmental circumstances (neurogenesis has normally ceased in the adult cortex) and instead differentiated specifically into that type of degenerating neuron, partially replacing that lost neuronal population. Pilot studies further suggest that some replacement neurons sent axons across the corpus callosum to appropriate targets in the contralateral hemisphere. Thus, this neurodegeneration may have created a 'milieu' which recapitulates normal embryonic developmental cues (e.g. for cortical neuronogenesis) to which NSCs can respond to therapeutic advantage.

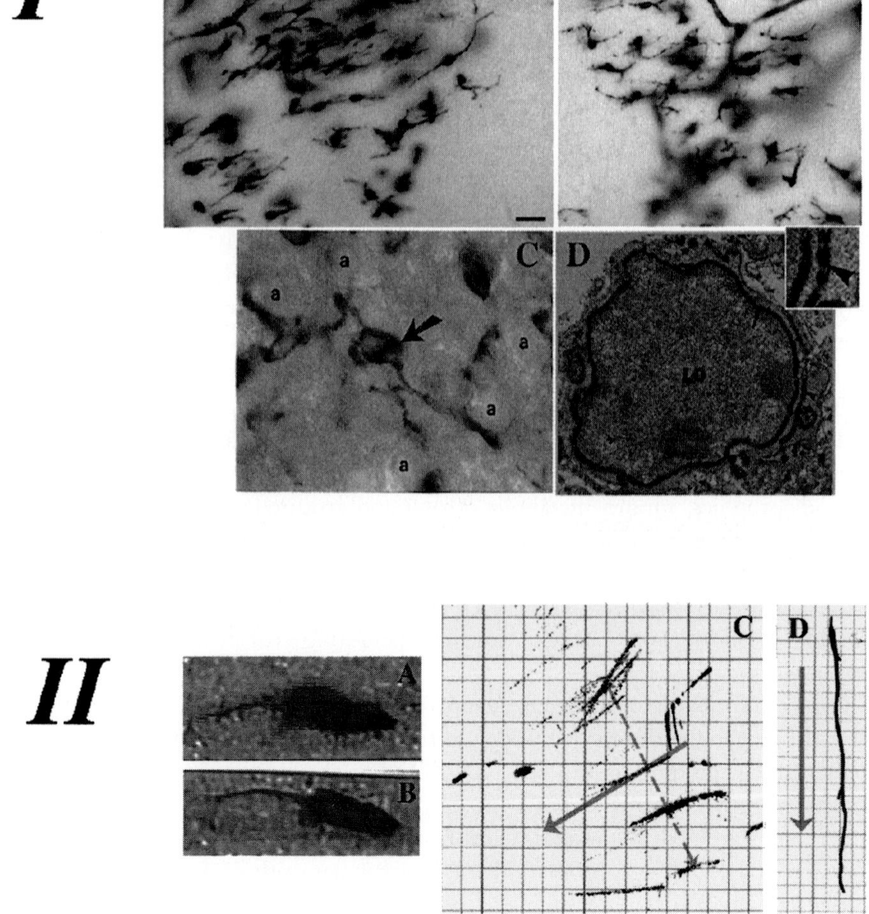

Evidence from experimental mouse models that even more closely emulate clinical situations further suggests that CNS injury or degeneration (of a certain type and/or during critical developmental time windows) might advantageously direct the migration, proliferation and differentiation of NSCs, both of host and donor origin. In a preliminary study, mice treated systemically with MPTP (1-methyl-4-phenyl-1,2,3,6-tetrahydropyridine), a drug selectively destroying dopaminergic cells in the brainstem, and subsequently grafted unilaterally with NSC clone C17.2 displayed a reconstituted dopaminergic cell population

---

FIG. 1.   Engrafted NSCs in recipient *shi* mutants differentiate into oligodendrocytes (I) and functional and behavioural assessment of transplanted *shi* mutants and controls (II). (I A,B) Donor-derived Xgal$^+$ cells in representative sections through the corpus callosum possess characteristic oligodendroglial features — small, round or polygonal cell bodies with multiple fine processes oriented in the direction of the neural fibre tracts. (C) Close-up of a representative donor-derived anti-β-galactosidase immunoreactive oligodendrocyte (arrow) extending multiple processes toward and beginning to enwrap large, adjacent axonal bundles viewed on end in a section through the corpus callosum. That cells such as those in A–C are oligodendroglia is confirmed by the representative electron micrograph in (D), demonstrating a donor-derived Xgal-labelled oligodendrocyte (LO) distinguished by the electron-dense Xgal precipitate that typically is localized to the nuclear membrane (arrow), endoplasmic reticulum (arrowhead), and other cytoplasmic organelles. The area indicated by the arrowhead is magnified in the inset to demonstrate the unique crystalline nature of individual precipitate particles. (II) The *shi* mutation is characterized by the onset of tremor and a 'shivering gait' by the second to third postnatal week. The degree of motor dysfunction in animals was gauged in two ways: (i) by blindly scoring periods of standardized videotaped cage behaviour of experimental and control animals and (ii) by measuring the amplitude of tail displacement from the body's rostral–caudal axis (an objective, quantifiable index of tremor). Video freeze-frames of representative unengrafted and successfully engrafted *shi* mice are seen in (A) and (B). The whole-body tremor and ataxic movement observed in the unengrafted symptomatic animal (A) causes the frame to blur, a contrast to the well-focused frame of the asymptomatic transplanted *shi* mouse (B). 60% of transplanted mutants evinced nearly normal-appearing behaviour and attained scores that were not significantly different from normal controls. (C) and (D) depict the manner in which whole-body tremor was mirrored by the amplitude of tail displacement (hatched arrow in C), measured perpendicularly from a line drawn in the direction of the animal's movement (solid arrow, which represents the body's long axis). Measurements were made by permitting a mouse, whose tail had been dipped in India ink, to move freely in a straight line on a sheet of graph paper as shown. Large degrees of tremor cause the tail to make widely divergent ink marks away from the midline, representing the body's axis (C). Absence of tremor allows the tail to make long, straight, uninterrupted ink lines on the paper congruent with the body's axis (D). The distance between points of maximal tail displacement from the axis was measured and averaged for transplanted and untransplanted *shi* mutants and for unaffected controls (hatched arrow). (C) shows data from a poorly engrafted mutant that did not improve with respect to tremor whereas (D) reveals lack of tail displacement in a successfully engrafted, now asymptomatic *shi* mutant. Overall, 64% of transplanted *shi* mice examined displayed at least a 50% decrement in the degree of tremor or 'shiver'. Several showed zero displacement. Bars: I. A,B, and C $=10\,\mu$m, D $=1.5\,\mu$m, II. A,B $=2.5$ cm. (Modified from Yandava et al 1999.)

I

II

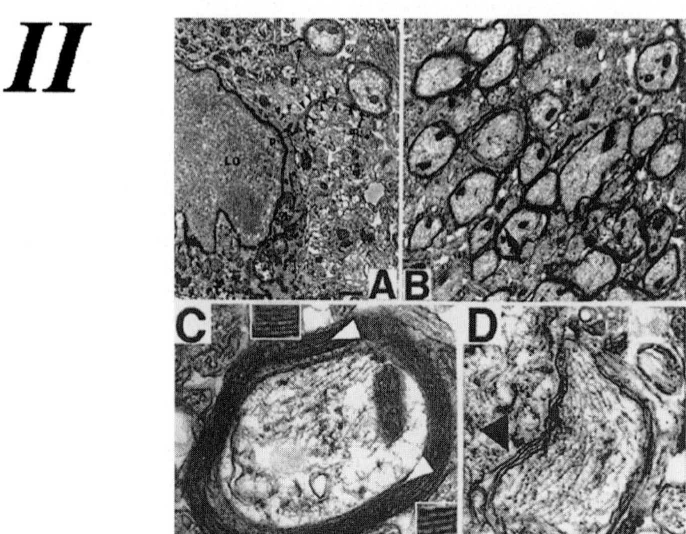

composed of donor and host. This suggests that NSCs not only replenished a defined pool of a missing cell type but also reactivated regenerative capacities within the aged host.

In a newborn mouse, unilateral carotid ligation combined with reduced ambient oxygen produces extensive hypoxic–ischaemic brain injury (HI) throughout the ipsilateral cerebral hemisphere. HI is an ideal prototype for a range of untreatable acquired and inherited neurodegenerative conditions and involves multiple cell types and regions in a devastatingly extensive manner. NSC clone C17.2 was used in two ways to help study the biology of NSC-based reconstitution of this large CNS lesion (Park et al 1997, 1999). In the first paradigm, NSCs are allowed to integrate during development into the representative cytoarchitecture of the normal brain prior to unilateral HI, creating virtually a chimeric brain of host and donor 'reporter stem cells'; the movements and responses of this 'reporter' NSC clone to HI (which can be reliably tracked by virtue of its *lacZ* reporter gene expression) would presumably mirror the behaviour of endogenous host progenitors and NSCs, with which it has intermixed, whose clonal relationships,

---

FIG. 2.   (I) Myelin basic protein (MBP) expression in mature transplanted and control brains. (A) Western analysis for MBP in whole brain lysates. The brains of three representative transplanted *shi* mutants (lanes 2–4) express MBP at levels close to that of an age-matched unaffected mouse (lane 1, positive control), and significantly greater than the amounts seen in untransplanted (lanes 7,8, negative control) or unengrafted (lanes 5,6, negative control) age-matched *shi* mutants. (Identical total protein amounts were loaded in each lane.) (B–D) Immunocytochemical analysis for MBP. (B) The brain of a mature unaffected mouse is immunoreactive to an antibody to MBP (revealed with a Texas red-conjugated secondary antibody). (C,D) Age-matched engrafted brains from *shi* mice similarly show immunoreactivity. Untransplanted *shi* brains lack MBP. Therefore, MBP immunoreactivity has also classically been a marker for normal donor-derived oligodendrocytes (C,D). II. NSC-derived 'replacement' oligodendrocytes appear functional as demonstrated by ultrastructural evidence of myelination of *shi* axons. In regions of MBP-expressing NSC engraftment, *shi* neuronal processes become enwrapped by thick, better compacted myelin. (A) At 2 weeks post-transplant, a representative donor-derived, labelled oligodendrocyte (LO) (recognized by extensive Xgal precipitate (p) in the nuclear membrane, cytoplasmic organelles, and processes) is extending processes (a representative one is delineated by arrowheads) to host neurites, and is beginning to ensheathe them with myelin (m). (B) If engrafted *shi* regions, such as that in A, are followed over time (e.g. to 4 weeks of age as pictured here), the myelin begins to appear healthier, thicker and better compacted (examples indicated by arrows) than that in age-matched untransplanted control mutants. (C) By 6 weeks post-transplant, it matures into even thicker wraps; ~40% of host axons are ensheathed by myelin. The higher power view of a representative axon shows its myelin to be dramatically thicker and better compacted than the *shi* myelin (an example of which is shown in D) (black arrowhead) from an unengrafted region of an otherwise successfully engrafted *shi* brain. In C, white arrowheads indicate representative regions of myelin that are magnified in the adjacent insets; major dense lines are evident. (Modified from Yandava et al 1999.)

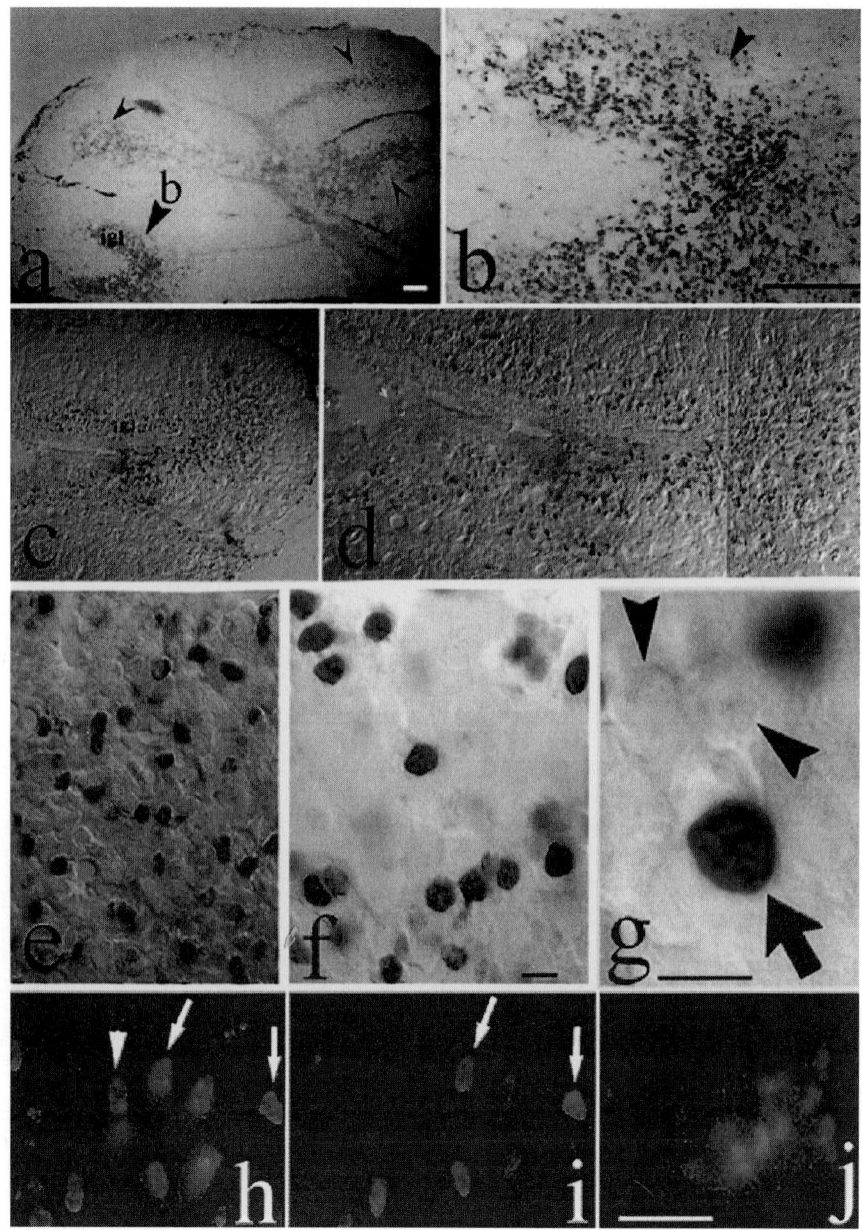

characteristics and degree of homogeneity are much less certain and which are otherwise 'invisible' to such monitoring. In the second paradigm, C17.2 'reporter cells' are implanted at various intervals following HI. In both paradigms, in response to HI, a subpopulation of 'reporter' and host cells transiently re-entered the cell cycle and migrated preferentially to the ischaemic site as if responding to newly elaborated cues. Donor-derived cells integrated extensively within the large infarcted areas that span the length of the brain; even cells implanted into the intact contralateral hemisphere migrated towards regions of injury. A subpopulation of both reporter- and host-derived cells (particularly in the penumbra) then once again became quiescent and differentiated into new neurons and oligodendrocytes, the neural cell types typically damaged following HI and least likely to regenerate spontaneously in postnatal CNS. In the injured postnatal neocortex there was a fivefold increase in donor-derived oligo-dendrocytes compared to the intact neocortex and, most significantly, NSCs now yielded neurons at a stage in mammalian development when no cortical neurons are normally born; 5% of engrafted NSCs on the injured side, compared to 0% on the intact contralateral side, now differentiated into neurons, an amount that translates into tens-of-thousands of replacement neurons. (While it is unknown how many neurons and how much circuitry are required to reconstruct a damaged system, older lesion data suggest that relatively little, even less than 10%, restoration may be sufficient.) As in the targeted apoptosis model, novel signals appear to be transiently elaborated following HI (three to seven days following HI appears

---

FIG. 3.   Neuronal replacement by a representative human neural stem cell (hNSC) clone following transplantation at birth into the cerebellum of the granule neuron-depleted *meander tail* mutant mouse model of developmental neurodegeneration. (a–g) BrdU-intercalated donor-derived cells identified three weeks following direct implantation into external germinal layer of the *meander tail* (*mea*) cerebellum by anti-BrdU immunochemistry. (a) hNSCs are present in the inner granular layer (igl, arrows) of all lobes of the cerebellum (granule neurons are diminished *throughout* the cerebellum with some prominence in the anterior lobe). (b) Higher magnification of the representative posterior cerebellar lobe indicated by arrow in panel a, demonstrating the large number of donor-derived cells present within the recipient igl. (c–g) Various magnifications of donor-derived cells within the igl of a *mea* anterior cerebellar lobe. (f,g) Nomarski optics are utilized to bring out the similarity in site and morphology of host BrdU-negative cerebellar granule neurons (arrow heads) and a BrdU-intercalated, donor-derived neuron (arrow). (h, i) Neuronal differentiation of a subpopulation of donor-derived, BrdU-intercalated cells is illustrated by co-labelling with BrdU in (h) and the mature neuronal marker NeuN in (i) (indicated with arrows). Adjacent, donor-derived cells are non-neuronal as indicated by their BrdU-positive, NeuN-negative phenotype (arrowhead). (j) Cells within the igl are demonstrated to be donor-derived human cells by FISH for a human-specific probe identifying the centromeres of all chromosomes, *all*. Other centromeres are present, but out of the plane of focus in this photomicrograph. Bars: a,b = 100 μm; c, d = 75 μm; e = 40 μm; f,g = 10 μm; h,i,j = 50 μm. (Modified from Flax et al 1998.)

optimal), to which NSCs (donor and host) respond by 'shifting' their normal fate to compensate for the loss of those particular cell types.

These phenomena are probably pervasive throughout the CNS. A similar tropism and trophism for NSCs by apoptotic neurodegenerative environments appears evident in the postnatal spinal cord (SC) during segmental motoneuron (MN) degeneration induced by neonatal sciatic axotomy, a classic experimental model of spinal neuron degeneration. Although MNs are normally born only in the fetus, in pilot studies where NSCs are implanted during active degeneration, a significant proportion of them will engraft, migrate toward and throughout the segments of MN-impoverished ventral horn and differentiate (20%) into cells that resemble the lost MNs (Himes et al 1995). Again, engrafted NSCs continue to express foreign reporter genes suggesting that, as in the asphyxiated brain, implantation of genetically engineered NSCs expressing trophic agents, cytokines or other factors might enhance neuronal differentiation, neurite outgrowth and proper connectivity.

NSCs and genetic engineering — combining cell replacement and gene therapy

Precisely what the stem cell-modifying signals are that are normally elaborated as a consequence of neurodegeneration is an area of active investigation. They no doubt are a complex mix of various mitogens, cytokines, trophic and tropic agents, adhesion and ECM molecules, chemotactic and angiogenic factors, etc., elaborated by reactive astrocytes, activated microglia, inflammatory cells, invading macrophages and damaged neurons and glia. Since the concentrations of these factors and their ratios change with time, they create a temporal 'window' of increased plasticity during the acute/subacute post-lesioning phase (first 2–3 weeks). Might this naturally established plastic phase in the injured brain, so favourable for successful engraftment of NSCs, be further prolonged and enhanced by augmenting some of those factors? Because in the paradigms described above, engrafted NSCs continue to express their marker transgene *lacZ* within the large infarcted areas, it appears feasible that such cells can be genetically manipulated prior to transplantation to express such agents, *in vivo* (much like a pump infusing growth factors).

Neurotrophin 3 (NT-3) is known to play a role in promoting neuronal differentiation (although its presence after HI remains unclear). An NSC clone secreting large amounts of NT-3 might not only have an impact on host cells, but, intriguingly, might itself respond to NT-3 in an autocrine/paracrine fashion. This, indeed, seems to be feasible. In preliminary studies, when a subclone of C17.2 NSCs, retrovirally transduced *ex vivo* to overexpress NT-3, are implanted into brains suffering from HI, the percentage of donor-derived neurons seems to be dramatically increased to 20% in the infarction cavity and to 80% in the penumbra (compared to the 5% when non-engineered NSCs are used) (Park et al 1997). As another example, we can again adduce the pilot experiments on parkinsonian mice we described above. A group of these mice were grafted with C17.2 cells overexpressing the neural cell adhesion molecule L1 (known to promote cell migration and neurite outgrowth; Burden-Gulley et al 1997). This resulted in an increased migration of donor-derived dopaminergic nerve cells and a quicker bilateral reorganization of the substantia nigra. Such observations suggest the use of NSCs for simultaneous, combined gene therapy and cell replacement in the same transplant using the same clone in the same recipient—an appealing NSC property with implications for therapies in other degenerative conditions involving other neural cell types.

The feasibility of a stem cell-mediated delivery system for therapeutic molecules was first affirmed by correcting the widespread neuropathology of a murine model of the genetic neurodegenerative lysosomal storage disease mucopolysaccharidosis type VII (MPS VII). Caused by a frameshift deletion of the β-glucuronidase gene (GUSB), this heritable condition causes progressive mental retardation in humans and inexorable neurodegeneration in mice (Snyder et al 1995). NSCs were genetically modified with a retrovirus encoding human GUSB to augment the mouse GUSB constitutively secreted by these cells. Transplantation of these GUSB-overexpressing cells into the cerebroventricular system of newborn MPS VII mice resulted in profuse incorporation of donor-derived cells throughout the mutant neuraxis. This brain-wide distribution of engrafted GUSB-secreting NSCs corresponded to the distribution of corrective levels of GUSB throughout the mutant brains devoid of that enzyme. The diffuse GUSB expression in turn resulted in widespread permanent correction of lysosomal storage in mutant neurons and glia, throughout mutant brains. While MPS VII may be regarded as 'uncommon', the broad category of diseases which it models (neurogenetic degenerative conditions) afflicts as many as 1 in 1500 persons. This approach is therefore being extended to other untreatable neurodegenerative diseases characterized by an absence of discrete gene products and/or the accumulation of toxic metabolites. For example, retrovirally-transduced NSCs, implanted into fetal and neonatal mice using the intracerebroventricular technique, have successfully mediated widespread expression throughout the brain of the α-subunit of β-hexosaminidase, a mutation of which leads to accumulation of GM2 ganglioside (Tay–Sachs disease, Lacorazza et al 1996).

With the stage having been set by experiments such as these, such *ex vivo* gene therapy strategies have been successfully employed in other experimental models of neurologic disease. These have included delivering tyrosine hydroxylase (TH) to the striatum of parkinsonian animals; nerve growth factor (NGF) to cholinergic systems of the septum and nucleus basalis magnocellularis to induce sprouting and to reverse cognitive deficits in models of Alzheimer's disease and ageing; NGF and brain-derived growth factor (BDNF) for neuroprotection against excitotoxic lesions in striatum mimicking Huntington's disease (Martínez-Serrano & Björklund 1996, Martínez-Serrano et al 1995a,b, 1996). In approaching metabolic diseases such as those above, there is an interesting point to be made that might be applicable to *ex vivo* gene therapy in general: NSCs, because they are normal CNS cells, often constitutively express baseline amounts of a particular enzyme or neuroactive factor. The extent to which this amount needs to be augmented by genetic engineering may vary from protein to protein and needs to be studied individually. Reassuringly, in most inherited metabolic diseases and in many neurologic diseases in general, the amount of enzyme required to restore normal metabolism and forestall CNS disease may be quite small. Also reassuringly, we affirmed that NSC expression of therapeutic levels of foreign genes (even if reduced) can persist lifelong and that transducing a given NSC multiple times with a retroviral vector, thus inserting multiple copies of a therapeutic transgene within the same cell, is a simple and immediately available method for blunting decrements in transgene expression.

Experiments like those described above have established a paradigm for the stem cell-mediated brain-wide distribution of other diffusible (e.g. synthetic enzyme, neurotrophin, viral vector) and non-diffusible (e.g. myelin, extracellular matrix) therapeutic or developmental factors, as well as the distribution of 'replacement' neural cells. In developing brains, the cells actually contribute to organogenesis of multiple CNS structures (Table 1). Because NSCs can populate widely disseminated developing or degenerating CNS regions with cells of multiple lineages, their use as graft material in the brain can be considered analogous to haematopoietic stem cell-mediated reconstitution and gene transfer in the body. Yet, unlike in bone marrow transplantation, this method of delivery does not preclude being able to transport gene products into the cytoarchitecture of circumscribed regions in order to effect selective manipulations and avoid extensive genetic alteration should the clinical context demand it. For some diseases, widespread gene product dissemination is not desired. In fact, solely by altering their mode of administration or implantation, NSCs can be selectively integrated into more focal and discrete regions in proximity to those neurons that require a given neuroactive factor without affecting cells at more remote locations for which the molecule might be problematic.

A recent unexpected use of the NSC takes advantage of its ability to migrate extensively and to 'home in' selectively on CNS pathology while continuing to express bioactive foreign genes. One of the impediments to the treatment of primary human brain tumours (e.g. gliomas) has been the degree to which they expand, infiltrate surrounding tissue and migrate widely into normal brain, usually rendering them 'elusive' to effective resection, irradiation, chemotherapy or gene therapy. In preliminary studies, we have observed that migratory NSCs, when implanted into experimental intracranial gliomas *in vivo* in adult rodents, distribute themselves quickly and extensively throughout the tumour bed and migrate uniquely in juxtaposition to widely expanding and aggressively advancing tumour cells while continuing to stably express a foreign gene. The NSCs, in effect, 'surround' the invading tumour border while 'chasing down' infiltrating tumour cells. Furthermore, when implanted intracranially at *distant* sites from the tumour bed in adult rodent brain (e.g. into normal tissue, into the contralateral hemisphere, or into the cerebral ventricles), the donor cells migrate through normal tissue targeting the tumour cells (including human glioblastomas). NSCs can deliver a bioactive therapeutically-relevant molecule — the oncolysis-promoting enzyme cytosine deaminase — such that *in vitro* and *in vivo*, upon activation, a dramatic, quantifiable reduction in surrounding tumour cell burden results. These data suggest the adjunctive use of inherently migratory NSCs as a delivery vehicle for more effectively targeting a wide variety of therapeutic genes and vectors to refractory, migratory, invasive brain tumour cells. More broadly, they suggest that NSC migration can be extensive, even in the adult brain and along non-stereotypical routes, if pathology (as modelled here by tumour) is present.

Getting closer to human therapy — establishment of human NSC clones

The ability of NSCs to migrate and integrate throughout the brain as well as to disseminate a foreign gene product is of great significance for the development of new therapies for neurodegenerative diseases in humans. Hereditary diseases like Tay–Sachs disease result in lesions throughout the CNS. Diseases of adult onset, too, e.g. Alzheimer's disease, can be diffuse in their pathology. Even acquired diseases such as spinal cord injury (SCI) are more extensive in their involvement than is typically assumed. Such trauma-related abnormalities may fully benefit from the multifaceted approach NSCs may enable: e.g. cell replacement to provide new neural connections as well as remyelination; gene therapy to support the survival of damaged neurons, to neutralize hostile milieu, to counter-act a growth-inhibitory environment and promote neurite regrowth, and the re-formation of stable and functional contacts. In the case of chronic SCI, an improved knowledge of the molecular barriers to SC remodelling is needed to optimize the plastic behaviour of NSCs in this otherwise foreboding terrain.

A better understanding of fundamental NSC biology may soon allow human NSCs to be transplanted with therapeutic efficacy and without concern for recipient safety. Progress in this regard is already being made. Several NSC clones have been established from the human fetal telencephalon (hNSCs) which seem to emulate many of the appealing properties of their rodent counterparts

(Flax et al 1998): they differentiate, *in vitro* and *in vivo*, into neurons, astrocytes and oligodendrocytes; they follow appropriate developmental programmes and migrational pathways similar to endogenous precursors following engraftment into developing mouse brain; they express foreign genes *in vivo* in a widely disseminated manner; and they can replace missing neural cell types when grafted into various mutant mice (Fig. 3).

Although very promising for ultimate human CNS therapy, these findings need first to be reproduced in animals that are closer to humans. As the analyses from our first studies indicate, hNSCs seem to respond to patterning signals from the developing monkey brain and intermingle with the endogenous cell populations following established migration streams (Ourednik et al 1999). If hNSCs behave in lesioned primate brains with respect to engraftment and foreign gene expression as they seem to do in mice, we soon might have a powerful and versatile therapeutic tool in hand for use in human trials to help address genuine clinical neurodegenerative diseases — the ultimate goal of experiments that started almost a decade ago.

Acknowledgements

Various aspects of the work reported in this review were supported by: Canavan Research Fund, Project ALS, A-T Children's Project, International Organization for Glutaric Aciduria (IOGA), March of Dimes, Paralyzed Veterans of America, American Paralysis Association and NINDS.

References

Auguste KI, Nakajima K, Miyata T, Ogawa M, Mikoshiba K, Snyder EY 1996 Neural progenitor transplantation into newborn reeler cerebellum may rescue certain aspects of mutant cytoarchitecture. Soc Neurosci Abstr 22:484

Breakfield X, Jacobs A, Wang S 1999 Genetic engineering for CNS regeneration. In: Tuszynski MH, Kordower JH (eds) CNS regeneration: basic science and clinical advances. Academic Press, San Diego, p 251–291

Burden-Gulley SM, Pendergast M, Lemmon V 1997 The role of cell adhesion molecule L1 in axonal extension, growth cone motility, and signal transduction. Cell Tissue Res 290:415–422

Dunnett SB, Björklund A (eds) 1994 Functional neural transplantation. Raven Press, New York

Fisher LJ, Gage FH 1993 Grafting in the mammalian central nervous system. Physiol Rev 73:583–616

Fisher LJ, Gage FH 1994 Intracerebral transplantation: basic and clinical applications to the neostriatum. FASEB J 8:489–496

Flax JD, Aurora S, Yang C et al 1998 Engraftable human neural stem cells respond to developmental cues, replace neurons, and express foreign genes. Nat Biotechnol 16:1033–1039

Gage FH, Ray J, Fisher LJ 1995 Isolation, characterization and use of stem cells from the CNS. Annu Rev Neurosci 18:159–169

Himes BT, Slowska-Baird J, Boyne L, Snyder EY, Tessler A, Fischer I 1995 Grafting of genetically modified cells that produce neurotrophins in order to rescue axotomized neurons in rat spinal cord. Soc Neurosci Abstr 21:537

Kordower JH, Tuszynski MH 1999 Fetal neural grafting for CNS regeneration. In: Tuszynski MH, Kordower JH (eds) CNS regeneration: basic science and clinical advances. Academic Press, San Diego, p 159–182

Kordower JH, Freeman TB, Snow BJ et al 1995 Neuropathological evidence of graft survival and striatal reinnervation after the transplantation of fetal mesencephalic tissue in a patient with Parkinson's disease. N Engl J Med 332:1118–1124

Lacorazza HD, Flax JD, Snyder EY, Jendoubi M 1996 Expression of human β-hexosaminidase α-subunit gene (the gene defect of Tay–Sachs disease) in mouse brains upon engraftment of transduced progenitor cells. Nat Med 2:424–429

Lundberg C, Martínez-Serrano A, Cattaneo E, McKay RD, Björklund A 1997 Survival, integration, and differentiation of neural stem cell lines after transplantation to the adult rat striatum. Exp Neurol 145:342–360

Marciano FF, Wiegand SJ, Sladek JR Jr, Gash DM 1989 Fetal hypothalamic transplants promote survival and functional regeneration of axotomized adult supraoptic magnocellular neurons. Brain Res 483:135–142

Martínez-Serrano A, Björklund A 1996 Protection of the neostriatum against excitotoxic damage by neurotrophin-producing, genetically modified neural stem cells. J Neurosci 16:4604–4616

Martínez-Serrano A, Snyder EY 1999 Neural stem cell lines for CNS repair. In: Tuszynski MH, Kordower JH (eds) CNS regeneration: basic science and clinical advances. Academic Press, San Diego, p 203–250

Martínez-Serrano A, Lundberg C, Horellou P et al 1995a CNS-derived neural progenitor cells for gene transfer of nerve growth factor to the adult rat brain: complete rescue of axotomized cholinergic neurons after transplantation into the septum. J Neurosci 15:5668–5680

Martínez-Serrano A, Fischer W, Björklund A 1995b Reversal of age-dependent cognitive impairments and cholinergic neuron atrophy by NGF-secreting neural progenitors grafted to the basal forebrain. Neuron 15:473–484

Martínez-Serrano A, Fischer W, Söderström S, Ebendal T, Björklund A 1996 Long-term functional recovery from age-induced spatial memory impairments by nerve growth factor gene transfer to the rat basal forebrain. Proc Natl Acad Sci USA 93:6355–6360

Ourednik W, Ourednik J 1994 Newly formed host cells in a grafted juvenile neocortex express neurone-specific marker proteins. Neuroreport 5:1073–1076

Ourednik J, Ourednik W, Van der Loos H 1993 Do foetal neural grafts induce repair by the injured juvenile neocortex? Neuroreport 5:133–136

Ourednik J, Ourednik W, Mitchell DE 1998 Remodeling of lesioned kitten visual cortex after xenotransplantation of fetal mouse neopallium. J Comp Neurol 395:91–111

Ourednik V, Ourednik J, Flax JD et al 1999 Transplantation of human neural stem cells (NSCs): insights from non-human primate experiments. Soc Neurosci Abstr 25:1310

Park KI, Jensen FE, Stieg PE, Fischer I, Snyder EY 1997 Transplantation of neural stem-like cells engineered to produce NT-3 may enhance neuronal replacement in hypoxia–ischemia CNS injury. Soc Neurosci Abstr 23:346

Park KI, Liu S, Flax JD, Nissim S, Stieg PE, Snyder EY 1999 Transplantation of neural progenitor and stem-like cells: developmental insights may suggest new therapies of spinal cord and other CNS dysfunction. J Neurotrauma 16:657–687

Renfranz PJ, Cunningham MG, McKay RD 1991 Region-specific differentiation of the hippocampal stem cell line HiB5 upon implantation into the developing mammalian brain. Cell 66:713–729

Reynolds BA, Weiss S 1992 Generation of neurons and astrocytes from isolated cells of the adult mammalian central nervous system. Science 27:1707–1710

Rosario CM, Yandava BD, Kosaras B, Zurakowski D, Sidman RL, Snyder EY 1997 Differentiation of engrafted multipotent neural progenitors towards replacement of missing granule neurons in meander tail cerebellum may help determine the locus of mutant gene action. Development 124:4213–4224

Snyder EY, Senut MC 1997 The use of nonneuronal cells for gene delivery. Neurobiol Dis 4:69–102

Snyder EY, Deitcher DL, Walsh C, Arnold-Aldea S, Hartwieg EA, Cepko CL 1992 Multipotent neural cell lines can engraft and participate in development of mouse cerebellum. Cell 68:33–51

Snyder EY, Taylor RM, Wolfe JH 1995 Neural progenitor cell engraftment corrects lysosomal storage throughout the MPS VII mouse brain. Nature 374:367–370

Snyder EY, Yoon C, Flax JD, Macklis JD 1997 Multipotent neural precursors can differentiate toward replacement of neurons undergoing targeted apoptotic degeneration in adult mouse neocortex. Proc Natl Acad Sci USA 94:11663–11668

Yandava BD, Billinghurst LL, Snyder EY 1999 'Global' cell replacement is feasible via neural stem cell transplantation: evidence from the dysmyelinated shiverer mouse brain. Proc Natl Acad Sci USA 96:7029–7034

DISCUSSION

Sinden: Were all the HI experiments done in adult rats?

Synder: The normal paradigm for doing this is to take a week-old mouse, ligate the common carotid artery, and then expose the animal for three hours to low oxygen tension, keeping the body temperature normal. This is a classic model for imposing a permanent injury that emulates a common cause of extensive, devastating cerebral palsy. (From an experimental point of view, by the way, this model comes as close as a neurobiologist will be able to come to emulating the haematopoietic stem cell biologist's test of ablating the bone marrow and looking for reconstitution.) Then we would selectively look at non-neurogenic areas; areas that, on the basis of clinical and animal data, never appear to 'repair' themselves.

Rosser: Have you put these cells into any adult models of injury?

Snyder: Yes. We are presently putting these cells in adult stroke and in adult SCI. Actually, one of the earliest examples of the response of NSCs to degeneration was observed in the adult in a series of experiments done with Jeff Macklis a number of years ago (Snyder et al 1997). Jeff has an intriguing model where he can selectively induce a subclass of pyramidal neurons in the adult neocortex to degenerate by apoptotic mechanisms. Cytolytic nanospheres are injected into one hemisphere. The subclass of pyramidal neurons in cortical layers 2 and 5 that send axons across the corpus callosum take up these nanospheres at their target regions and retrogradely transport them back to their cell bodies. If those cells are exposed to a laser beam of a prescribed wavelength, they will die an apoptotic death, leaving the rest of the cortex intact. If we implant an NSC clone into this 'depyramidized' area, a significant proportion will now become pyramidal neurons, although cortical neurogenesis has normally ceased. A subpopulation of these stem cell-derived pyramidal neurons will send their axons back across the corpus callosum to the appropriate target. Outside of that circumscribed area of neuronal loss, NSCs will *not* yield neurons at all; they will produce the 'normal' post-fetal developmental profile of cells; glial or undifferentiated cells. In other words, the exogenous NSCs seem to mirror faithfully the normal developmental processes prevalent at a given time in a given region; where neurogenesis is ongoing, NSC-derived neurons will be found; where neurogenesis has ceased and gliogenesis predominates, NSC-derived glia will be found. However, we find that if the same terrain is injured, a different scenario unfolds. In the mouse there seems to be a 'window' of one week following injury during which there seems to be a 'resetting' of the 'clock' transiently back to an embryonic environment; then the window closes again.

Gray: In stating that this was apoptotic cell death, is that simply the model you use, or are you implying that signals from apoptotic cell death are critical, and that from necrosis you would get a different set of signals?

Snyder: That is a great question. When Jeff and I first did that experiment, because the results were somewhat unexpected, we thought that, perhaps, it was something particular to apoptosis. It was because of those data that I subsequently approached the spinal cord to investigate the apoptotic degeneration of another selected neural cell type outside its normal period of neurogenesis — the α MN. As we started employing other injury models such as infarcts, I was a little less certain about the singular role of apoptosis. Although we are learning that 'paraptosis' or 'apoptosis' play a prominent role in many degenerative processes, including those that have classically been thought of as predominantly 'necrotic', such as an infarct, and although I can't rule out that it is those apoptotic components that are causing the effects we see, I am beginning to suspect that the altered responses of NSCs to degeneration and injury reflect a broader phenomenon.

Reier: In the MN replacement study, am I right in thinking that you did neurectomies and grafting of the cells at the same time, in the neonate?

Snyder: It is important to recognize that MNs are not normally born beyond fetal life. The model entails first performing a sciatic nerve transection in the neonatal period, but then allowing the animals to mature by which time the MNs degenerate irreversibly. We started implanting NSCs at 4 weeks. Interestingly, the closer the implantation was performed to the actual active degeneration of the MNs, while they were undergoing apoptosis, the more robust the differentiation 'shift' by NSCs to yield MNs was.

A ebischer: Sciatic nerve axotomy is a rather acute model. There are many chronic models for MN degeneration: have you looked at these?

Snyder: We are starting to do this now. Initially, we wanted to examine a model that had a well-characterized, controllable onset and caused a robust, synchronized neuronal death, ideally by an apoptotic mechanisms in a well-defined region. This is why we chose sciatic nerve axotomy. We are now starting to approach models that perhaps emulate amyotrophic lateral sclerosis (ALS) better, but where the mechanism may be less clear. In early studies in the SOD transgenic mouse, we have observed preliminary suggestions of a prolonged lifespan and diminished symptoms. These preliminary results, of course, require more detailed analysis.

Lindvall: Is there any functional recovery provided by these cells you inject into the penumbra zone or into the infarcted area?

Snyder: We are starting to look at this now. At this initial stage it is probably better to think of these experiments as cell biology that happened to be performed *in vivo*. Second, anyone who has worked with mice knows that even that kind of dramatic experimental defect in the cortex does not give a dramatic functional phenotype. We have not yet done more subtle cognitive testing.

Lindvall: The cortical deficit can be assessed by neurological tests.

Snyder: I agree, and we are starting to do some of those tests. We, however, want to make sure that we do tests that don't just reflect global behaviour. We want to do functional tests that key in specifically to the cells that we were trying to replace, to see whether our cells are being integrated into the circuitry, as opposed just to turning up the gain on parallel systems, or just providing a cellular source of released trophic factors. We are trying to be selective in the tests we employ.

Perry: The glioma seems to be full of interesting puzzles. The phenomenology is clear, but how do you interpret it from the cell biology? Why would a progenitor cell hitch a ride on tumour cells that go wandering off across the brain? Why are the cells migrating towards a tumour?

Snyder: The simple answer is that I don't know. I can come up with the same kind of hypotheses that any of us would entertain. A number of investigators think that tumours are progenitor cells that have gone awry, yet retain some of the same biological properties. One of these is robust migratory behaviour. It may be that the tumour cells infiltrate normal tissue by the same mechanisms that progenitor cells migrate through normal tissue. It may not be that one is 'hitching a ride' on the other, even though it looks like that; they could instead both be responding to similar cues. A second possibility is that the tumour is secreting factors that draw cells to it. This is suggested by some of our *in vitro* work in which tumour cells are permitted to confront stem cells. A third option is that the tumour is causing tissue damage that, in turn, produces signals that attract the progenitors. The migration of these donor NSCs seems to be highly directed. In an adult cortex without a tumour, the cells will engraft well but remain relatively restricted in their distribution and don't have this robust migration. However, the introduction of pathology appears to prompt directed migration to the affected area.

Gray: Does this offer a means of targeting something to a tumour in a manner that might then destroy the tumour cells?

Snyder: That is our hypothesis. The hope is that this could be an adjunctive therapy for gene therapy or other types of interventions against brain tumours.

Blakemore: You have to be very careful to determine whether you are looking at migration or survival. It may just be that you have produced a survival trackway, and this is the only place the cells can go. If this was the case, you could mistake this for directed migration.

Snyder: That is a good point. The total number of cells doesn't appear to change, so we do not believe we are losing cells. It doesn't say that there is not migration; it raises the question of what is causing the migration.

Gray: It is not even about what the causes are — I think Bill is saying that what appears to be a causal process could just be a selective process.

Snyder: We do not appear to be losing cells, such that the appearance of a given population of cells is merely a selection for survival. The distribution of the same number of cells seems to be altered. The real question, as mentioned before, is identifying the forces driving or directing this migration. For example, in the model of spinal MN degeneration in which stem cells implanted into dorsal horn migrate ventrally, one could remark that this is a long way for a diffusible factor to attract cells. An alternative intriguing explanation might hold that the 'inclination' of NSCs to migrate is not altered but rather as the SC starts developing, barriers to migration are progressively established as a normal part of regional specification. With an injury, especially with the selective loss of a particular cell type, there may be a loss of these barriers, a disinhibition, such that exogenous NSCs that ordinarily would have been excluded from migration to that ventral horn region now have the opportunity to enter it and encounter cues that they had been excluded from seeing that led to α MN differentiation.

Blakemore: This is my point: we must not mistake survival for migration.

Finsen: Do any of your cells differentiate into microglial cells?

Snyder: Microglial cells are derived from the bone marrow. We have no evidence that NSCs, when implanted into the brain *in vivo*, can give rise to haematopoietic lineages.

Price: Yesterday we discussed the transient developmental mechanisms, which are involved in generating cells during embryogenesis, but which are absent later on during the process of regeneration. Your MN model is a beautiful system with which you could start to address some of those issues, particularly with regard to the hypothesis you just posed that there might be some sort of barrier. What I would have thought was more likely, rather than some barrier being removed (for which there is currently no evidence), would be thinking about what is taking place of the floorplate during development. The floorplate is crucial in determining the fate during development of exactly the population of cells that you have killed and then replaced. One could hypothesize that somehow the mechanism the floorplate uses is being reactivated in the absence of the floorplate. Isn't an obvious experiment to ask whether sonic hedgehog is being turned on again during repair? If so, which cells are taking on the role of producing that factor? You might find that you are able to manipulate expression.

Snyder: That is an excellent speculation and we are looking at that. The netrins or the semaphorins may be appropriate candidates for the 'attractants' in this model, but the recapitualted differentiation of MNs is very 'floorplate-esque', and hence suggestive of a role for sonic hedgehog or a related factor.

Rosser: Have you seen any differences between the oncogenically transformed and non-transformed stem cells.

Snyder: Those cells are not transformed, and the term 'oncogenesis' would be totally misused in such a context. For me, as for oncobiologists, 'transformation' has a specific rigorous definition, which is synonymous with the loss of growth control mechanisms (by meeting such established criteria as loss of contact inhibition, ability to grow in soft agar, ability to give rise to tumours in the nude mouse, the inability to respond to normal signals to withdraw from the cell cycle). In stem cell clones in which propagation is assisted by a cell cycle regulatory gene, as soon as the cells enter the brain, that gene product constitutively and spontaneously disappears. To help answer your question, we now have various clones of human NSCs that are either propagated solely with exogenous mitogens (e.g. fibroblast growth factor [FGF] 2) or are propagated by mitogens augmented by the non-transforming propagating gene v-*myc*. V-*myc* operates downstream of and within the same signal transduction pathway as FGF2. It appears to be regulated in the same manner as endogenous cellular *myc* by normal developmental mechanisms including being down-regulated by the cell as it becomes quiescent during mitotic arrest and/or differentiation. Though the cells contain v-*myc*, they are nevertheless dependent on FGF2 for their propagation; in the absence of FGF2, the cells exit the cell cycle and differentiate. We suspect that the function of *myc* may be to prevent the cells from senescing or losing their multipotent phenotype after multiple passages. We are trying to compare these variously propagated clones 'head to head' in all of these paradigms. In every aspect that we have examined so far, the human NSCs with v-*myc* and those without seem to behave identically, even after multiple passages. It frankly remains a matter of speculation in the stem cell field the best way to identify, expand and employ human NSCs. In the absence of reliable, unambiguous, universally agreed upon and widely verified cell surface or other markers, the field still relies upon operational definitions. As indicated in my paper, in collaboration with Richard Mulligan and Lou Kunkel at my institution, we are devising prospective FACS-based methods for isolating NSCs from neural tissue (both rodent and human) that appear to be based on cell cycle properties common to stem cells from all organ systems. (Indeed the established and proven murine and human NSC clones described in the experiments I have referred to in my presentation segregate to and virtually engorge the 'bin' that selects stem cell populations, and cells in this bin have been shown to be NSCs by criteria employed by even other investigators, e.g. 'sphere formation', etc.)

The loss of v-*myc* expression spontaneously and constitutively from stably engrafted NSCs following transplantation is consistent with the invariant absence of brain tumours derived from implanted v-*myc*-propagated NSCs, even after several years *in vivo* in mice. With human NSCs, as with mouse NSCs, expanded in this manner, neoplasms are never seen. We have begun to entertain the hypothesis that v-*myc* may help to maintain cells in the cell cycle — hence holding their differentiation in abeyance — just long enough for them to exit the cell cycle within the transplanted brain as opposed to the culture dish and hence engraft and integrate optimally having been influenced maximally by their environment. (Cells that exit the cell cycle and pre-differentiate in the dish rather than in the recipient brain tend to engraft quite poorly.) We are also beginning to hypothesize, based on our observations, that v-*myc* may both preclude senescence of NSCs even after multiple passages as well as insuring that the cells maintain their NSC character — i.e. preventing phenotypic 'drift' — from passage-to-passage over prolonged periods of time. If you put v-*myc*-containing mouse cells or human cells into serum-free medium without a defined mitogen, they will come out of the cell cycle and differentiate, so v-*myc* alone is not sufficient to maintain cells in the cell cycle.

Price: The issue surely would be whether the cells are more susceptible to becoming transformed. This is slightly different, and would be the crucial issue if one is thinking in terms of therapy. Transformation is thought to be a multistep process, and you have pushed your cells at least one step closer to transformation. Therefore the probability that a subpopulation of the cells can emerge that were transformed is raised.

Snyder: I actually don't believe that such cells have been pushed a step closer to 'transformation'. As you have indicated, we now appreciate that the development of a neoplasm is a much more complex, multifactorial process than was originally believed in the 1980s. It entails a number of aberrations, beyond just the presence of one or even multiple genes. There are fundamental cellular processes that must go awry. (Indeed, even the term 'oncogene' has become passé — at least among oncobiologists; indeed most of the 'oncogenes' of the 1980s — *bcl-2*, *trk*, *wnt*, *erbB4*, *myc* — have lost that designation as a better understanding of their fundamental cellular role has unfolded.) My bias is that, if the correct genes are used to permit maintenance in the cell cycle while *in vitro* but not *in vivo* — genes that are controlled constitutively and in self-regulated manner by the normal cellular processes that routinely chaperone cell cycle regulatory processes — then there is no more risk (and perhaps less risk) than taking a cell and 'bathing' it chronically in a mitogen. Probably our notions of what it takes to really 'transform' a cell are somewhat naïve. Over 14 years, both in our lab and in the labs of multiple collaborators throughout the world, there have been thousands and thousands of mice transplanted with genetically propagated cells without a single neoplasm, actually a better track record than some growth factor-perpetuated cells after prolonged passages.

It probably bears discussing that, although the term 'transformation' is casually and usually incorrectly tossed about by non-oncobiologists in the NSC field, even manipulated NSC clones never meet the established, rigorous criteria that properly define that term *in vitro* or *in vivo;* such clones respond to and respect all appropriate growth control signals for cell cycle withdrawal, differentiation and interaction with host cells. In culture, they become contact-inhibited, cannot grow in soft agar, contain normal arrestable actin stress fibres and have a normal cell cycle length. When tested in nude mice, neoplasms never develop. In normal grafting studies, brain tumours are never seen; donor-derived cells insinuate themselves seamlessly and non-disruptively into the host cytoarchitecture. They never form inappropriate cell types. Furthermore, the total number of cells (host-plus-donor) observed in a given engrafted region always equals that observed in an analogous region of an untransplanted animal (i.e. host cells alone), suggesting that donor NSCs do not abnormally augment or deform their region of integration, but rather compete equally for space with host progenitors. These observations are in agreement with the finding that, when recipient animals are 'pulsed' with BrdU, the proportion of donor cells that are still mitotic falls to zero by 48–72 h post-engraftment in non-lesioned, non-neurogenic regions, a phenomenon that mirrors their behaviour in culture following contact inhibition. Accordingly, transplanted mice never exhibit neurological dysfunction and CNS regions within which donor cells engraft develop normally. In fact, recent studies have shown that they function in concert with host cells in a physiologically appropriate manner. Indeed, some of the clones of murine NSCs we have used (which happen to be genetically propagated) have been most useful in helping to delineate fundamental stem cell properties (in addition to being among the safest and most efficacious to date).

It actually still remains uncertain the best way to expand and propagate stem cells. There appears to be little doubt that expansion by some technique of the relatively small NSC population that exists in the brain will be required at some stage in the process in order to make therapeutic interventions practical. Our data, especially with human NSCs, that clones propagated by one technique or the other seem to behave virtually identically, suggests that the door has been thrown open for investigators and/or clinicians to pick the technique that best serves their clinical or research demands. Importantly, these findings have helped unify various research directions in this field: insights from studies of NSCs perpetuated by one technique can now be legitimately joined to those derived from studies employing others, providing a more complete picture of NSC biology and its applications. (In fact, for some needs, because the key to exuberant engraftment is insuring that NSCs exit the cell cycle at precisely the right time — within the parenchyma, not outside it — self-regulated genetic means may actually prove to be the easier, safer, more cost-effective and reliable of strategies. Furthermore Svendsen has begun to marshal evidence that mitogen-mediated expansion alone may confront a Hayflick-like phenomenon of inherent senescence that may require blunting by genetic means.)

Whether re-deriving stable, well-characterized clones for each clinical situation is prudent or effective by whatever means remains to be empirically determined. While the field has been contemplating of late the value and feasibility of isolating adult NSCs from a given prospective recipient for subsequent autologous grafting, it should be noted that, for neurodegenerative diseases of possible genetic aetiology or predisposition — among them, Parkinson's disease — one clearly would *not* employ such a strategy. Indeed, the most effective and safest NSC clones (human or otherwise) — and the tacit goal within the stem cell community — is to derive human NSCs that can serve as 'off-the-shelf' reagents and behave like established, stable, physiologically normal, well-characterized, homogeneous, readily accessible, abundant and *universally tolerated* cell lines. Regardless of how these debates settle out over the next few years of empirical study, the human NSC clones described by us here — if not the cells that actually go to clinical trials — can clearly serve as prototypes and the experiments in which they are used as proofs-of-principle for reporting on the efficacy of NSCs in these neurodegenerative environments. Based on our results to date using such murine and human NSCs in various disease models, they certainly can help establish a therapeutic standard that should be at least met by any method proffered for generating NSCs for clinical use. To achieve less may mean failing to truly realize or unlock the capabilities of the NSC.

Reference

Snyder EY, Yoon C, Flax JD, Macklis JD 1997 Multipotent neural precursors can differentiate toward replacement of neurons undergoing targeted apoptotic degeneration in adult mouse neocortex. Proc Natl Acad Sci USA 94:11663–11668

Functional repair with neural stem cells

John D. Sinden, Paul Stroemer, Gregory Grigoryan, Sara Patel, Sarah J. French and Helen Hodges

ReNeuron Limited, Europoint Centre, 5–11 Lavington Street, London SE1 0NZ, UK

Abstract. Approval to commence phase I/II clinical trials with neural stem cells requires proof of concept in well-accepted animal models of human neurological disease or injury. We initially showed that the conditionally immortal MHP36 line of hippocampal origin (derived from the H-2K^b-tsA58 transgenic mouse) was effective in repopulating CA1 neurons in models of global ischaemia and repairing cognitive function, and have now shown that this line is multifunctional. MHP36 cells are effective in restoring spatial memory deficits in rats after excitotoxic lesions of the cholinergic projections to cortex and hippocampus and in rats showing cognitive impairments due to normal ageing. Moreover, grafts of MHP36 cells are effective in reversing sensory and motor deficits and reducing lesion volume as a consequence of occlusion of the middle cerebral artery, the major cause of stroke. In contrast, MHP36 cell grafts were unable to repair motor asymmetries in rats with unilateral 6-hydroxydopamine lesions of the nigrostriatal dopamine system, the prototype rodent model of Parkinson's disease. These data show that conditionally immortal neuroepithelial stem cells are multifunctional, being able to repair diverse types of brain damage. However, there are limitations to this multifunctionality, suggesting that lines from different regions of the developing brain will be required to treat different brain diseases. ReNeuron is currently developing human neuroepithelial stem cell lines from different brain regions and with similar reparative properties to our murine lines.

2000 Neural transplantation in neurodegenerative disease. Wiley, Chichester (Novartis Foundation Symposium 231) p 270–288

Neural transplantation has spawned a new generation of therapeutics

Chronic diseases of the CNS are now among the commonest causes of ill health in the industrialized world. Disorders such as Alzheimer's disease (AD) and Parkinson's disease (PD) affect an increasing proportion of the rapidly expanding older segment of the population. In the UK alone, Department of Health statistics indicate there are 750 000 cases of AD, 350 000 cases of epilepsy, 200 000 cases of PD and 50 000 cases of multiple sclerosis. In addition, each year 140 000 people suffer the consequences of a stroke. Brain-related disorders account for the majority of the Western world's long-term care costs.

In all of the chronic neurological diseases, there are either no successful treatments, or only partially effective palliative treatments with a range of unpleasant side-effects. Novel therapeutic approaches are therefore badly needed and much of the stimulus for these has come from neural transplantation research. The degenerative and traumatic neural diseases cited above involve loss of neural cells as a cause or consequence of the disease, so cellular replacement therapies offer a rational and attractive therapeutic solution. Additionally, a number of valid strategies employing delivery systems including cellular transplantation for the purposes of targeting neurotransmitters or growth factors to the sites of neural dysfunction are discussed elsewhere in this symposium and therefore will not be considered here.

Neural transplantation has already made a relatively successful transition from the research laboratory to human neurosurgery for the treatment of PD. This symposium will address the increasingly positive evidence that implantation of human fetal ventral mesecenphalic dopaminergic cells into basal ganglia can retard or reverse the motor deficits of this disease, along with increasing dopaminergic surrogate marker activity in the graft region. These fetal transplant trials have been extensively reported in detailed case studies in Sweden (Lindvall et al 1994, Freeman et al 1995) and have recently received positive attention following the first public announcements of early results in a placebo-controlled large-scale study in the USA (Freed et al 1999). However, the use of primary fetal tissue as the transplant source raises difficult practical and ethical issues. Hence the trials of neural transplantation have been confined to relatively small patient populations, such as late-stage PD and Huntington's disease. These difficulties are likely to impede the widespread use of this otherwise promising therapy, particularly in indications with large patient populations such as stroke and AD. The future scale-up of transplantation therapies using more readily available, off-the-shelf transplant sources to overcome the practical and ethical issues surrounding the use of primary tissue has brought the approach under regulatory scrutiny. This has meant that the preclinical and clinical development of potentially suitable transplantation products has become more vigorous and organized and that commercial involvement is therefore obligatory to covering the cost of such development. So far, only a few small bioscience companies have entered the field, and have in general met with constructive responses from the regulators (notably the US Food and Drug Administration; FDA) concerning the requirements for and conduct of early clinical trials. Large pharmaceutical companies appear to be waiting on the sidelines for the first human efficacy results to emerge.

Various alternative approaches to primary human tissue transplants have therefore been proposed and are currently under both preclinical and early clinical testing, largely led by small biotechnology companies. These include fetal primary neural tissue xenografts. Genzyme/Diacrin are currently in Phase II trials for PD, Huntington's disease and intractable epilepsy and have now begun a Phase I/II in stroke with fetal porcine tissue grafts. A xenograft approach is controversial, largely for reasons of concern about horizontal transmission of porcine retroviruses into human hosts. However, a recent study has not revealed any such transmission in patients with porcine tissue grafts (Paradis et al 1999). Nevertheless, ethical doubts and issues relating to immunosuppression of xenografts or genetic modification of donor pigs so as to reduce rejection may enhance porcine retrovirus transmission and render this approach unattractive.

The most promising alternative to primary fetal tissue grafts is clonal cellular therapy from human origins. The furthest advanced cell system in testing is the Pittsburgh trial (sponsored by Layton Biosciences Inc.) of a human terato-carcinoma cell line (NT2 cells). The trial is an open, uncontrolled study of 12 lacuna stroke volunteers conducted by the same neurosurgeon. The cells, from their teratoma origin, are pluripotent and if grafted to animals in an undifferentiated state will grow unchecked (as malignantly transformed) but will also differentiate into cells of a variety of tissue lineages (Andrews et al 1984). To control the fate of these cells, they are first differentiated into a neuronal population by treatment with retinoic acid and a selection process (Pleasure & Lee 1993). In the Pittsburgh trial they have been implanted into penumbral regions of the stroke infarct area identified by magnetic resonance imaging (MRI) using stereotaxic methods. The first trial patient received her implant in June 1998 and the final patient by the end of the same year. The first full reports of this trial are anticipated in the last quarter of 1999. As a background to this first human CNS cell trial, preclinical efficacy data with neuronally differentiated NT2N cells showed that the grafted cells produced relatively long-lasting improvements in passive avoidance learning and memory and body swing bias (modelling cognitive deficits and motor asymmetries, respectively, in stroke) in rats following middle cerebral artery occlusion (MCAo) (Borlongan et al 1998a). The graft effects were also cell-dose dependent: the larger the number of viable cells implanted and the greater the number of surviving graft cells post-mortem, then the better the stroke recovery (Borlongan et al 1998b).

In spite of the satisfaction of the FDA's likely stringent requirements for safety testing prior to the trial being approved, there are many critics of the use of teratocarcinoma cells as a source for transplantation. In particular, concerns have arisen over both the 'research laboratory' history of the cell line and the cells' likely long-term stability, since they are unlikely to be normal, diploid and with no additional or deleted chromosomes. There is thus a strong impetus for a new generation of cells with both a more 'natural' origin and with a more controlled provenance that will have advantages over cancer-derived cells.

Neuroepithelial stem cells as therapeutic agents

Neuroepithelial stem (NES) cells are neural precursor cells that have the cardinal properties of stem cells: they are capable of self-replication under appropriate environmental stimulation and they are multipotential. In the context of the CNS this latter property means they can generate the three major neural cell types: neurons, astrocytes and oligodendrocytes, as well as copies of themselves. This capacity has been demonstrated in series of tissue culture studies, using neural stem cells isolated by a variety of techniques. Neural stem cells have been immortalized by the introduction of an oncogene. This means that cell lines can be cloned and expanded as robust cells that will survive handling, freezing, thawing, etc. For the purposes of introducing cells with a potential for cellular differentiation into a host brain, conditional immortality is preferred. An example is the temperature-sensitive (ts) mutated allele (A 58) of the SV40 large T antigen (TAg). This is stably expressed in cells cultured at temperatures below mammalian body temperature (e.g. 33 °C) but the oncogenic protein is readily denatured at normal body — or brain — temperature (37–39 °C). Cells into which this gene has been introduced may therefore be maintained, expanded and efficiently cloned *in vitro* at the permissive temperature of 33 °C; upon culturing at the higher temperature or, indeed, implantation into a host brain, however, they cease dividing and enter the pathway to differentiation. Human fetal neural cell lines have recently been generated by infection with a retroviral vector in which expression of v-*myc* is tetracycline-regulated (Sah et al 1997). In the presence of tetracycline v-*myc* is turned off, and in some of the lines this results in neuronal and glial differentiation. Therefore, cultures of human neural progenitor cells can be generated and retrovirally infected with oncogenes. Furthermore, extrinsic signals could prevail over intrinsic determinants by redirecting the phenotypic fate of a particular cell.

More recently human neural stem cell populations and lines have been generated by epigenetic expansion in serum-free defined media with a cocktail of mitogenic growth factors (Flax et al 1998, Vescovi et al 1999). In addition, lines of multipotential and self-renewing neural stem cells have been generated by immortalization with v-*myc* (Flax et al 1998). Clonal lines could be passaged for at least a year *in vitro*. Upon engraftment into newborn mouse brain, v-*myc* expression was down-regulated constitutively and spontaneously, and clones gave rise to cells in all three fundamental neural lineages.

Therefore, cultures of human NES lines can be generated and expanded, in proliferative growth conditions, to provide a renewable, homogenous source of multipotential neural stem cells. The advantages of conditional immortalization of human NES cells are manifold: (1) The cells can be readily cloned, taking advantage of the selectable marker gene, such as *neo*[R], to select for stably infected colonies. (2) Addition of an immortalization step allows for subversion or extension of the replicative senescence that is a feature of serial cultivation of human cell systems (Jha et al 1998), permitting several orders of magnitude greater expansion of cells beyond the point of crisis and subsequent senescence than in epigenetically expanded cell populations. (3) From a product development point of view a clonal line will have a single identical gene insertion site, thereby assuring product consistency across the cell line's clinical life, avoiding the prospect of changes in cell mix in a polyclonal population with increasing passage number. Finally, (4), the derivation of multiple cell lines with a similar origin and phenotype allows for rational tests of identity, purity and bioactivity that will ensure the best cell product is made available to the clinician for each particular target condition.

Proof of clinical potential with neuroepithelial stem cells

Expansion of NES cells and the generation of conditionally immortal cell lines from the human fetal brain could therefore represent a viable and indeed preferable alternative to both human fetal primary tissue and established cancer-derived cell lines, offering an unlimited and consistent source of relatively normal cells with the capacity to generate all of the CNS cell types on demand.

However, to develop such cells as therapeutics means overcoming a series of major scientific hurdles. One as yet relatively unchallenged hurdle is to demonstrate the clinical potential of these cells, through testing the cells in predictive animal models of human neurological diseases.

To help bridge this data gap, our group has focused on the functional efficacy of conditionally immortal NES cells in transplantation experiments using a variety of animal models. Our starting point was to take advantage of a set of clonal NES cell lines directly derived from the H-2K^b-tsA58 transgenic mouse, the 'immortomouse' (Jat et al 1991). This transgenic mouse constitutively expresses the tsA58 TAg gene in all cells under the control of the interferon-inducible H-2K^b promoter, and has allowed us to generate a range of NES cell lines from a number of fetal brain regions at different developmental ages (Sinden et al 1997, this volume: Hodges et al 2000a, Price et al 2000). The first key finding was that a particular clonal NES cell line (MHP36), derived from the immortomouse hippocampus at embryonic day (E) 14, was capable of integrating into the global ischaemia-lesioned rat hippocampus. A major functional deficit produced by the four-vessel occlusion (4VO) damage, namely loss of spatial learning and memory, was reversed by the clonal MHP36 grafts, in a similar fashion to allografts of primary CA1 cells (Sinden et al 1997). The graft cells, labelled by a *lacZ* genetic marker or by [³H]thymidine autoradiography, were fully integrated into the principal cell layer of CA1, demonstrating the potential for seamless structural and functional integration of the grafted cells (Sinden et al 1997, Gray et al 1999). More recently, we have demonstrated that the MHP36 cells are equally capable of functional reconstruction of the hippocampus following an excitotoxic lesion of the CA1 field in marmoset monkeys (Virley et al 1999).

The hippocampal origin of the MHP36 cell line might suggest its capacity to act as an effective transplant source is confined to cell death in the hippocampus. An alternative hypothesis is that the functional activity of the cell line may cross the regional boundary, but the limitation is to the nature of the behavioural function recovered, i.e. cognition. We therefore have set out to investigate a wider range of animal models to test the extent to which a multipotential cell line such as MHP36 may also be 'multifunctional' (Gray et al 2000). The questions we therefore asked were whether certain NES cells (such as MHP36) have the ability to repair brain damage across: (i) a wide range of brain areas; (ii) not only acute (ischaemic and/or excitotoxic) damage, but also degenerative damage such as occurs in brain ageing; and (iii) in both cognitive and motor function.

NES cells repair cognitive deficits in aged impaired rats

To address the issue of whether NES cells would be effective in restoring a 'natural' ongoing degenerative process in the CNS, we have recently studied the effects of MHP36 cell grafts on aged rats (Hodges et al 2000b). We pretrained a large group of aged rats (22 months) to locate a hidden platform in Morris water maze. On the basis of their performance we divided them at the median into two groups of faster and slower learners. The group that learned more quickly was seen as 'unimpaired'. The best of the aged animals, which learned normally, just like a group of young (6 month old) rats, were used as unimpaired controls. The impaired group were carefully matched on their pretraining performance into groups that received either grafts of MHP36 cells in three brain regions bilaterally (frontal cortex, hippocampus and striatum, $3\,\mu l$ containing 75 000 cells in each site) or the equivalent grafts of cell vehicle. Rats were tested for their ability to find the submerged platform in a different position in the pool for 12 days, starting 6 weeks after surgery. On day 13 the platform was removed to test memory for its position. We compared four groups of 9–15 rats: old impaired rats with control grafts, old impaired rats with MHP36 cell grafts, old unimpaired controls and young controls — these latter two groups also receiving control grafts.

As shown in Fig. 1, the old impaired rats with MHP36 grafts performed as well as old unimpaired rats. They found the platform as quickly, but also spent as much time in the area where the platform was located and headed out in the right direction when placed in the pool. Impaired old control rats with control grafts

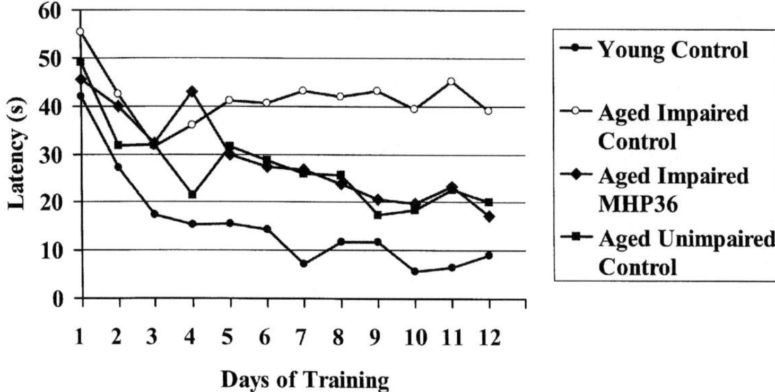

FIG. 1. Mean acquisition latency to reach the platform in aged impaired controls, aged impaired rats with MHP36 grafts, aged unimpaired rats and sham-operated young controls. The aged impaired rats showed substantial deficits relative to all other groups. Aged unimpaired and aged impaired rats with transplants took longer to find the platform than the young controls, but this reflected slower swim speed, because they were as efficient as the young controls in terms of distance swum.

still performed poorly, taking longer to find the platform, swimming further distances and spending less time searching in the correct area than either the unimpaired old or impaired old with MHP36 graft groups (Hodges et al 2000b). Labelled MHP36 cells were found well differentiated and integrated in all three grafted forebrain areas and had the distinct morphological appearance of neurons (including, for example, hippocampal pyramidal neurons) and glial cells.

Hence, MHP36 cells are able to restore function in chronic degeneration that is frequently a consequence of ageing, equally as well as following acute ischaemic damage, such as after 4VO. Perhaps most significantly, unlike the case with fetal primary cell implants, the graft cells did not clump at the site of implant but migrated and dispersed extensively to integrate into frontal cortex, striatum and hippocampus, penetrating and differentiating into, e.g. hippocampal principal cells (Hodges et al 2000b).

NES cells restore cognitive function in rats with
excitotoxic lesions of the basal forebrain

If NES cell grafts are able to reverse progressive deterioration of cognitive function in ageing rats, we sought to investigate whether grafts of MHP36 cells are effective in rats with excitotoxic lesions of the nucleus basalis magnocellularis and the medial septal area, a partial model for cognitive deficits associated with dementia in AD (Grigoryan et al 2000). We used rats that had sustained small bilateral infusions of α-amino-3-hydroxy-4-izoxazole propionic acid (AMPA) via

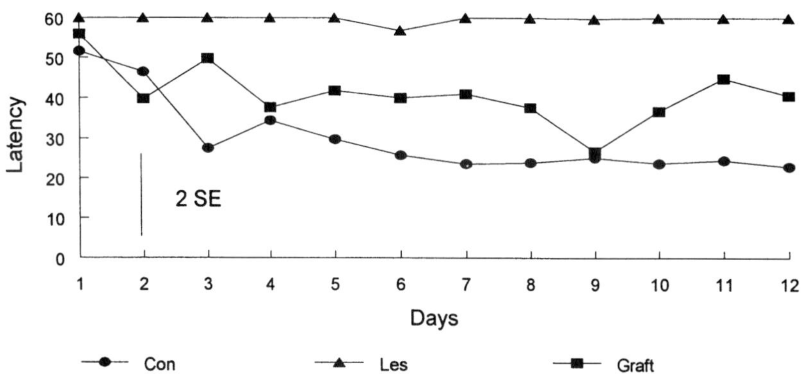

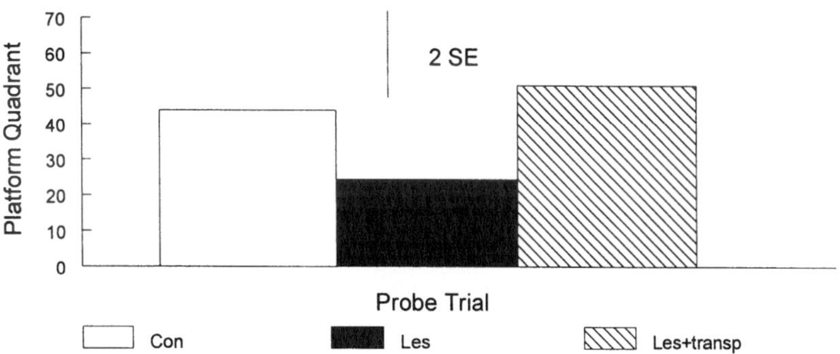

FIG. 2.   Effects of transplants of MHP36 cells bilaterally into the fronto-parietal cortex and hippocampus in rats with bilateral excitotoxic lesions of the nucleus basalis and the medial septal area/diagonal band complex, on performance in the Morris water maze. Con, intact animals given sham surgery; Les, rats with lesions and control grafts; Les+transp, rats with both lesion and transplanted cells. (*Above*) Latency to find the hidden platform over 12 training days. (*Below*) % time in the training quadrant with the platform absent during the probe trial on day 13.

multiple microinjections into both the above regions, producing relatively discrete loss of the forebrain cholinergic projection neurons in these areas and stable deficits in the performance of spatial tasks such as the water maze. Six months after lesioning, rats were bilaterally grafted with MHP36 cells into frontal and parietal cortex and hippocampus. Controls received equivalent infusions of cell vehicle. Five months after grafting, the rats were trained to find a hidden platform in the water maze. The rats with lesions and control grafts showed marked deficits in a range of spatial learning measures, such as escape latency. The MHP36-grafted rats, on the other hand, located the platform as efficiently as unlesioned control rats

(Fig. 2). The pattern of distribution of the labelled grafted cells was less clear following this lesion than in the older rats. However, cells were distributed throughout the hippocampal formation (Grigoryan et al 2000). We are currently determining to what extent these graft cells have a cholinergic phenotype. Whatever the action of these cells, their efficacy in both normal age-related deficits as well as following experimental lesions involving the forebrain cholinergic system encourages the development of NES cells for the treatment of dementia in Alzheimer's and related neurodegenerative diseases.

NES cells resolve sensory and motor deficits following stroke

Transient intraluminal occlusion of the middle cerebral artery (MCAo) provides a reproducible and clinically relevant model for the effects of thromboembolic stroke. The efficacy of rehabilitation in stroke patients appears to reach its limit at 3–6 months post-infarct, and some 25% of all surviving patients suffer some form of serious residual disability for which no products are available. Thus the possibility of promoting recovery by neural transplantation appears attractive, particularly in younger victims who may suffer decades of disability. We have recently examined the potential of grafts of MHP36 cells in an animal model of MCAo stroke (Veizovic et al 2000).

Focal MCAo ischaemia in the rat produces extensive areas of forebrain damage on the occluded side (Fig. 3). Effective cell grafting requires targeting sites away from the core of the lesion, in adjacent 'penumbra'. To avoid injecting cells into areas undergoing dense cavitation, we infused our cell grafts into cortex and striatum on the side *contralateral* to the infarct, taking advantage of the key property of MHP36 cells to migrate towards lesioned areas.

Rats were subjected to transient intraluminal MCAo in the left hemisphere for 60 minutes (Ginsburg & Busto 1998). The control procedure consisted of exposure of the left carotid only. Transplant surgery was undertaken 2–3 weeks later. 3 μl of cell suspension containing 75 000 cells were infused into eight sites in cortex and striatum on the side contralateral to the infarct. Control rats received vehicle infusion only. The rats were tested over a 10 month post-graft period as follows: (1) from 6–18 weeks on the bilateral asymmetry test, a test of sensorimotor neglect; (2) at 26 weeks on the water maze; and (3) at 38 weeks on spontaneous and amphetamine-induced rotation. Histological analysis examined both volume of lesion as well as disposition of the labelled cells in all groups. In the bilateral asymmetry test, standard strips of tape were wound around each of the two forepaws and the rats were timed for latency to contact and remove each tape. As shown in Fig. 4, rats subjected to MCAo showed a marked disparity between the two paws, with the right paw contacted and the tape removed significantly more slowly than the left. In the control grafted MCAo group, this deficit persisted through the 18 weeks of

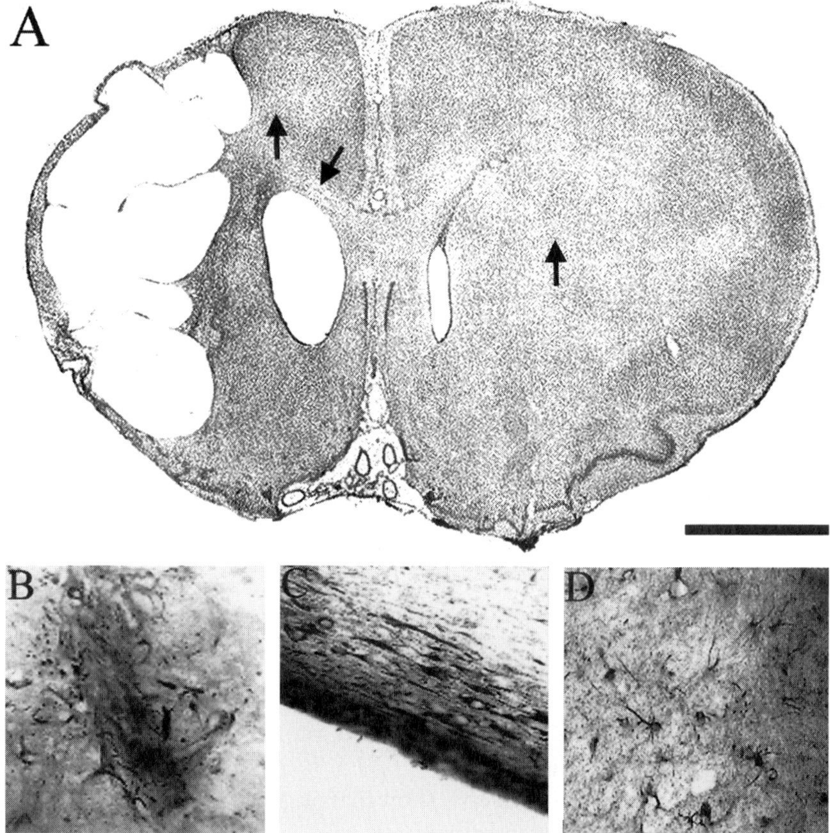

FIG. 3. (A) Photomicrograph of a cresyl fast violet stained coronal section through the MCAo lesioned brain. The occlusion caused a unilateral infarct with primary tissue damage to the cortex and striatum, leaving the external surface of the cortex/meninges intact, and a widening of the lateral ventricle. The arrow on the contralateral side indicates the positioning of the transplanted cells, which are visualized in (B) by β-galactosidase immunohistochemistry. At the site of transplant the cells have a fibrous appearance. The β-galactosidase-positive transplanted cells in (C) were photographed from the region illustrated by the arrow in the ipsilateral corpus callosum; these cells are elongated as they pass along the corpus callosum fibre bundles. The transplanted cells were also seen in the ipsilateral cortex, as indicated in (A), and shown in (D), the cells within the cortex are highly processed and differentiated. Scale bar = 2 mm (A); 100 μm (B, C and D).

testing. In rats that received MHP36 grafts, the stroke-induced forepaw disparity was not significant by 8 weeks after grafting, and this improvement persisted thereafter. Hence grafted animals did not differ from unlesioned controls. Thus, sensorimotor neglect was effectively reversed by the MHP36 grafts. In a similar fashion, MHP36 grafts normalized the amphetamine-induced rotation seen in the

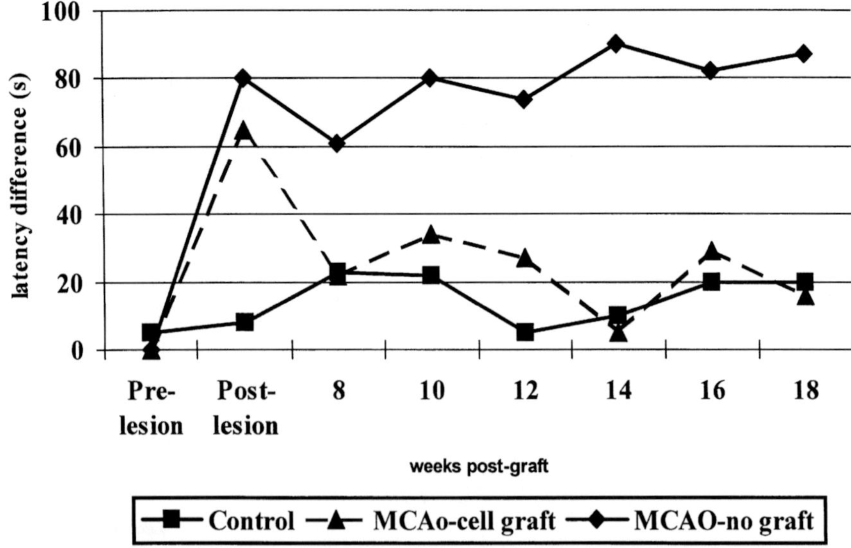

FIG. 4. Difference in latency to remove tape from both paws in Sprague–Dawley rats following sham MCAo ($n=11$), MCAo plus vehicle transplant ($n=10$) and MCAo plus MHP36 cell transplant ($n=11$). The contralateral sensory neglect in MCAo rats is highly significantly reversed by MHP36 cell grafts.

control-grafted MCAo rats. However, MHP36 grafts failed to ameliorate water maze deficits produced by the MCAo.

The results of this experiment clearly show that our conditionally immortal NES cells are effective in repairing sensorimotor (but not cognitive) function following stroke, demonstrating further the degree of multifunctionality of these cells. Perhaps the most striking outcome of this experiment, providing a clear explanation of these positive behavioural results, was found in the histology data. The volume of the infarct in the grafted group was reduced by 35% (Fig. 5). Note that this result was seen in rats with grafts placed contralaterally to the infarct. In addition, immunohistochemical staining for the β-galactosidase marker revealed the presence of graft cells on both sides of the brain, along with migratory profiles within the corpus callosum (Fig. 3). These data provide further evidence for the 'multifunctionality' of NES cells and demonstrate that deficits in motor, as well as cognitive, function are amenable to NES graft therapy.

NES cells do not reverse motor asymmetries in the hemi-parkinsonian model

We have been able to show that motor asymmetries in rats subjected to MCAo stroke are normalized by grafts of MHP36 cells. Therefore the potential of these

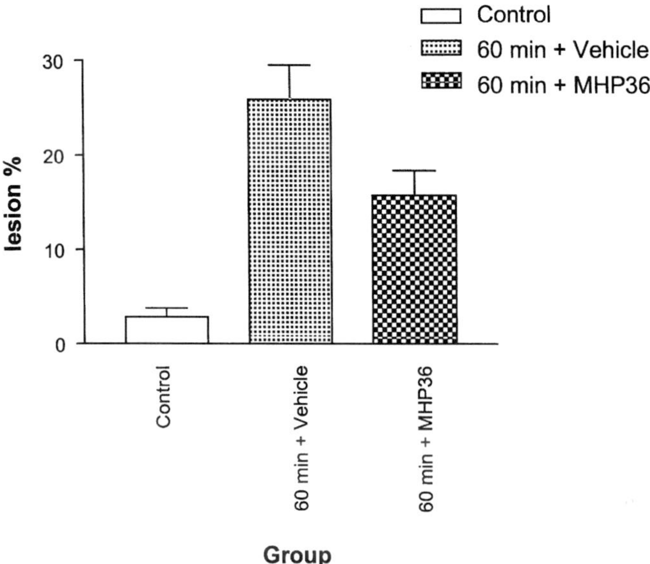

FIG. 5.   Effects of MHP36 grafts on MCAo lesion volumes as a percentage of whole brain. The lesion volumes were calculated from serial sections using image analysis software. MHP36 grafts significantly reduced lesion volumes by 34%.

cells in reversing motor deficits in an animal model of PD was investigated in collaboration with Dr Stephen Dunnett of Cambridge University. In rats with unilateral 6-hydroxydopamine lesions of the nigrostriatal bundle, grafts of MHP36 cells were implanted in ipsilateral striatum, substantia nigra and both regions. In contrast to the results in MCAo stroke, amphetamine-induced rotation was not normalized by MHP36 grafting, although graft cells were identified in both implanted regions. We are currently investigating NES cell lines derived from the immortomouse fetal striatum and ventral mesencephalon for their efficacy in the same PD model. Recent experiments suggest that expression of the *nurr1* gene in neural precursor cells may be a requirement for generating a sufficient number of dopaminergic neurons to effect repair (Wagner et al 1999). It would therefore be of interest to determine the level of this gene expression from NES cells in different fetal brain regions.

Prospects for clinical transplantation with NES cells

Taken together our data have demonstrated that NES cell lines conditionally immortalized by the SV40 tsA58 Tag oncogene have significant potential in restoring function across a wide range of ischaemic and neurodegenerative CNS diseases. The prototype MHP36 cell line has retained its phenotype, multipotentiality and effectiveness in repair over multiple passages and is sufficiently robust to survive freezing, thawing and handling. Other data from our laboratory (Price et al 2000, this volume) show that a number of other multipotential NES cell lines derived from the immortomouse neuroepithelium, including one line derived from the same immortalized E14 hippocampal population as MHP36, do not show the same capacity for neural repair. Therefore, neural stem cells show marked heterogeneity in their capacity to act as an effective graft source.

The effectiveness of MHP36 cells over a range of animal models of neurological dysfunction is the first evidence that repairing NES lines have a remarkable degree of 'multifunctionality' (Gray et al 2000) across both the loci and cause of the lesion or degeneration as well as the type of function (cognitive or sensorimotor) implicated. The failure of MHP36 cells to repair in a model of Parkinson's disease suggests that regional specificity of the NES cells may also be important to their functional effectiveness.

ReNeuron is currently developing conditionally immortalized NES cells derived from the human fetal brain. Our success in developing lines that have the capacity to produce both functional and structural repair will depend on our ability to mirror what we believe to be the key characteristics of MHP36 cells: multipotentiality, migration to areas of damage and capacity to differentiate *in vivo*.

References

Andrews PW, Damjanov I, Simon D et al 1984 Pluripotent embryonal carcinoma clones derived from the human teratocarcinoma cell line NTera-2. Differentiation *in vivo* and *in vitro*. Lab Invest 50:147–162

Borlongan CV, Tajima Y, Trojanowski JQ, Lee VMY, Sanberg PR 1998a Transplantation of cryopreserved human embryonal carcinoma-derived neurons (NT2N cells) promotes functional recovery in ischaemic rats. Exp Neurol 149:310–321

Borlongan CV, Saporta S, Poulos SG, Othberg A, Sanberg PR 1998b Viability and survival of hNT neurons determine degree of functional recovery in grafted ischemic rats. Neuroreport 9:2837–2842

Flax JD, Aurora S, Yang C et al 1998 Engraftable human neural stem cells respond to developmental cues, replace neurons, and express foreign genes. Nat Biotechnol 16:1033–1039

Freed CR, Breeze RE, Greene PD et al 1999 Double-blind placebo-controlled human fetal dopamine cell transplants in advanced Parkinson's disease. Soc Neurosci Abstr 86.5, p 212

Freeman TB, Olanow CW, Hauser RA et al 1995 Bilateral fetal nigral transplantation into the postcommissural putamen in Parkinson's disease. Ann Neurol 38:379–388

Ginsberg MD, Busto R 1998 Small animal models of global and focal ischemia. In: Ginsberg MD, Bogousslavsky J (eds) Cerebrovascular disease, vol 1. Blackwell Science, Malden, MA, p 14–35

Gray JA, Hodges H, Sinden J 1999 Prospects for the clinical application of neural transplantation with the use of conditionally immortalized neuroepithelial stem cells. Philos Trans R Soc Lond B Biol Sci 354:1407–1421

Gray JA, Grigoryan G, Virley D, Patel S, Sinden JD, Hodges H 2000 Conditionally immortalized, multipotential and multifunctional neural stem cell lines as an approach to clinical transplantation. Cell Transplant 9:153–168

Grigoryan G, Gray JA, Rashid T, Chadwick A, Hodges H 2000 Conditionally immortal neuroepithelial stem cell grafts restore spatial learning in rats with cholinergic system damage. Submitted

Hodges H, Sowinski P, Virley D et al 2000a Functional reconstruction of the hippocampus: fetal versus conditionally immortal neuroepithelial stem cell grafts. In: Neural transplantation in neurodegenerative disease. Wiley, Chichester (Novartis Found Symp 231) p 53–69

Hodges H, Veizovic T, Bray N et al 2000b Conditionally immortal neuroepithelial stem cell grafts reverse age-associated memory impairments in rats. Submitted

Jat PS, Noble MD, Ataliotis P et al 1991 Direct derivation of conditionally immortal cell lines from a H-2K^{b}tsA58 transgenic mouse. Proc Natl Acad Sci USA 88:5096–5100

Jha KK, Banga S, Palewala V, Ozer HL 1998 SV40-mediated immortalization. Exp Cell Res 245:1–7

Lindvall O, Sawle G, Widner H et al 1994 Evidence for long-term survival and function of dopaminergic grafts in progressive Parkinson's disease. Ann Neurol 35:172–180

Paradis K, Langford G, Long Z et al 1999 Search for cross-species transmission of porcine endogenous retrovirus in patients treated with living pig tissue. Science 285:1236–1241

Pleasure SJ, Lee VMY 1993 NTera 2 cells: a human cell line which displays characteristics expected of a human committed neuronal progenitor cell. J Neurosci Res 35:585–602

Price J, Uwangho D, Peters S, Galloway D, Mellodew K 2000 Neurotransplantation in neurodegenerative disease: a survey of relevant issues in developmental neurobiology. In: Neural transplantation in neurodegenerative disease. Wiley, Chichester (Novartis Found Symp 231) p 148–165

Sah DWY, Ray J, Gage FH 1997 Bipotent progenitor cell lines from the human CNS. Nat Biotechnol 15:574–580

Sinden JD, Rashid-Doubell F, Kershaw TR et al 1997 Recovery of spatial learning by grafts of a conditionally immortalized hippocampal neuroepithelial cell line into the ischaemia-lesioned hippocampus. Neuroscience 81:599–608

Veizovic T, Beech J, Straemar P, Watson W, Soiruski P, Hodges H 2000 Resolution of stroke deficits following contralateral grafts of conditionally immortal neuroepithelial cells. Submitted

Vescovi AL, Parati EA, Gritti A et al 1999 Isolation and cloning of multipotential stem cells from the embryonic human CNS and establishment of transplantable human neural stem cell lines by epigenetic stimulation. Exp Neurol 156:71–83

Virley D, Ridley RM, Sinden JD et al 1999 Primary CA1 and conditionally immortal MHP36 cell grafts restore conditional discrimination learning and recall in marmosets after excitotoxic lesions of the hippocampal CA1 field. Brain 122:2321–2335

Wagner J, Åkerud P, Castro DS et al 1999 Induction of a midbrain dopaminergic phenotype in Nurr1-overexpressing neural stem cells by type 1 astrocytes. Nat Biotechnol 17:653–659

DISCUSSION

Gray: Could you say more about migration in the light of Evan Snyder's paper (Ourednik et al 2000, this volume)?

Sinden: In our stroke model, where clearly we are doing something that requires migration because we injected the cells into the contralateral side, we still found many β-galactosidase positive cells at the point of implantation in striatum and cortex, so we saw cells engrafting in the contralateral side. These could be the critical cells for the recovery of function. They could be involved in the process of reorganization that goes on in the contralateral side. We also saw profiles in corpus callosum moving across, and a large number of differentiated cells in infarcted regions on the lesion side.

Perry: How do you measure lesion size in something 12 weeks after you have made this huge lesion and now injected cells?

Sinden: We took serial sections through the brain. We used a computer macro where we took the image of these tissue sections and generated a set of data that allowed us to compare the volume.

Perry: What are you comparing it with? You have a brain with a chunk missing and another one with a transplant.

Sinden: You don't actually see the transplant: it is seamlessly integrated into the tissue.

Björklund: Could you elaborate on the mechanisms you assume to operate here. You have used quite different lesion models. The assumption is, of course, that the lesions interfere with different parts of the brain, so the mechanism underlying behavioural impairment would not be the same in the different models. Do you think there is a common mechanism that may be equally relevant in all models?

Sinden: The best evidence we have is in hippocampal damage, in the sense that we know that the cells fully integrate into the CA1 area. We know quite a lot about what happens in the 4VO ischaemic model. The only other feature that we see in the other models that is common to all is a degree of cell replacement. We see that graft cells make all of the normal cell types in the areas we would expect to see them.

Lindvall: In the stroke model, 30–40 min ischaemia leads to relatively selective damage in the striatum of rats. With 60 min duration the cortex also becomes involved. How does the grafting of these cells reconstruct the striatum versus the cortex? Have you seen more striatal neurons, or is it just a mess of neurons?

Sinden: We see cells in both cortex and striatum that we think have migrated over from the contralateral side.

Lindvall: I'm talking about striatal projection neurons versus cortical neurons.

Sinden: We haven't done that level of phenotyping.

Raisman: How do you get 24 μl into the brain without causing an enormous amount of damage? 1 μl is 1 mm^3 in volume.

Sinden: We see no damage, other than the typical needle track.

Raisman: Do you have any controls to ensure that the cells with the reaction product are in fact donor cells?

Sinden: Yes.

Björklund: When was the grafting done relative to the insult?

Sinden: Two to three weeks afterwards.

Gage: These are mouse cells from a transgenic mouse. Will you use these cells in humans?

Sinden: These are a model system for a human product. We would use the same conditionally immortalized oncogenes, but in human cells. We would use the nestin-positive human stem cell type.

Perry: Coming back to the issue of the mechanism of repair, is this an increase in the ability of the nervous system to express plasticity, or is there specificity? I think this comes back to the nature of the behavioural task you use. In the recovery of function literature, there is this whole issue of what are we using as our parameters of recovery of function. If you use a particular set of tasks, there is always the problem that the animal finds different ways to solve the task, and does need an absolutely specific pathway. I don't know much about the behavioural tasks that you are using, but I would suggest that animal does have the opportunity to solve the task in certain different ways. The only way in the recovery of function literature where it ever became absolutely clear that there were no differences between infant-lesioned and adult-lesioned animals, for example, was to go to a sensory threshold. Under those conditions, it was not possible to demonstrate that the infant brain was any more or less plastic than the adult. Getting at the mechanism requires the use of behavioural tasks where there is only one pathway. In contrast, if you use tasks for which are many different routes you are left with the problem that you never know whether the mechanisms that the cells are expressing are allowing a global plasticity, or actually that those cells that turned into neurons are now doing a good job.

Gray: I commented in my introductory remarks on the lack of good electrophysiology in this field. One way of answering your question would be to record from, for example, the pyramidal neurons in a behavioural task.

Perry: Or work in a system where there are absolute thresholds.

Sinden: The answer that I would give to your question goes back to our 4VO ischaemia, where our original experiments were to look at grafts of hippocampal tissue from different fields of the hippocampus. We were able to show that CA1 cells could repair that function, but CA3 cells wouldn't, and nor would dentate gyrus cells. However, these stem cells would. Using this argument, it would suggest that our cells are essentially recapitulating the function of CA1 cells.

Price: We are missing the point over the MCAo results that John Sinden presented. What John says is correct—with the 4VO hippocampus/CA1 damage, the hypothesis could be that you are reconstructing the circuits that have been destroyed. That is not a tenable hypothesis in MCAo. To state the obvious: there is a hole in the brain before the cells are put in, and afterwards there is still a big hole in the brain. It is conceivable that the missing circuits have been reconnected. Surely the crucial data are those John showed showing that there is an apparent reduction in the lesion size, even though the cells were grafted considerably after the lesion took place. I'm not an expert in this, but surely what we are looking at is what you were suggesting: the induction of some mechanism that has prevented secondary degeneration. More brain is being saved, not in the primary lesion, but in a series of knock-on effects. I don't think we want to try to restrict the models and test for specific pathways, as Hugh Perry suggests.

Perry: I think there are good reasons to do so. In the clinical studies it is clear that there are behavioural measures that are repaired and those that are not. Until one understands precisely what the transplant does, in the context of its specificity or lack of specificity, you can't bias it either way. In parkinsonian patients, tremor is not improved. If one really wanted to tap into that, you would like to understand the mechanisms by which you could make a transplant that would improve tremor as well, if this was a major clinical issue.

Price: The point I am making is that you have to understand first what effects you can produce, and then try to dissect how they are working. I don't think there is any point in demanding a repair that you can't get, as it were.

Freeman: Do you have a map of the time-course of migration across the corpus callosum? How does this correlate to the time-course of improvement in the passive avoidance and sensory neglect in the rotometer testing?

Sinden: Our first preliminary data show that by two weeks there is migration across the corpus callosum.

Hodges: In the 4VO model there is migration across the corpus callosum within 2 weeks, but in the MCAo model the earliest we have killed the animals is about 12 weeks. There, in rats with grafts in the striatum opposite to the infarct, fewer cells have migrated to the site of injury and fewer cells are seen in the corpus callosum than in rats with contralateral grafts that were killed 11 months after transplantation.

Freeman: So only a minority of cells have reached the lesioned side by 12 weeks. When did the recovery start?

Sinden: In the tape paradigm its started at about 8 weeks. In the other behavioural tasks it is also around about that time.

Hodges: There is no recovery of asymmetry in rotometer testing at 8–10 weeks, but there is at 10 months.

Raisman: You say that the lesion size goes down. But if you are telling me that the lesion is a hole full of cerebrospinal fluid, wouldn't you just reduce the lesion size just by aspirating this? What is the significance of its size going down? It is just a cyst.

Price: A better way to think of this is not that the lesion volume decreases, but that there is more brain saved.

Raisman: Do you mean that the lesion would have been progressive?

Price: That is my guess.

Sinden: The next stage is to do some regional volume measures.

Dunnett: We are trying to tease out the mechanism. Are the cells you are putting in replacing and repairing the neural circuitry at the lesion site, or does the graft provide a protection mechanism? The histology that we all look at focuses on the advanced stage of degeneration, many months after the lesion. Presumably it doesn't look like that at the time that you are grafting the cells or when the tests are done. The lesion itself has a natural history. We need to see the acute and progressive histology if we are to interpret the mechanism about whether there is less death of the intrinsic striatal cells or the intrinsic cortical cells at the time when you are doing behavioural testing and before the MHP cells have migrated across.

Annett: I am surprised that the improvement in the sensory motor neglect was back to normal on the first test, since the neglect task is quite sensitive. This was with only a 35% decrease in the infarct size. Therefore, there was still a big lesion. Have you compared neglect data from animals with the infarct alone and with grafts that have comparable size lesions? I would predict that you would still get a big deficit on this task. The implication of these neglect data is that the recovery is not due to a simple replacement mechanism — you are not putting back sufficient tissue.

Sinden: We haven't done that experiment.

Annett: You could look at the lesioned controls, to see how the size of the damage affects task performance.

Isacson: Some very important issues are being raised here. Each lesion that we are discussing is different. A degeneration of a specific cell type like the dopamine cells in PD is a different lesion model than an ischaemic global tissue destruction. The other issue is whether we accept that there could be dynamic and parallel ways in which different mechanisms could be active at the same time. There could be both global and specific neuroprotective mechanisms operating at the same time. Even if we accept that, I still think it is incumbent upon us scientifically to ask, as Lucy Annett has done: if it is another mechanism that is operating, do we really need to transplant cells into an ischaemic lesion, or do we need to find a neuroprotective factor and a plasticity-inducing factor that will then do the same job in a rational pharmacological and medical sense?

Perry: Mark Peschanski told me yesterday that if you take enough care with your Huntington patients before you transplant them, and help them overcome their depression, what is remarkable is the amount of recovery seen even before transplant. Whether transplantation is the biological basis of this placebo effect seems to be very important. This is why I think it is worthwhile finding out whether this is a mechanism that is specific to cells in specific places, or 'global growth factor effects' that need to be discovered.

Gray: I think at the very least this kind of placebo effect can be eliminated with regard to the experiments with rats!

Perry: Handling animals clearly makes a fantastic difference.

Hodges: The controls were handled just as much.

Reference

Ourednik V, Ourednik J, Park KI et al 2000 Neural stem cells are uniquely suited for cell replacement and gene therapy in the CNS. In: Neural transplantation in neurodegenerative disease. Wiley, Chichester (Novartis Found Symp 231) p 242–269

Remyelinating the demyelinated CNS

W. F. Blakemore, P. M. Smith and R. J. M. Franklin

Department of Clinical Veterinary Medicine, University of Cambridge, Madingley Road, Cambridge CB3 0ES, UK

Abstract. The CNS has an inherent capacity to generate remyelinating cells following episodes of myelin loss. However, persistent demyelination is the major pathology of multiple sclerosis and the leucodystrophies, and is also a feature of spinal cord trauma. There are potentially two approaches for achieving remyelination in situations where it fails; enhancement of the inherent remyelinating capacity of the CNS, or transplantation of an exogenous source of myelin forming cells. In experimental animals it is possible to remyelinate demyelinated CNS axons by transplanting cultures containing central or peripheral myelinogenic cells. Glial cell transplantation may thus provide a therapeutic strategy for remyelinating areas of chronic demyelination as well as for stimulating axon regeneration. This presentation will review four issues that have to be addressed before glial transplantation can be undertaken in humans: is the procedure safe, what cells would be used, where would the cells come from and can we predict how much remyelination will be achieved? It concludes that the most promising approach will be to use multipotent neural precursor cells that have been committed to oligodendrocyte lineage differentiation prior to implantation. However, even with such preparations, which have considerable myelinating potential, the extent of remyelination that would be achieved can not yet be predicted with any degree of certainty.

2000 Neural transplantation in neurodegenerative disease. Wiley, Chichester (Novartis Foundation Symposium 231) p 289–301

Persistent demyelination, in addition to being the major pathology of multiple sclerosis and the leucodystrophies, is also a feature of spinal cord trauma where there is evidence that it contributes to the functional deficit (Bunge et al 1993, Shi et al 1997). In experimental animals it is possible to remyelinate demyelinated CNS axons by transplanting cultures containing central or peripheral myelinogenic cells (Blakemore et al 1995). Myelin sheaths made by transplanted glial cells enhance action potential conduction (Honmou et al 1996, Imaizumi et al 1998, Utzschneider et al 1994) and we have shown that both normal and transplant-mediated remyelination results in restoration of function lost as a consequence of demyelination (Jeffery & Blakemore 1997, Jeffery et al 1999). Glial cell transplantation may thus provide a therapeutic strategy for remyelinating areas of chronic demyelination. However, before glial transplantation can be undertaken in humans a number of issues have to be resolved. The most

289

important are, will the procedure be safe and will it be effective in restoring function lost as a consequence of chronic demyelination?

Will introduction of glial cells into areas of demyelination be safe?

The experience of human and xenogenic tissue grafting for the treatment of Parkinson's disease would indicate that the introduction of exogenous cells into the human brain is not an inherently hazardous procedure, providing donor tissue is monitored for potentially harmful pathogens. It has been our experience that injection of suspensions of immature glial cells into areas of acute demyelination does not lead to axon damage, while others who implant cells into myelin mutants have not commented on any adverse consequences. However, there is some evidence that injections of cultures containing large numbers of astrocytes can lead to an increase in axon damage and it should also be remembered that injection of embryonic tissue has the potential to form classical neural grafts consisting of discrete populations of neurons and glia. If such grafts develop in white matter tracts they will act as space-occupying lesions and are likely to have deleterious effects. Thus, provided the injected cell suspension can generate myelinogenic cells, glial cell transplantation would appear to be a safe procedure. One must add, however, that prolonged expansion of multipotent cells *in vitro* may result in formation of cell lines that could fail to respond to environmental signals. It will be important therefore to examine the behaviour of any cell preparations intended for human use in a variety of animal models prior to any clinical application.

As glial cell transplantation appears to be a safe procedure the central issue to be addressed is the ability of transplanted glial cells to remyelinate large areas of demyelination. Predictions on this matter revolve around three linked questions: what cells to use, where would the cells come from, and can we predict how much remyelination there will be following the introduction of different types of cells?

What cells would be most appropriate to transplant?

Oligodendrocyte lineage cells, Schwann cells and olfactory bulb ensheathing cells all remyelinate axons following transplantation. This presentation will concentrate on oligodendrocyte lineage cells since our understanding of Schwann cell remyelination of CNS axons suggests that these cells would have a very restricted ability to remyelinate CNS axons following transplantation (reviewed in Blakemore et al 2000, Franklin & Blakemore 1993). Within the oligodendrocyte lineage, the oligodendrocyte progenitor (OP) cell has been the focus of much attention, primarily because it produces more myelin over a larger area than later stages of the lineage when transplanted into the myelin-deficient shiverer mouse

(Warrington et al 1993). This result was to be expected given the greater capacity for division and migration of the immature cell *in vitro* (Pfeiffer et al 1993). Recent data suggest that cells earlier in the oligodendrocyte lineage than the A2B5+ progenitor may have an even greater capacity for extensive transplantation-derived remyelination (Avellana-Adalid et al 1996, Crang & Blakemore 1997, Keirstead et al 1999, Zhang et al 1998a).

Self-renewing multipotential neural stem cells that can differentiate into neurons, astrocytes and oligodendrocytes can be isolated from both the embryonic and adult rodent brain and can be expanded *in vitro* as clusters of cells in serum-free medium containing epidermal growth factor (EGF) or fibroblast growth factor (FGF) 2. A more restricted differentiation occurs when these multipotent neural stem cell clusters are expanded under the influence of medium conditioned by the B104 neuroblastoma cell line (Avellana-Adalid et al 1996, Zhang et al 1998a). Such clusters are termed oligospheres and it is significant that implantation of oligospheres into the spinal cord of the myelin-deficient rat results in larger areas of myelination than implantation of neurospheres (Zhang et al 1998b).

Availability of human cells

Although oligodendrocytes can be obtained from the adult human CNS in relatively large numbers, these cells fail to generate myelin sheaths when transplanted into demyelinated rat CNS (Targett et al 1996). On the other hand, implantation of fetal human CNS tissue into the developing rodent brain results in the generation of myelination competent cells (Seilhean et al 1996). Until recently this meant that if glial cell transplantation using CNS cells was to be developed clinically, it would be necessary to use human fetal tissue, a prospect that posed a number of problems. Not only would the ethical issues and availability of human fetal tissue have to be confronted, it would also be necessary to develop methods to generate large numbers of oligodendrocyte progenitors from such tissue. Although, some oligodendrocytes can be generated *in vitro* from early human embryonic CNS tissue (Murray & Dubois-Dalcq 1997, Satoh & Kim 1994), injection of such cultures into areas of demyelination in immunosuppressed rats is not followed by extensive remyelination (S. Chandran & W. F. Blakemore, unpublished observations).

The problem of generating large numbers of myelination competent cells from human fetal CNS tissue has recently been resolved using human multipotential neural stem cells expanded *in vitro* as neurospheres (Brüstle et al 1998) or as immortalized cell lines (Flax et al 1998). In addition, *in vitro* conditions have been established for the generation of tissue-specific embryonic stem cell lines from human blastocytes (Thomson et al 1998). This ability to generate large numbers of neural stem cells from a single aborted fetus or a blastocyte removes one of the major obstacles to considering oligodendrocyte progenitors as the cell of choice for developing glial cell transplantation as a clinical therapy in humans. However, unlike the situation with the rodent, the *in vitro* conditions required for commitment of human neural multipotential stem cells to the oligodendrocyte lineage have yet to be established.

Recent experience with implanting porcine tissue rich in neural precursors into areas of acutely demyelinating lesions in immunosuppressed rats has highlighted the need to commit cells to the oligodendrocyte lineage prior to transplantation if remyelination is to be achieved and the production of space-occupying tissue masses avoided. Thus, when freshly isolated porcine periventricular cells from newborn piglets are transplanted into areas of acute demyelination little if any oligodendrocyte remyelination is observed and the area of demyelination is filled with groups of undifferentiated neural precursors and astrocytes (Fig. 1). However, when the same preparation is grown in medium conditioned by the B104 neuroblastoma cell line for 7 days prior to transplantation—a procedure that induces oligosphere formation from neural progenitors (Zhang et al 1998b)—extensive oligodendrocyte remyelination is achieved (Fig. 1). The need for commitment to the oligodendrocyte lineage is also demonstrated by the failure of transplanted human or porcine embryonic tissue-derived cultures to achieve significant remyelination. Instead following transplantation such cultures generate large numbers of immature neurons that greatly expand the lesion area causing compression of surrounding tissue (Fig. 2). Such experiments indicate that without commitment to the oligodendrocyte lineage, the introduction of multipotent neural progenitors into areas of acute demyelination may not only fail to generate the large numbers of oligodendrocytes necessary for remyelination, but may also be deleterious. However, no deleterious effects have been reported following the introduction of multipotent cells into the developing or neonatal nervous system and it is reported that more extensive myelination is

FIG. 1.   The appearance of an area of demyelination created by the injection of 1 μl of 0.1% ethidium bromide into spinal cord white matter exposed to 40 Grays of X-irradiation. In (A), there is no evidence of remyelination 3 weeks following transplantation of 10^4 neonatal porcine SVZ cells exposed to B104 conditioned medium for 7 days into an animal that received no immunosuppression, whilst in immunosuppressed animals (B) extensive oligodendrocyte remyelination is present. (C) and (D) illustrate features of lesions in immunosuppressed animals transplanted with similar numbers of freshly isolated SVZ cells. (C) Shows the area of demyelination contains clusters of undifferentiated cells and astrocytes and no evidence of oligodendrocyte remyelination. (D) The cells in the clusters illustrated in (C) have the appearance of undifferentiated cells normally present in the SVZ. Scale bar$=25\,\mu$m (A, B and C) and $2\,\mu$m (D).

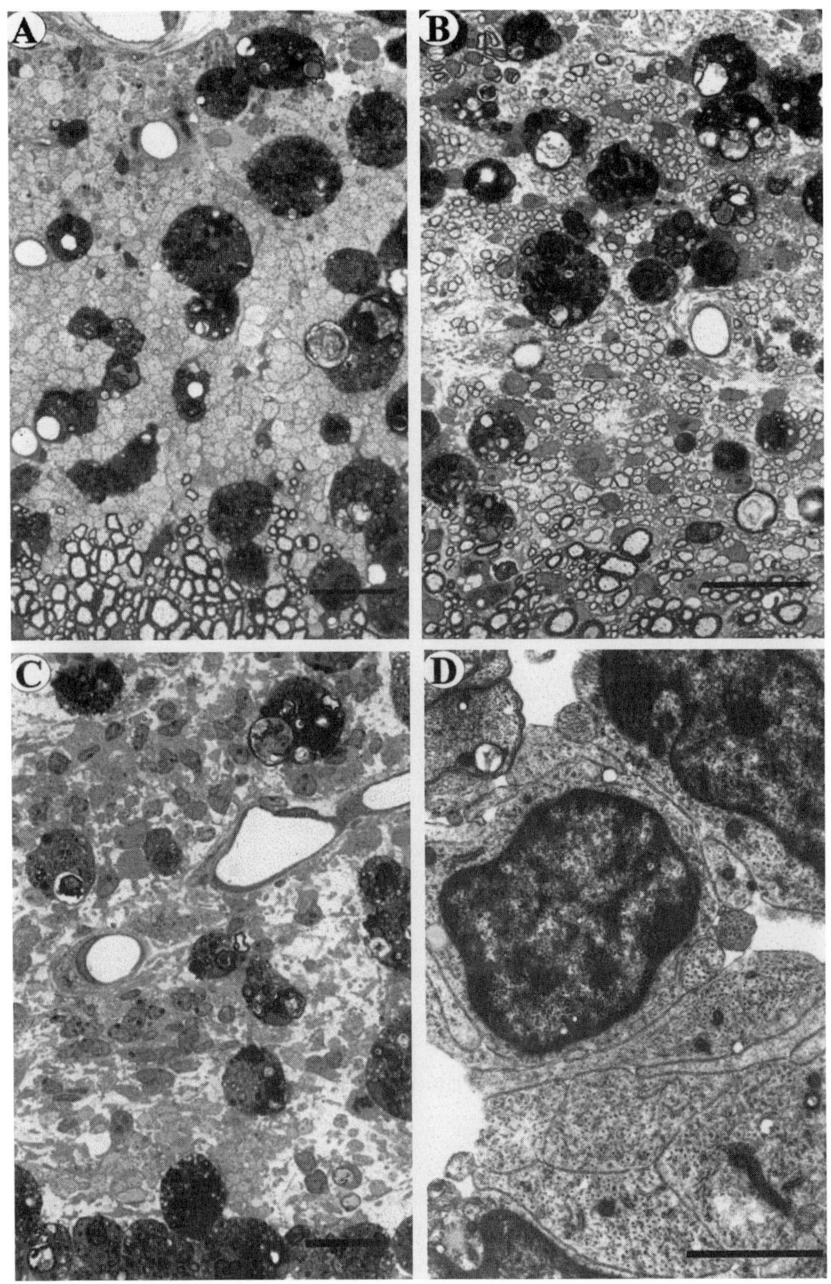

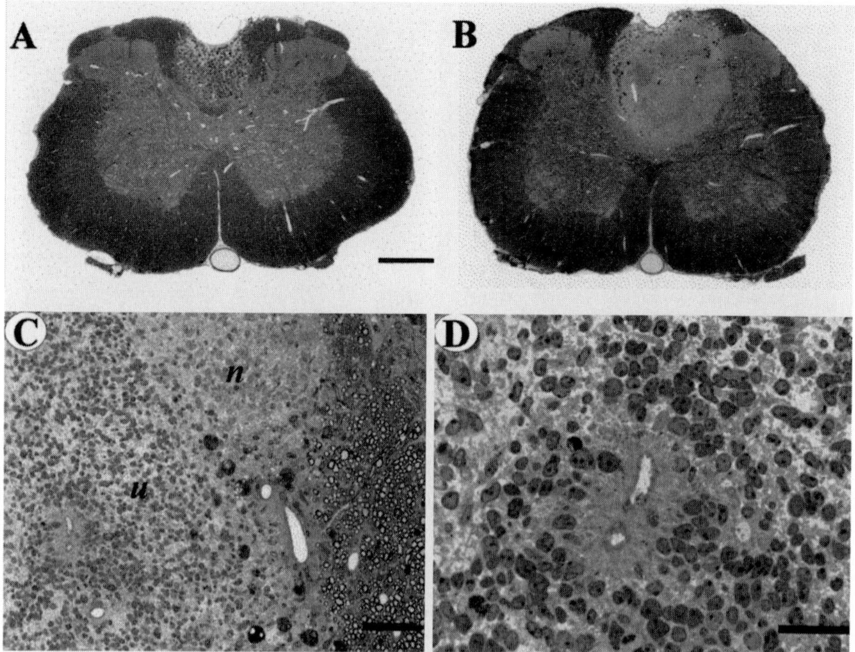

FIG. 2.　Following the injection of freshly prepared suspension of fetal CNS cells into areas of acute demyelination, proliferation of cells results in the development of an expanding tissue mass that compresses adjacent tissue. Compare the appearance of the non-transplanted ethidium bromide lesion in X-irradiated spinal cord after one month (A), with a lesion into which 10^4 cells prepared from the ganglionic eminence of a 25-day-old pig fetus had been injected (B). (C) Within the transplanted lesion some areas contain undifferentiated cells (u) whilst in places evidence of neuronal differentiation (n) is apparent. (D) Undifferentiated cells associated with an ependymal cell rosette. Scale bar = 1 mm (A, B) and 25 μm (C, D).

achieved following the introduction of oligospheres than when neurospheres are used (Zhang et al 1998b).

Can we predict how much remyelination will be achieved?

To date most transplantation studies have been conducted either in developing animals or using models of acute demyelination in which the area available for myelination by the transplanted cells is small, approximately 1–2 mm³. These lesions do not mimic the pathology found in potential target situations in humans. Here the areas of demyelination are chronic and/or the areas to be myelinated are large. Multiple sclerosis (MS) is characterized by multiple areas of chronic demyelination with axons set within an astrocyte environment, while in the leucodystrophies there is loss of myelin throughout the neuraxis. Thus if widespread remyelination, a requirement for restoration of function, is to be achieved, implanted cells will have to migrate extensively. Whether this will be achieved is by no means clear because of our incomplete knowledge of CNS remyelination and limitations imposed by the models currently used for transplantation experiments.

Most of the studies that have demonstrated the oligodendrocyte generating potential of mutipotent neural stem cells and extensive migration of transplanted myelinogenic cells have been conducted in the immature nervous system. It is clear from our own work that progenitor cells behave very differently when introduced into the adult CNS. Thus, despite their capacity to migrate *in vitro*, during development and after implantation into the developing CNS, transplanted oligodendrocyte progenitors do not survive following implantation into normal adult white matter (Franklin et al 1996, O'Leary & Blakemore 1997). They do however survive and differentiate into oligodendrocytes when implanted into areas of demyelination and will migrate in normal white matter if it has been subjected to doses of X-irradiation sufficient to deplete the tissue of endogenous precursors (Franklin et al 1996, O'Leary & Blakemore 1997). This latter observation demonstrates that although the adult CNS cannot support OP survival and migration in its native state, it is amenable to modification to enable it to do so.

There have been only a very limited number of studies that give an indication of the extent of remyelination that might be achieved following the introduction of a given number cells into an area of chronic demyelination in adult individuals. This paucity of information arises for two reasons. Firstly, the survival time following transplantation is usually short because the animals into which they have been introduced do not live long. Thus, most experiments using the myelin-deficient rat have to be terminated after 2–3 weeks, while those using adult animals subjected to the X-irradiated ethidium bromide protocol are terminated after one month because of the potential for developing radiation necrosis. This lack of data is important as it is now clear from studies on endogenous remyelination that contrary to our previous understanding remyelination can be a protracted process. As much myelin sheath formation occurs during the second month following demyelination as there is during the first month (Franklin et al 1997, Shields et al 1999). Secondly, it is not always appreciated that the tissue into which cells have been implanted may be having a beneficial effect on the remyelinating ability of the transplanted cells. Thus, when cells are introduced into young animals they are being introduced into a situation primed for myelination. A similar situation pertains when cells are placed into acute demyelinating lesions, an environment where remyelination would normally be occurring. These environments do not resemble potential clinical situations in humans. There, cells would be introduced into tissue where endogenous remyelination has failed and where axons are set in a matrix of astrocyte processes. The properties of the astrocytes that occur in chronic MS plaques are not fully understood. However, it is clear from *in vitro* studies that astrocytes can have an inhibitory effect on movement of progenitors (Fok-Seang et al 1995), influence process formation by oligodendrocytes (Morley et al 1997) and in some experiments actually inhibit myelination by reducing oligodendrocyte numbers (Rosen et al 1989). If these properties were exhibited by the astrocytes of the chronic MS plaque then it would clearly be a very unfavourable environment for remyelination.

Prospects

Currently, we can restore function by transplantation in experimental models and have identified the pre-OP as the cell with the greatest remyelinating potential. It is also reasonable to expect to be able to generate large numbers of such cells from human tissue in the near future. However, although intriguing results from Ian Duncan's laboratory indicating that transplant-mediated myelination can be very extensive (Archer et al 1997), we still lack the quantitative information to predict the extent of remyelination that could be achieved following transplantation of such cells into an area of chronic demyelination. Once these final hurdles have been overcome the experimental data will be complete for the formulation of clinical trials.

Acknowledgements

PMS holds a Wellcome Trust Research Training Award and RJMF holds a Wellcome Trust Research Career Development Fellowship. Financial support of the Wellcome Trust and the Multiple Sclerosis Society of Great Britain and Northern Ireland is gratefully acknowledged.

References

Archer DR, Cuddon PA, Lipsitz D, Duncan ID 1997 Myelination of the canine central nervous system by glial cell transplantation: a model for repair of human myelin disease. Nat Med 3:54–59

Avellana-Adalid V, Nait-Oumesmar B, Lachapelle F, Baron-Van Evercooren A 1996 Expansion of rat oligodendrocyte progenitors into proliferative 'oligospheres' that retain differentiation potential. J Neurosci Res 45:558–570

Blakemore WF, Crang AJ, Franklin RJM 1995 Transplantation of glial cells. In: Kettenmann H, Ranson BR (eds) Neuroglia. Oxford University Press, New York, p 869–882

Blakemore WF, Franklin RJM, Noble M 2000 Restoring CNS myelin by glial cell transplantation. In: Jessen KR, Richardson WD (eds) Glial cell development: basic principles and clinical relevance. Oxford University Press, Oxford, in press

Brüstle O, Choudhary K, Karram K et al 1998 Chimeric brains generated by intraventricular transplantation of fetal human brain cells into embryonic rats. Nat Biotechnol 16:1040–1044

Bunge RP, Puckett WR, Becerra JL, Marcillo A, Quencer RM 1993 Observations on the pathology of human spinal cord injury. A review and classification of 22 new cases with details from a case of chronic cord compression with extensive focal demyelination. Adv Neurol 59:75–89

Crang AJ, Blakemore WF 1997 Attempts to produce astrocyte cultures devoid of oligodendrocyte generating potential by the use of antimitotic treatment reveal the presence of quiescent oligodendrocyte precursors. J Neurosci Res 48:64–71

Flax JD, Aurora S, Yang C et al 1998 Engraftable human neural stem cells respond to developmental cues, replace neurons, and express foreign genes. Nat Biotechnol 16:1033–1039

Fok-Seang J, Mathews GA, ffrench-Constant C, Trotter J, Fawcett JW 1995 Migration of oligodendrocyte precursors on astrocytes and meningeal cells. Dev Biol 171:1–15

Franklin RJM, Blakemore WF 1993 Requirements for Schwann cell migration within CNS environments: a viewpoint. Int J Dev Neurosci 11:641–649

Franklin RJM, Bayley SA, Blakemore WF 1996 Transplanted CG4 cells (an oligodendrocyte progenitor cell line) survive, migrate and contribute to repair of areas of demyelination in X-irradiated and damaged spinal cord, but not in normal spinal cord. Exp Neurol 137:263–276

Franklin RJM, Gilson JM, Blakemore WF 1997 Local recruitment of remyelinating cells in the repair of demyelination in the central nervous system. J Neurosci Res 50:337–344

Honmou O, Felts PA, Waxman SG, Kocsis JD 1996 Restoration of normal conduction properties in demyelinated spinal cord axons in the adult rat by transplantation of exogenous Schwann cells. J Neurosci 16:3199–3208

Imaizumi T, Lankford KL, Waxman SG, Greer CA, Kocsis JD 1998 Transplanted olfactory ensheathing cells remyelinate and enhance axonal conduction in the demyelinated dorsal columns of the rat spinal cord. J Neurosci 18:6176–6185

Jeffery ND, Blakemore WF 1997 Locomotor deficits induced by experimental spinal cord demyelination are abolished by spontaneous remyelination. Brain 120:27–37

Jeffery ND, Crang AJ, O'Leary MT, Hodge SJ, Blakemore WF 1999 Behavioural consequences of oligodendrocyte progenitor cell transplantation into experimental demyelinating lesions in the rat spinal cord. Eur J Neurosci 11:1508–1514

Keirstead HS, Ben-Hur T, Rogister B, O'Leary MT, Dubois-Dalcq M, Blakemore WF 1999 PSA-NCAM positive CNS precursors generate both oligodendrocytes and Schwann cells to remyelinate the CNS following transplantation. J Neurosci 19:7529–7536

Morley M, Pleasure D, Kreider B 1997 Quantification of the effects of astrocytes on oligodendroglial morphology. J Neurosci Res 49:219–228

Murray K, Dubois-Dalcq M 1997 Emergence of oligodendrocytes from human neural spheres. J Neurosci Res 50:146–156

O'Leary MT, Blakemore WF 1997 Oligodendrocyte precursors survive poorly and do not migrate following transplantation into the normal adult central nervous system. J Neurosci Res 48:159–167

Pfeiffer SE, Warrington AE, Bansal R 1993 The oligodendrocyte and its many processes. Trends Cell Biol 3:191–197

Rosen CL, Bunge RP, Ard MD, Wood PM 1989 Type 1 astrocytes inhibit myelination by adult rat oligodendrocytes *in vitro*. J Neurosci 9:3371–3379

Satoh J, Kim SU 1994 Proliferation and differentiation of fetal human oligodendrocytes in culture. J Neurosci Res 39:260–272

Seilhean D, Gansmüller A, Baron-Van Evercooren A, Gumpel M, Lachapelle F 1996 Myelination by transplanted human and mouse central nervous system tissue after long-term cryopreservation. Acta Neuropathol (Berl) 91:82–88

Shi RY, Kelly TM, Blight AR 1997 Conduction block in acute and chronic spinal cord injury: different dose-response characteristics for reversal by 4-aminopyridine. Exp Neurol 148:495–501

Shields SA, Gilson JM, Blakemore WF, Franklin RJM 1999 Remyelination occurs as extensively but more slowly in old rats compared to young rats following gliotoxin-induced CNS demyelination. Glia 28:77–83

Targett MP, Sussman J, O'Leary MT, Compston DAS, Blakemore WF 1996 Failure to achieve remyelination of demyelinated rat axons following transplantation of glial cells obtained from the adult human brain. Neuropath Appl Neurobiol 22:199–206

Thomson JA, Itskovitz-Eldor J, Shapiro SS et al 1998 Embryonic stem cell lines derived from human blastocysts. Science 282:1145–1147

Utzschneider DA, Archer DR, Kocsis JD, Waxman SG, Duncan ID 1994 Transplantation of glial cells enhances action potential conduction of amyelinated spinal cord axons in the myelin-deficient rat. Proc Natl Acad Sci USA 91:53–57

Warrington AE, Barbarese E, Pfeiffer SE 1993 Differential myelinogenic capacity of specific developmental stages of the oligodendrocyte lineage upon transplantation into hypomyelinating hosts. J Neurosci Res 34:1–13

Zhang SC, Lundberg C, Lipsitz D, O'Connor LT, Duncan ID 1998a Generation of oligodendroglial progenitors from neural stem cells. J Neurocytol 27:475–489

Zhang SC, Lipsitz D, Duncan ID 1998b Self-renewing canine oligodendroglial progenitor expanded as oligospheres. J Neurosci Res 54:181–190

DISCUSSION

Price: Do you know anything about the migration potential of the B104 conditioned medium-treated subventricular zone cells in undamaged tissue?

Blakemore: One would predict that in undamaged normal tissue they would behave like cells from that region of brain, in other words they would not migrate. The subventricular cells migrate within their tracts: they are locked into those channels, and so they only migrate down these pathways. The exception is when there is pathology: then they break out of the pathway and go towards the damaged site. Usually, they go into areas where there is high expression of PSA-NCAM. One then has to ask whether this is expansion into a permissive environment or migration to an attractive signal. One has to be a little careful about this concept of attraction, because if you are an expanding population and this bit is the only permissive channel, that is the way you go.

Björklund: In the experiment where you compared the intact rat and irradiated rats you saw more migration in the latter case. What is the pathology caused by the irradiation?

Blakemore: There is a slight astrocytic hypertrophy, the blood–brain barrier is intact, and the growth factor profile is unchanged. However, the number of microglia is reduced by half as is the number of NG-2-positive cells.

Björklund: Are the myelin sheaths intact?

Blakemore: Yes.

Björklund: If the poor migration in the intact animal is due to lack of space, how do you explain the increased migration in the irradiated tissue? It doesn't seem that you have created any more space in the irradiated tissue.

Blakemore: We have: we have taken out half the NG-2-positive population.

Gage: The NG-2-positive cells are actually dividing cells, and if you label with BrdU just in the normal cord, 95% of the BrdU-labelled cells that you find long-term are in fact NG-2-positive.

Blakemore: That is very exciting information. There is work from Canada that says that a population of cells is turning over constantly, and these cells really are turning over because they can be killed by just 2 Grays of radiation (Li & Wong 1998).

Björklund: Do these cells occur throughout the brain and spinal cord? Are they present in both white and grey matter?

Blakemore: Yes, at least in the rat and mouse, throughout the CNS. The NG-2-positive cells, or at least some of them, are the tissue-specific multipotent cells which are different from the multipotent cells in the subventricular zone. In culture people have shown that they behave very differently.

Gray: How multipotent are they? Do they generate neurons as well as oligodendrocytes?

Blakemore: We are not sure at the moment. When you culture adult tissue and generate cells, one has to ask, where are these cells coming from? We always assume that oligodendrocytes have come from the adult OP, which is well documented in tissue culture.

Gray: A clear difference between what you are reporting and what Evan Snyder and John Sinden have described at this meeting is that, in these models of spinal cord demyelination, you have to commit progenitors first to the oligodendrocyte lineage in order to get repair whereas, in the other CNS models, we were seeing uncommitted stem cells turning into a variety of cell types. What is it that accounts for this difference?

Blakemore: I don't know. We do know that all these multipotent cells in tissue culture will make oligodendrocytes and astrocytes, but they don't like making oligodendrocytes, which usually form just 2–3% of the cells. If you are going to use these cells therapeutically, it would appear to be an advantage to commit them to what you want.

Gray: Is this a difference between spinal cord and the brain?

Blakemore: It could be.

Smith: Is it possible that with all the macrophages you have in there providing cytokines, that there is a specific suppression of oligodendrocyte commitment?

Blakemore: It could be, but this again highlights the fact that acute pathology is different from chronic pathology and development.

Snyder: I agree: this could reflect more the difference of how the pathology evolves and its source. It is very complex. We need to know as much about the abnormal terrain into which these cells are being implanted as we need to know about the cells themselves. In our shiverer mice, a multipotent cell can shift and yield more oligodendrocytes. Had we precommitted them to become more oligodendrocytes, we might have found a more robust effect. We were looking for multiple cell types.

Gray: Where did you implant in that experiment?

Snyder: Into the ventricles of newborns.

Blakemore: This is where the problem arises. These experiments are done in development. If we take a rat that is equivalent to the shiverer mouse and transplant into that animal when it is three months old, we don't get very much myelination, because although this animal has abnormal myelination, it has a population of oligodendrocytes that are relating to the axons and the relationship established is sufficiently robust not to allow the transplanted cells to form normal myelin to myelinate those axons. In other words, there is no space for them to get into the system. To remyelinate the adult shiverer, we would have to demyelinate it first.

Isacson: There is some confusion even among experts about this. Even where we transplant into the striatum, if we do it into a neonate, we see migration and integration which we do not see in the adult or adult lesioned nervous system. Bill's data are very important. One cannot generalize graft behaviour by implanting developing nervous system into only one host condition.

Blakemore: There is another bit of data I didn't present. We have done these migration studies using the CG4 cell line, which is a nice OP cell line. When these cells are transplanted into normal white matter, there is no migration, but when introduced into an irradiated white matter we get extensive migration over a long distance and have more cells integrating than when we use primary OPs. There appears to be a difference in the migratory behaviour of this cell line compared to expanded endogenous cells. This may be either a good thing or a bad thing: it really depends how well the cells differentiate. Therefore, one of the strategies we are thinking about for repair of large demyelinated regions is that we want to develop cells that are more invasive and migrate further than normal cells. As long as such cells differentiate appropriately and respond to the appropriate signals they will be good repairers.

Price: This is an area where embryology may help us out. During development, all multipotential cells are not truly multipotential, even though in a culture dish we can manipulate them to do anything we like. *In vivo*, not all of them have the capacity to generate oligodendrocytes. The best data on this come from Bill Richardson, who has shown that in the spinal cord, oligodendrocytes appear to arise from a tiny population of the ventricular zone cells (Pringle & Richardson

1993). The general conclusion that seems to follow from what everyone has said is that in the lesioned adult, multipotential precursor cells will go on to regenerate whichever population of neurons have gone missing, whereas what you are showing is that those cells, although one can get them to make oligodendrocytes, don't have a predisposition to make them. Going back to the embryological situation, we shouldn't be surprised by this.

Gray: There is an interesting experiment coming out of this. That is, to put the Evan Snyder/John Sinden type of cell into Bill Blakemore's models. We know that these cells make oligodendrocytes.

Blakemore: I would like to take issue with what Jack Price has said. You can take embryonic stem cells and make oligodendrocytes from them. Development is very ordered. In repair and regeneration, this order is absent, so we have to try to reimpose some order on cell differentiation. This is the challenge.

Price: My point is, if you take a multipotential neuroepithelial cell out at random, you will be lucky to get one that would have been fated to generate oligodendrocytes. The evidence suggests that although such a cell can make oligodendrocytes if you mess with it, it wouldn't tend to do that. What you are seeing is this reticence of these multipotential cells to give rise to oligodendrocytes. From the neuroembryology, this is probably what we would have expected.

References

Li YQ, Wong CS 1998 Apoptosis and its relationship with cell proliferation in the irradiated rat spinal cord. Int J Radiat Biol 74:405–417
Pringle NP, Richardson WP 1993 A singularity of PDGF alpha-receptor expression in the dorsoventral axis of the neural tube may define the origin of the oligodendrocyte lineage. Development 117:525–533

General discussion II

The embryonic stem cell approach

Smith: The primary interest of my laboratory is in embryonic stem (ES) cells rather than with brain repair. However, the possibility of using ES cells as a system for cell therapy is increasingly becoming apparent (Smith 1998, Thomson et al 1999) (Fig. 1 *[Smith]*). An ES cell is a cell derived from a mouse blastocyst. These are pluripotent cells, which means that they can generate every fetal cell type. The second key property of these cells is that they are genuinely immortal and can be expanded indefinitely. We can demonstrate that these are normal cells by putting them back into a mouse embryo. The concept is straightforward: given that ES cells have the capacity to make any cell type, we should be able to harness this potential to make just nerve cells. Such a system would be useful for studying neural development and for transplantation (Okabe et al 1996, Brüstle et al 1999, Svendsen & Smith 1999).

The problem is that despite the rapid advances that have been made over the last few years in developmental biology, we are not yet able to instruct a pluripotent cell to make any one cell type. When we differentiate ES cells, therefore, we end up with a mix of different cell types in a disorganized fashion. Because of the lack of morphogenic organization, we can't even dissect out the different types of cells. Obviously, we would not want to take this mixture of cells and stick them in the brain. The question then is, in the absence of directed differentiation, is there a way to pull out the types of cells that we require? One method for doing this is a strategy pursued by Meng Li, a postdoctoral fellow in our lab, who has used a selective approach (Li et al 1998) (Fig. 2 *[Smith]*). This involves the ablation of non-neuroepithelial cells. Differentiation is induced by a protocol which gives about 50% neuroepithelial cells. The strategy is to integrate a marker into a gene that is only expressed in neural precursor cells. This then allows a drug selection or fluorescence-activated cell sorting (FACS) to eliminate other lineages from the population. From this selected population we can attempt to amplify the cells we are particularly interested in, namely the multipotent neural stem cells. The gene we have used to do this is called *Sox2*. Certain of the Sox transcription factors are expressed only in the neuroectoderm in the early embryo. They are expressed along the entire length of the neural axis but only in dividing neuroepithelial progenitors (Pevny et al 1998). They come on very early in the neural plate, and remain on in the

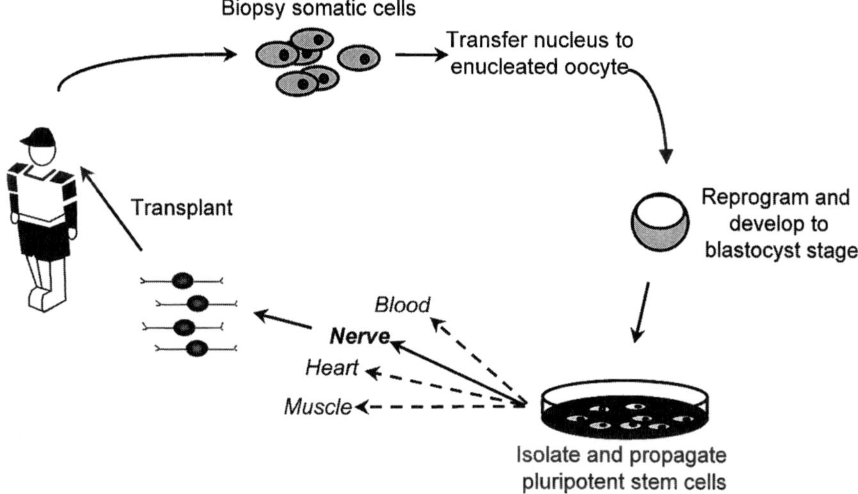

FIG. 1.   (*Smith*) Stem cell therapy via somatic cell reprogramming.

dividing neuroepithelial precursors. The beauty of the mouse ES cells is that it is possible to do sophisticated genetic manipulations. We can integrate our selectable marker by homologous recombination into the *Sox* gene. We then induce differentiation and subsequently eliminate all the cell types that we don't want. In the absence of any added mitogen we then obtain populations of cells which are essentially completely neuronal. The cells that we are really interested in are the precursors to these differentiated cells. We can amplify these as morphologically homogeneous populations of neuroepithelial cells using fibroblast growth factor (FGF) plus chick embryo extract. The key question we would now like to ask is how these cells relate to the types of cells that we have heard about at this meeting from other people.

Isacson: We have published on this (Deacon et al 1998, Isacson 1999). We were surprised. We started down the *in vitro* route, taking ES cells in leukaemia inhibitory factor (LIF)-containing culture and using retinoic acid to try to differentiate the cells into nerve cells. We transplanted the retinoic acid-treated cells into the brain as controls. We reluctantly put in non-treated ES cells, which then ended up becoming largely neuronal. We then went from there to ask whether that was a brain-specific induction, and transplanted these cells to the kidney capsule with the same results.

Smith: It has been known for a long time that embryo-derived tumours, either directly from the ectopically grafted embryos, from EC cells (which are tumour cells derived from those primary tumours), or from ES cells, form teratocarcinomas, of which neurectoderm is generally a major component. It is

(A) Target marker into neural precursor-specific gene in ES cells

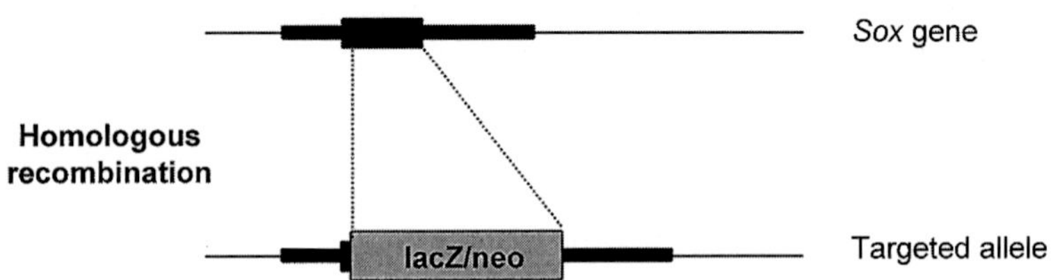

(B) Elimination of non-neural cells from differentiating ES cell cultures

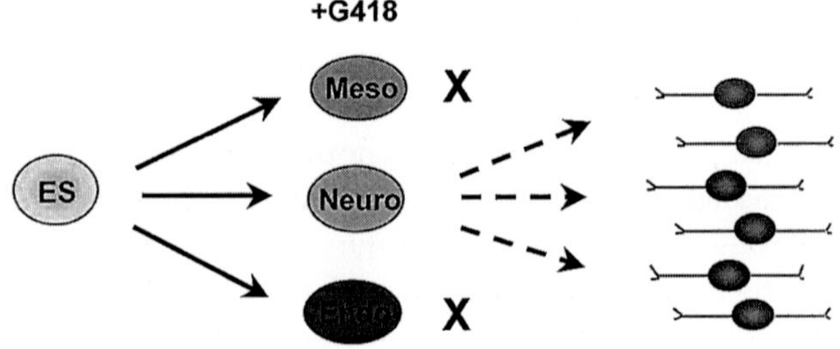

(C) Expansion and differentiation of tripotential neural stem cells

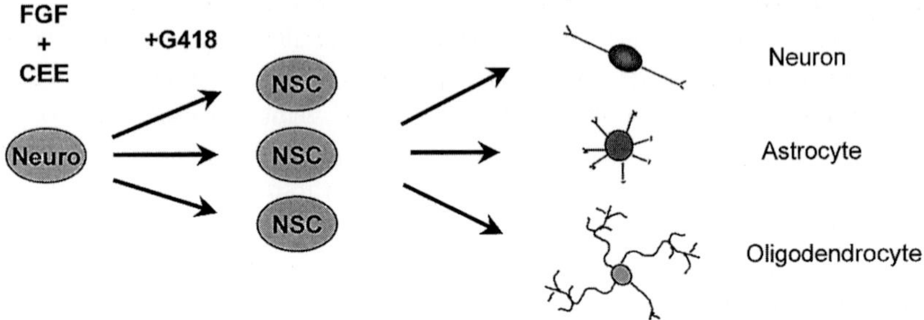

FIG. 2.   (*Smith*) Lineage selection strategy. NSC, neural stem cell.

interesting that you see these in the brain. It is quite an alarming development if you are thinking about using these cells for transplantation. The key thing that this tells us is that we have to select a lineage-restricted precursor out of the ES cells, otherwise we will end up with unwanted cell types.

Isacson: The important observation is that the ES-derived neurons that did survive had the capacity to innervate adult brain regions.

Smith: Did you say that you actually saw that this was more effective, just taking the undifferentiated ES cells rather than differentiating them?

Isacson: Yes.

Smith: One might argue that this is because plastic neuroepithelial stem cells are being generated *in situ* in the brain after the transplant. When you differentiate the cells *in vitro* you may have gone past that phase.

Isacson: Yes, these neurons may not have developed in the normal developmental sequence or into the typical phenotypes. We have some dopaminergic neurons developed from ES cells which are not at all the same morphological type as seen in the normal substantia nigra.

Björklund: In your selection procedure, do you have a particular protocol for inducing neuronal phenotypes?

Smith: We make embryoid bodies which form an aggregation of ES cells. The protocol we use is that after 4 days we add retinoic acid (Bain et al 1995). Whether retinoic acid is essential, and what it is doing is uncertain. People glibly say that retinoic acid is a neural inducer, but one of the main things it does is to induce a lot of cell death. It is not clear to me that it is acting as a specific neural inducer. However, under this protocol we get a high proportion of neural committed cells.

Björklund: In the selection phase, do you continue to culture them in dispersed cultures?

Smith: The selection phase is done by adding G418 in the final 48 h of the aggregate phase. Then the embryo bodies are dissociated and plated as dispersed cells in DMEM/F12+N2, and grown as monolayer cultures. In order for differentiating neurons to survive, the G418 selection must be removed. If we want to expand the precursor cell population, we generally do that by maintaining selection and adding FGF plus chick embryo extract.

References

Bain G, Kitchens D, Yao M, Huettner JE, Gottlieb DI 1995 Embryonic stem cells express neuronal properties *in vitro*. Dev Biol 168:342–357

Brüstle O, Jones KN, Learish RD et al 1999 Embryonic stem cell-derived glial precursors: a source of myelinating transplants. Science 285:754–756

Deacon T, Dinsmore J, Costantini LC, Ratliff J, Isacson O 1998 Blastula-stage stem cells can differentiate into dopaminergic and serotonergic neurons after transplantation. Exp Neurol 149:28–41

Isacson O 1999 The neurobiology and neurogenetics of stem cells. Brain Pathol 9:495–498

Li M, Pevny L, Lovell-Badge R, Smith A 1998 Generation of purified neural precursors from embryonic stem cells by lineage selection. Curr Biol 8:971–974

Okabe S, Forsberg-Nilsson K, Spiro AC, Segal M, McKay RD 1996 Development of neuronal precursor cells and functional postmitotic neurons from embryonic stem cells *in vitro*. Mech Dev 59:89–102

Pevny LH, Sockanathan S, Placzek M, Lovell-Badge R 1998 A role for Sox1 in neural determination. Development 125:1967–1978

Smith A 1998 Cell therapy: in search of pluripotency. Curr Biol 8:R802–R804

Svendsen CN, Smith AG 1999 New prospects for human stem-cell therapy in the nervous system. Trends Neurosci 22:357–364

Thomson JA, Itskovitz-Eldor J, Shapiro SS et al 1998 Embryonic stem cell lines derived from human blastocysts. Science 282:1145–1147 (erratum 1998 Science 282:1827)

Final discussion

The future for fetal grafts

Gage: I don't know whether we have had enough discussion yet about the possibilities for using fetal tissue in neural transplantation. I would conclude that while there is great hope for cell types from different sources, there is no evidence of any cell type that I know of other than primary fetal tissue from mesencephalon that can give rise to authentic dopaminergic neurons in the striatum, and give behavioural recovery. Before we cast off fetal tissue, we need to recognize this.

Lindvall: I have a similar comment to make. At least in Parkinson's disease (PD), we have a specific mechanism that we want to restore, i.e. striatal dopamine neural transmission. With primary fetal cells we have been able to do this to a significant extent in both animals and humans. The problem is that the alternatives have hitherto not been shown to be effective, even in animal models. There is a problem when you don't know the mechanism of a partial recovery in a clinical trial. How can you improve the symptomatic relief if you don't know what is causing it?

Snyder: If we are talking about substitutes for fetal tissue, we have to at least do as well as fetal tissue, and understand exactly what it is we are trying to substitute. It is still the gold standard.

Gray: It is worth commenting here that if we had been waiting to understand the mechanisms by which fetal grafts act, no one would have gone into clinical trials because those mechanisms are still obscure.

Lindvall: I disagree. The mechanisms of how fetal grafts work in PD were quite well understood when we went to clinical trials.

Gray: My recollection is that when the first trials started there was very little evidence regarding how fetal grafts produced recovery of function in very good animal models of PD. I remember hearing Steve Dunnett give papers at that time in which there was a long list of possible mechanisms of action, and the jury was still out. It may be that the jury is no longer out.

Dunnett: There is quite a contrast between the history of clinical adrenal transplantation, where there was a clear rush to try it out without the scientific basis (and it didn't work), against the history of fetal tissue transplantation, where the models were well established. Although there were some ambiguities about the precise mechanism of the latter, a variety of alternatives had certainly been ruled out and the scientific principles of placement, integration and tissue handling had been worked out.

Price: We must not set the hurdle too high. Consider the stroke work we heard about earlier. The therapeutic potential is clearly enormous. None the less, we have no idea how it works, and it is likely to be so complex that it may take 20 years before we do have a clear idea. If we argue that we need to have a fundamental understanding of how the rewiring is taking place before we would conceive of going into patients, I think we would be seen as being much too conservative.

Sinden: The reality is that any scale-up of neural transplantation will necessarily involve one of these other approaches that can effectively substitute for primary fetal tissue.

Gage: I don't think the argument is to say that we should stop looking at the cell lines. I'm just saying that we have passed over fetal tissue and given this impression that we are marching forwards with cell lines and that fetal tissue is in the past. Rather, we have set a very good standard with fetal grafts that we need to meet with the newer cells. None of the cell lines that we are talking about at this meeting have even got close to the effects of fetal tissue. And in talking about the mechanism, we are not talking about whether or not it is point–point contact. All we know about the mechanism is that dopaminergic neuronal replacement is key in this phenomenon.

Lindvall: I agree. We are beginning to understand that the mechanism of action of successful neurografts in patients with PD is more than just simple dopamine delivery.

Aebischer: What you have said about the lack of understanding of mechanism may be true for cell transplantation, but in terms of gene therapy we can be mechanistic at the molecular level, for instance in Huntington's disease or amyotrophic lateral sclerosis.

Freeman: I agree that we may be setting the standard too high for the new cell lines. Even if fetal tissue is a gold standard, if it is not viable epidemiologically and if another therapy comes along that is viable epidemiologically and has a better safety profile, or can be upscaled so that multiple patients can receive it, it doesn't necessarily have to be as efficacious. There may be diseases where fetal tissue transplants are not feasible because of their lack of migrational capacity, and the migratory capacity of certain types of cell lines may be advantageous. I would be a little cautious in trying to overgeneralize fetal tissue as a gold standard.

Reier: At this stage I feel like I'm preaching to the choir, but from a broad perspective we are still trying to learn how to rebuild the nervous system. We have a building block in fetal tissue, and we can learn from that. As we look at alternatives to fetal tissue, we have to ask what components do we need to have for optimal functional repair. We still have a template in that regard in primary fetal grafting. When new technologies come, we have to face the reality that however well groomed we are for being systematic about things, all too often the new technology comes and the old one goes out of the picture. Then, 20 years later someone who reads the literature more than five years back suddenly rediscovers the old technology!

Primary fetal tissue is very important. We keep arguing about fetal tissue in terms of the ethics and practicalities. However, there are cases where two fetuses can be enough to achieve repair in a certain type of spinal cord lesion in humans. Even if fetal grafts are not going to be a widespread therapy, there is a framework where this could be valuable and where there is a proof of principle at the human level that we shouldn't overlook. All the therapies we are discussing at this symposium are going to be based on proof of principle. No matter what you do in an animal, until you carry it to the human it is only a proof of principle.

Isacson: To phrase this differently, the idea that we are 'moving beyond' fetal cells is a dangerous one. We are learning a lot from fetal grafts. Each cell is different in the brain, even in the substantia nigra, where even neighbouring dopamine cells have functional differences. Maybe one goal is to be able to generate cells from other sources than fetal that do the same thing. I want to make a comment to those who are clinically oriented: the pragmatic aspect of getting any cell that works is a useful clinical goal, but gaining a full understanding of now these transplanted cells develop and function is the scientific and medical goal.

Blakemore: One area that is advancing quickly is glial cell transplantation.

Gray: How close is that to going into the clinic?

Blakemore: If it was the rat clinic it would be today! This is why it is exciting, because the starting material for doing the same thing with human tissue is available now. We either have to start with human fetal tissue or human embryonic stem (ES) cells. We know that what we do not want is to implant primary fetal tissue, because this is dangerous stuff for glial cell therapy.

Stem cell strategies

Gray: I would like to move the discussion to Fred Gage's work. Can you stimulate those endogenous stem cells that you have so beautifully described? Do you see that as a potential avenue forward, and if so how is one going to stimulate the brain to do more than it does already in response to injury?

Gage: My perspective is to understand how this process occurs normally. There are areas of the brain where neurogenesis occurs, and there are areas where myelinating events are occurring naturally. We can't begin thinking about activating these cells endogenously to migrate and replace missing cells in a rational manner until we understand that process. The goal would be to understand what activates the cells to begin proliferating, what controls their migration and what controls their differentiation. If we achieve this goal, then we can do the experiments of expressing those molecules with vectors that can be regulated endogenously in specific cell types. Using specific cell type promoters to drive specific genes within specific cells, we can get these cells to express genes on the surface so that the local endogenous cells can respond to those cues and migrate to new locations that they wouldn't go to otherwise. All this will require a better understanding of the endogenous molecules that are involved in the spontaneous process. I concur with the idea of using directed delivery as a tool, not so much for using growth factors to protect cells from dying, but also to activate the endogenous process.

Gray: Are there any realistic prospects, or even thought experiments, of how one might do this in a way that would allow your approach or Austin Smith's to provide autologous grafts, i.e. something that is taken from the patient and then expanded and given back?

Gage: One experiment which we published last year was in a spinal cord injury, where we grafted autologous skin fibroblasts that were engineered to express NT-3. We injected these into a lesion cavity. We had previously shown that we could induce corticospinal regenerative responses within these grafts and in the surrounding areas. But the surprising thing was that the axons were myelinated with NT-3 grafts as opposed to control cells. And when we pulsed with BrdU and did a time-course, we found that the NT-3-induced myelination of the regenerating axons was coming from host cells. With NT-3 secretion, which induced an axonal event, a secondary effect of the NT-3 was for induction of proliferation and migration of the oligodendrocytes into the grafts where they myelinate. We don't know the exact mechanism behind this, but we do know that the myelination was derived from the host cells.

Raisman: This fits with Raff's work, that the signal for myelination is an axonal signal.

Gage: It is a combination of NT-3 plus an axonal signal.

Raisman: The NT-3 may be acting on the neurons to produce that axonal signal.

Smith: On the issue of autologous transplants, the thing people are excited about is the possibility of deriving ES cells by nuclear transfer directly from the patient (see Fig. 1 [*Smith*], p 303). This is currently just a vision, but it is potentially a promising avenue.

Blakemore: It is an important issue. Most countries are considering changing their law to allow or prohibit these types of procedures.

Gray: As I see it we have been talking about three types of stem cell approaches. First, there are stem cells that are partially differentiated prior to implantation, then cells that are immortalized and not pre-differentiated, and thirdly conditionally immortalized cells.

Snyder: I'm not sure that these are different approaches. What I talked about was simply a model demonstrating the potential of a cell with these capabilities. For me, it illustrates what could be achieved if we could harness this biology. The questions left open remain the best way to expand the cells, whether we need to expand them, and whether we need to predifferentiate them prior to grafting. These are all open questions. The work we have all been doing simply says that there is potential in a cell of this type. From an epistemological point of view there is one truth — one type of stem cell — we need to explore how to harness that biology.

Sinden: We think that there is more than one type of stem cell, from the point of view of brain repair.

Gage: When we graft cells harvested from the dish, they are a mixed population. It is not a purified stem cell population. In fact, we don't know that there are any stem cells that remain from the original population. Furthermore, we don't know whether or not the cells that differentiate into neurons hadn't already been committed in the dish. When we graft cells and observe differentiation, there seems to be an attribution that it is the most primitive cells among the stem cells that has the most potential. But it may be that this cell becomes quiescent upon entering an adult milieu, and it is only the committed cells in the population that are appropriately committed and can recognize the cues in that local environment. One of our goals is therefore to try to purify populations by methodologies like fluorescence-activated cell sorting, and then graft identified populations of cells at defined lineages, using homogeneous populations to see the optimal cell type for grafting in different conditions.

Snyder: It is possible to synchronize clones. It still leaves the question you pose open, but it minimizes that kind of problem.

Gage: These cells would be committed to specific lineages.

Price: Fred, I understand your point, but how are you going to deal with that? I don't see what you are going to be able to do. I don't see how you can prove that a population of 10^7 cells in a plate are all identical.

Gage: I'm pointing out the converse: that you can't say at present which cell is the appropriate cell to graft for any one indication.

Price: My point is that you never will be able to do this. In our MHP cells, if we switch them from the permissive to the non-permissive temperature, they start to diversify very quickly. We can see subpopulations that label with embryonic N-CAM, where there weren't any before, for example. But at permissive temperature, we can't see any difference between the cells.

Gage: You have identified that there is a problem; it doesn't mean that there is not a solution. One of the major problems in this work is that we lack adequate markers to identify cells of different ages. A major effort is underway to identify local temporal and spatial markers that will help predict the fate of individual cells.

Gray: As we draw to the end of this meeting, what are the clinical prospects of the approaches that we have been talking about?

Aebischer: The stem cell work raises some interesting issues. If we can go into the clinic with conditionally immortalized cells, we may be able to do phase I trials, but if we want to scale up we will have to be more sophisticated, and regulatory agencies would be very concerned about the presence of oncogenes in implanted cells, even if they are conditionally immortalized. We would need excision systems or suicide genes built-in before we could consider using them. They are fantastic tools, but it is premature to start talking about going to the clinic. We have worked with genetically engineered cells with regulatory agencies, and the amount of things that you need to do to please them is immense.

Gray: Does anyone have any insight as to how Layton Bioscience managed to get to the clinic?

Aebischer: In a phase I trial the conditions are not as strict. When you get to phase III it is very different. Getting authorization for a phase I trial does not indicate that there is a good chance of approval. They may allow you to do a phase I trial with a cell line immortalized with an oncogene, but this doesn't mean that they will approve it as a product.

Freeman: The FDA initially looks primarily at safety and tolerability issues. As long as there is a rationale for the programme, an understanding of the mechanism is not one of the criteria for the initiation of a phase I trial.

Perry: The issue that is of key interest to the wider public is whether there are going to be more experiments in people. The PD patients that have received grafts have been a fantastic step forward showing that this sort of treatment can work. Experiments in people will continue because there are people who are willing or desperate enough to have it done to them, and there are enough clinically minded scientists who want to do it.

Snyder: The issues that Patrick Aebischer raised about the FDA apply not just to genetic manipulation, but to any kind of manipulation of the cells, including bathing them in growth factors. Any manipulation of the cells needs to pass a rigorous examination. The only clinical trial right now with cells that would be permissible in the USA is using fresh primary cells with no manipulation at all of any kind. This may or may not be the best approach. This is a huge obstacle.

Freeman: The FDA has very recently claimed regulatory authority over even unmodified fetal tissue. As to where this work is going clinically, there are at least 30 on-going or approved cellular therapy trials for neurological disorders alone (Table 1). We can't escape the fact that whether the science is there or not, these things are happening.

Gray: Our discussion could clearly continue for many hours or even days longer, but the time has come to wind it up. In my introduction to the symposium, I said that this was likely to be a timely meeting, and the discussion has clearly demonstrated this to be the case. We are at a crossroads between, on the one hand, the scientific and clinical work that has led to the demonstrations,

TABLE 1 **Recently completed, on-going or approved cellular therapy trials for neurological disorders**

Number of trials	Details	Location/sponsor
Parkinson's disease		
5	Phase I human fetal nigral grafts, unmodified tissue	Colorado, France, Los Angeles, Sweden, Tampa
1	Phase I human fetal double grafts to striatum and nigra	Halifax
1	Phase I human fetal trials with trophic factors	Halifax
1	Phase I human fetal nigral/striatal cografts	Taiwan
1	Phase I human fetal nigral grafts with antioxidants	Sweden
1	Phase I human cervical ganglia transplants	Japan
2	Human fetal nigral prospective double-blind, surgical placebo-controlled trials	Colorado/New York, Tampa/ New York/Chicago
1	Human RPE cells on microcarriers	Titan
2	Porcine (cross-species) nigral transplant trials (one phase I, two prospective double-blind)	Genzyme/Diacrin LLC
Huntington's disease		
4	Phase I human fetal striatal grafts, unmodified	France, England, Los Angeles, Tampa
1	Encapsulated BHK cells genetically engineered to secrete hCNTF	Pitras, Cytotherapeutics, Astra
1	Phase I cross-species fetal striatal	Diacrin
Stroke		
1	Phase I porcine striatal grafts with Fab	Diacrin
1	Phase I hNT neurons	Layton Biosciences
1	Phase II hNT neurons	Layton Biosciences
Other		
1	Encapsulated BHK cells genetically engineered to secrete hCNTF in ALS	Cytotherapeutics/Astra
2	Phase I/II trials of encapsulated chromaffin cells for terminal cancer pain	Cytotherapeutics/Astra
1	Phase I trial of non-encapsulated human adrenal medullary cells for cancer pain	Toulouse, France
1	Phase I porcine striatal grafts for spinal cord injury pain	Diacrin
1	Phase I porcine striatal grafts for epilepsy	Diacrin
2	Spinal cord syringomyelia, human fetal transplants	Gainesville, Sweden

Totals are trials ongoing or to be started within six months. Does not include adrenal transplants for PD, or fetal transplant programmes in China, Poland, Mexico or Cuba.

documented in our meeting, that transplants of primary fetal grafts into the damaged human brain are capable of bringing real benefit to patients with serious brain disease and, on the other, the exciting new developments in developmental neurobiology that we have heard about and which are opening up a whole range of new and promising clinical applications.

Primary fetal neural grafts have proved their worth clinically, and they have been a vital stepping stone to the novel approaches to which much of our symposium has been devoted. There is much work that remains to be done, in both the laboratory and the clinic, to bring these approaches to fruition, and it will take time to do it; but we seem to be on the verge of a transition to a whole new technology for the treatment of the diseased and damaged brain. Thank you all for your superb contributions to this absorbing meeting.

Index of contributors

Non-participating co-authors are indicated by asterisks. Entries in bold indicate papers; other entries refer to discussion contributions.

Subject index